Applied Oral Physiology

Second edition

To Eileen, Maria and Bridget

Applied Oral Physiology

Second edition

Christopher L. B. Lavelle PhD, DSc, DDS, MRCPath, FRCD
Professor, Department of Oral Biology, University of Manitoba, Winnipeg, Manitoba, Canada

WRIGHT
London Boston Singapore Sydney Toronto Wellington

Wright
is an imprint of Butterworth Scientific

First edition 1975 published by John Wright and Sons Ltd, Bristol
Second edition 1988

British Library Cataloguing in Publication Data

Lavelle, Christopher L.B.
Applied oral physiology.—2nd ed.
1. Man. Oral region. Diseases—Questions & answers—For dentistry
I. Title
612′.92

ISBN 0-7236-0818-0

Library of Congress Cataloging-in-Publication Data

Applied oral physiology/[edited by] Christopher L.B. Lavelle —2nd ed.
p. cm.
Rev. ed. of: Applied physiology of the mouth. 1975.
Includes bibliographies and index.
ISBN 0-7236-0818-0
1. Mouth—Pathophysiology. 2. Teeth. I. Lavelle, Christopher L.B.
[DNLM: 1. Mouth—physiology. 2. Applied physiology of the mouth. WU 102 A6517]
RK280.A65 1988
616.3′1—dc19 88-12

Phototypeset by Scribe Design, Gillingham, Kent
Printed and bound in Great Britain by Butler and Tanner, Frome, Somerset

Preface

Dental treatment and treatment planning hinge upon a thorough understanding of the underlying physiological processes and principles. It is therefore unfortunate that undergraduate and graduate dental training is not more successful in bridging the hiatus between the basic sciences and clinical dentistry; yet, with the changing patterns of dental practice consequent upon the declining prevalence of dental caries, the more complex needs and expectations of the patient will hinge upon a much greater knowledge of oral physiology.

Dentistry is changing at an alarming rate, primarily driven by the results of modern research. Only by constantly updating our data base will we be able to keep pace with current trends. This work has been compiled after a rigorous scrutiny of the literature, and only those subjects with an adequate scientific base are included. The topics selected have a direct bearing upon oral diagnosis and treatment planning. The references, quoted at the end of each chapter, are selected to provide a basis for future in-depth topic evaluation rather than as a comprehensive literature compendium.

Acknowledgements

Many thanks are due to A. Domokas, Mrs Anna Stein, Linda Delmage, Darryl Backman and David Wong for all their help and to the University of Manitoba for providing facilities and weekends free from teaching.

Contents

1

Pain

Introduction

Dentistry owes its very beginnings to the quest for pain relief, and the identification, diagnosis and early elimination of pain remain important foundations to the dental profession.

Pain is a symptom in the completely subjective sense. It is a complex experience that includes a sensory–discriminatory component. Pain also includes the accompanying responses or reactions elicited by the stimulus. For instance, some of the reactions to a noxious stimulus include pain, startled response, muscle reflex, vocalization, sweating, increase in heart rate, in addition to blood pressure and behavioural changes. Such reactions will in turn be modified by a number of factors, including the emotional status of the patient, past experience and memories of pain, magnitude of tissue damage or stimulus, other concomitant sensory experiences, ability to comprehend the causes (aetiology) and consequences (pathogenesis) of the pain, and ethnic group and culture. Thus pain is both complex and multidimensional, with the result that accurate diagnosis and appropriate treatment is often difficult.

What is pain?

Neuroscience is characterized by two major rules:

(1) The more sensory nerves that supply a region of the body, the more acute the sensibility in the area.
(2) The higher the ratio of motor nerves to muscles, the greater the possible control finesse.

On both accounts, the oral cavity and face exceed most other bodily regions. The number of patients who have orofacial discomfort and pain is therefore not surprising. Unlike other sensations, however, pain is an experience that cannot be shared: it is wholly personal, belonging to the sufferer alone. Different individuals therefore feel and react to pain and suffering in different ways. One person cannot possibly sense exactly the feelings of another. Patients in pain therefore require individualized treatment.

The ability to diagnose and treat a patient suffering from pain depends largely on an intimate knowledge of the mechanisms and behavioural characteristics of pain. But here there is a problem, since much of our knowledge concerning the physiology of pain is largely conjectural. Nevertheless, acute pains are generally associated with tissue damage or threat of damage. By contrast, chronic pains may persist for long periods of time, and are often associated with a variety of factors, including:

(1) Some definite past event (e.g. accident, infection).
(2) Some ongoing disease process (e.g. rheumatoid arthritis, temporomandibular dysfunction).
(3) An unknown cause in many cases.

In contrast to acute pain, chronic pain, characteristically, serves no useful purpose in providing a warning of impending pathology. Rather the severity of chronic pain is more of a measure of the suffering it induces rather than the actual perception of noxious stimulation. For instance, low intensity pain may result from very serious causes, whereas excruciating pain may arise from some imperceptible cause, e.g. tic douloureux. Pain intensity may, therefore, provide an index of the urgency of treatment rather than the severity of its cause. Pain intensity is, however, directly correlated with duration. The higher the intensity, the shorter the period of tolerance: low-intensity pain can be sustained for several hours, whereas maximum-intensity pain can be tolerated for only a few seconds. Also, the higher the intensity of a pain, the more likely is the pain to be intermittent. In fact, intractable pain may not be pain in the true sense of the word but simply an unpleasant or unwanted sensation.[1]

The onset of pain may be described by different characteristics. For instance, spontaneous pain occurs without provocation, whereas some provocative factor can usually be identified with induced pain. Alternatively, a pain may be triggered out of proportion to the actual stimulus. A single painful experience may last either for a few seconds or many months, during which time the pain may recur with sufficient frequency to establish a temporal relationship. Pains of short duration, separated by wholly pain-free periods, are defined as intermittent; pains of longer duration, even though variable in intensity, are termed continuous. A painful episode that lasts for several days is described as protracted, whereas intractable pain signifies that the symptoms do not respond to therapy. Two or more similar painful episodes signify recurrent pain, with intermittent pain-free intervals being termed remissions. Periodic pain is characterized by regularly recurring episodes.

A steady pain describes an unpleasant sensation, whereas paroxysmal pain comprises a volley of jabs. Bright pain has a stimulating quality, whereas dull pain is depressing. Both may be punctuated by sharp or radiating exacerbations. Pain may also be described as a function of the area where the symptom is felt, i.e. localized, spreading, migrating of referred.

Terms used to describe pain

The characteristics of a pain are difficult to define, although an 'ache' is the term most frequently used. Other terms include:

(1) *Burning pain*: a connotation of warmth.
(2) *Deep pain*: from deep visceral or somatic structures, with the symptoms being generally diffuse, often associated with symptom referral to other regions and/or muscle spasms.
(3) *Itch*: a subthreshold pain, which may have a warm or burning quality, but may become intractable.
(4) *Pricking pain*: a sharp intermittent character of short duration.
(5) *Stinging pain*: a more or less continuous high-intensity characteristic.
(6) *Superficial pain*: usually precisely localizable to a superficial lesion, with the timing, location and intensity of symptoms often being accurately described by the patient.
(7) *Throbbing* or *pulsatile pain*: an intermittent quality coincident with cardiac systoles.
(8) *Tickle*: a sensation induced by light superficial movement.

The level of suffering may increase with the duration of pain, even though the input intensity remains either the same or actually decreases. All pains, regardless of initial type or aetiology, appear to take on the clinical characteristics of psychogenic intensification with time, e.g. chronic orofacial pain syndromes are ultimately associated with chronic depression.

Somatic pain often reflects a pathological lesion in a specific organ or tissue, whereas neurogenous pain may indicate a disease process affecting a particular nerve fibre. The site where pain is felt, however, may or may not identify the location of the pain source. A primary nociceptive input characterizes pain emanating from the structures that hurt, whereas secondary pain may comprise pain felt some distance from the actual lesion, e.g. deep somatic pain input. All deep somatic pains are not alike, however, in that pain emanating from bones, joints, ligaments, muscles, soft connective tissues and tendons may be closely related to biomechanical functional demands. By contrast, high-threshold receptors innervate visceral structures so that pain is not usually felt until a certain threshold level is reached. Tissue injury (and healing) is generally associated with an inflammatory reaction that includes pain, although the symptoms depend on the location, type and phase of the inflammatory process. Most pains result from stimulation of nerves that innervate the site although some pains occur spontaneously apparently without stimulation. Pain is therefore a complex series of phenomena that may be described as unpleasant emotional and sensory experiences, associated with either actual or potential tissue damage or described in terms of such tissue damage.

Neural pain mechanisms

Classically, pain was considered a specific sensation with its own anatomically distinct receptors, primary afferent fibres, nerve tracts, relay systems and cortical reception areas. This theory contended that only free unmyelinated nerve endings in the orofacial area were activated by noxious stimuli. More recently, the anatomical specificity of receptors, has been discarded, as most receptors, if sufficiently stimulated, can respond to noxious irritation.

An alternative theory postulates that pain does not depend on specific pathways but on excessive stimulation involving all types of receptors, with the resultant central neural summation and/or convergence of activity. This summation theory was subsequently replaced by the pattern theory whereby the pattern of neural impulses set up by the noxious stimuli were considered important. Another theory (sensory interaction theory) contended that pain resulted from the interaction of both nociceptive and non-nociceptive afferent fibres on central neurones, the resulting excitatory or inhibitory interactions determining whether or not pain was perceived. Such a plethora of theories serves to emphasize the complexity of the neuronal components of pain sensation.

In fact, the central and peripheral mechanisms for pain (nociception) are both extremely complex and only partially understood. In fact, approximately 50% of sensory fibres and up to 20% of the spinal motor roots can transmit pain. Also, most pain receptors are poly- rather than unimodal. There is no central pain centre in the central nervous system analogous to the respiratory or vasomotor centres. This adds to the complexity of the nervous pathways serving pain.

The sensory (pain) receptors serving nociception may be divided into three main groups, although there is a considerable degree of functional overlap.

Pain receptors

Exteroceptors

These receptors are stimulated by the immediate external environment, with most of the impulses being sensed at conscious levels. Such receptors include:

(1) *Free nerve endings*: tactile and superficial pain.
(2) *Krause's corpuscles*: cold receptors.
(3) *Meissner's corpuscles*: tactile skin receptors.
(4) *Merkel's corpuscles*: tactile receptors in the oral mucosa and submucosa of the tongue.
(5) *Ruffini's corpuscles*: pressure and warmth receptors.

Interoceptors

Located in the body cavities, these serve involuntary bodily functions below conscious levels. These receptors include:

(1) *Free nerve endings*: perception of visceral pain and other sensations.
(2) *Pacinian corpuscles*: perception of pressure.

Proprioceptors

These receptors are chiefly involved in automatic functioning, and perceive movement, pressure and position. They include:

(1) *Free nerve endings*: perception of deep somatic pain and other sensations.
(2) *Golgi tendon organs*: mechanoreceptors in muscle tendons relaying data concerning muscle length and tension.
(3) *Muscle spindles*: mechanoreceptors between muscle fibres responsive to passive muscle stretch.
(4) *Pacinian corpuscles*: perception of pressure.
(5) *Periodontal receptors*: perception of tooth movement.

Free (unencapsulated) receptors

Free unencapsulated nerve endings are therefore the predominant form of nociceptor, especially in the cutaneous tissues, oral mucosa and periodontal tissues. But although these free nerve endings are associated with pain sensation, similar responses can also be elicited from other specialized nerve endings.

Central connections for pain

Oral or facial pain sensation is mediated centrally by afferent primary neurones that pass through the following:

(1) The posterior roots of the Vth (trigeminal), VIIth (facial), IXth (glossopharyngeal) and Xth (vagus) cranial nerves.
(2) The first, second and third cervical spinal nerves.
(3) The visceral afferents that descend through the cervical sympathetic chain to pass through the posterior roots of the upper thoracic spinal nerves.

The nerve cell bodies of the primary sensory neurones are located in the posterior root ganglion of the respective nerves through which they pass (with the exception of the proprioceptive fibres of the trigeminal, which are located in the mesencephalic nucleus in the midbrain).[2]

Subsequently, the pain fibres from the maxillofacial region terminate in the nucleus caudalis. This is the lower portion of the trigeminal spinal-tract nucleus.

The second order trigeminal neurones begin in the substantia gelatinosa of the nucleus caudalis and project to the thalamus. Third order neurones then project from the thalamus to the cerebral cortex. During this transition from first to second and from second to third-order neurones, considerable neural convergence occurs.

During the transmission of nerve impulses through these tracts, however, they are subjected to numerous inhibitory and facilitatory impulses from the higher cerebral centres. This is illustrated by the fact that the general intensity of suffering relates to a number of factors, including attention, attitude, preconditioning experience and temperament, all of which exert presynaptic inhibitory influences on the painful stimuli reaching the nucleus caudalis.[3] Thus, pain transmission from the face and mouth is not just a simple neural pathway: a variety of intermediate influences may be exerted on the neural transmission. Such a modulating system may involve the following:

(1) A change in the character of the evoked discharge.
(2) Alteration of the modalities to which the neurone responds.
(3) Alteration of the characteristics of its receptive field.[4]

There appears to be a general relationship between nerve fibre diameter and conduction velocity:[5] large fibres conduct impulses more rapidly than small ones. There also appears to be some relationship between fibre size and the type of impulse transmitted, in that Aδ and C fibres appear to convey pain impulses, in addition to other sensory modalities, whereas the fast conducting Aα, β and γ fibres primarily convey tactile and propioceptive impulses but not pain. Aδ fibres also conduct warmth, touch and cold, whereas C fibres conduct itch, warmth and cold.[6] It seems therefore that the larger peripheral nerve fibres have functional specificity that excludes pain, whereas pain sensations are predominantly carried by small fibres in addition to other sensations.[7]

Sensory information may be rapidly conducted to the CNS by transmission of nerve impulses, or more slowly by means of neurochemical substances passing through the axonal transport system.[8] Nociceptive neurones range from high-threshold mechanosensitive and mechanothermoreceptive afferents to slowly adapting low-threshold polymodal afferents. Although a significant proportion of afferent fibres enter the central nervous system via the dorsal root ganglion and brain stem, a number also travel in the ventral root. For instance, approximately 20% of the fibres in the motor root of the trigeminal may be sensory and related to nociception.[4]

Chemical mediators (transmitters)

A number of biochemical factors are also associated with the transmission of pain, some act as algogenic agents, some as neurotransmitters and some in both capacities.

Bradykinin

Bradykinin is an endogenous polypeptide released from the inflammatory reaction or from ischaemic tissues. This serves as a powerful vasodilator in addition to increasing vascular permeability. Bradykinin also excites all types of receptors, sensitizing some high-threshold receptors to respond to otherwise innocuous stimuli.[9] Bradykinin acts only in the presence of prostaglandins.[10]

Histamine

Histamine is a vasoactive amine that not only acts as a vasodilator but also increases small vessel permeability. Conceivably, histamine also functions as a central nervous system neurotransmitter.

Prostaglandins

Prostaglandins sensitize nociceptors to different types of stimuli, thus lowering their pain thresholds to all types of stimulation.[11] Prostaglandins are also required for the action of bradykinin;[10] bradykinin also stimulates the release of prostaglandins.[12] In addition, prostaglandin E increases the response of slowly adapting Aδ mechanoreceptors to non-noxious stimuli.[13]

Serotonin

Peripherally, serotonin is associated with vascular pain syndromes as an algogenic agent.[14] Centrally this monoamine appears to be an important endogenous antinociceptive mechanism.[15]

Substance P

This polypeptide acts centrally as an excitatory neurotransmitter for nociceptive impulses.[16] It is also released from spinal cord cells by Aδ and C fibre afferent stimulation and excites dorsal horn neurones that are activated by noxious stimuli.[17] Substance P modulating action on pain is both rapid and short-lived.[18]

Other agents

Acetylcholine[4], potassium[19] and a variety of endogenous toxic substances[20] serve as algogenic agents.

Mechanics of pain

At one time pain was considered to be evoked by noxious stimulation of neural structures, with the pain reaction involving a cerebral level modified by prior conditioning, memory, emotional response and evaluative significance of the pain. Pain is now considered to be a much more complex process, with neural impulses being altered, changed and modulated on passing to the higher centres, in addition to being affected by excitatory and inhibitory influences.

Gate theory

The gate control theory of pain is still the most accepted mechanistic theory of pain. It was devised by Melzack and Wall.[21–23] It proposed that noxious stimulation of the substantia gelantinosa functions as a gate control system that modulates the afferent patterns before they influence the transmission cells. The afferent patterns in the dorsal column system therefore function in part as a control trigger which activates selective brain processes that influence the modulating properties of the gate control system. The transmission cells activate neural mechanisms that comprise the action system responsible for response and perception.

On noxious stimulation of the skin, impulses are transmitted centrally by both large Aδ and small C fibres. The nerve impulses passing in the large Aδ fibres arrive at the substantia gelatinosa before those transmitted by the C fibres. These latter activate the transmission cells initially, in addition to activating a negative feedback mechanism which reduces their effect on the transmission cells. Nerve impulses in small C fibres therefore activate a positive feedback mechanism, which exaggerates the effect of impulses arriving on the transmission cells. Large-fibre impulses therefore close the gate, whereas small-fibre impulses open the gate.

Continuous ongoing bombardment by afferent nerve impulses by C fibres serves to hold the gate in a relatively open position, i.e. pre-sets the gate before the arrival of noxious stimulation. This is a critical part of the gate control theory. If this activity is accentuated by inflammation or hyperaemia, the stimulus will stimulate the transmission cells more effectively. It will also be perceived as pain.

On noxious stimulation, the activity of the large fibres increases disproportionately to that of the small fibres, and the stimulus is received as pain. Large-fibre activity also partially closes the synaptic gate, thus shortening the transmission cell barrage. The perception of, and the reaction to, the noxious stimulus are thereby shortened and reduced, as the stimulus disproportionately affects the large fibres. Thus the synaptic gate, which permits the nerve impulses of the primary afferent neurones to fire the secondary transmission cells, is affected or reset by the noxious stimulus itself. With stimulation, more receptor fibre units will be recruited. This results in both counteractive positive and negative effects, and the transmission cell output slowly rises. Thus as the noxious stimulus is increased, pain perception and reaction slowly increase, although other factors modulate the response, i.e. the response is not necessarily proportionate to its cause. If the stimulation is prolonged, the large fibres begin to adapt, decreasing large-fibre activity. This will result in a shift in the balance in favour of small fibre activity, allowing the gate to open more widely. Thus, even though the intensity of the noxious stimulus may not increase, the fact that it is continuous tends to gradually increase the perception of the reaction to the stimulus. In effect, the duration of pain normally increases its intensity.

Large-fibre activity therefore modifies the degree of gate opening. Decreased large-fibre activity will result in gate opening, whereas there will be increased pain perception if there is disproportionate small-fibre activity. A critical level of gate activity is therefore set by the large-fibres. When this critical level is set high, pain is not perceived until the firing level is reached, causing a delay between stimulus and perception, termed temporal summation. After reaching this critical firing level, a transmission cell barrage may occur explosively, causing pain that is wholly disproportionate to stimulus intensity. This is termed spatial summation. Deficient large-fibre activity may therefore elevate the critical firing level of the gate control system reflected by summation effects. Deficiency in large-fibre activity may also result in the gate being opened, with the effect that lower-intensity stimulation is perceived as pain. Gate-setting and critical firing levels are therefore different facets of the pain mechanism, even though both affect the gate control system. Presetting of the gate is also determined by higher central nervous system centres, as illustrated by the following:

(1) Past experience.
(2) Conditioning.
(3) Attention directed to suffering.
(4) The emotional status of the individual at a given time.

Such inputs may individually or collectively serve to modulate the gate. When the gate is open, the patient will not only suffer more from the same noxious stimulus but may also perceive as pain stimuli those that normally should not be painful. A calm, placid and emotionally well-adjusted individual perceives and reacts to pain differently from a distraught, anxious, emotional patient.

Presetting of the gate is also dependent on the stimulus. When stimulation occurs, certain extremely fast-conducting fibres bypass the substantia gelantinosa to synapse first in the thalamus and then to the sensory cortex. These very rapidly transmitted impulses convey data concerning the location and nature of the noxious stimulus before the same stimulus reaches the synaptic gate. Such very rapid impulses have two effects:

(1) Setting the receptivity of cortical neurones for the subsequent afferent impulse volley from the transmission cells fired from the gate control system.
(2) Resetting the gate itself by nerve impulses transmitted by descending efferent fibres from the higher cortical centres to the gate control mechanism.

There may therefore be central modulation of the gate before the noxious impulses have had time to reach the gate. If such central inhibitory feedback control on the gate is total, no pain will be felt, regardless of the intensity of the noxious stimulus. If the central inhibitory system fails, however, all sensation may be perceived as pain.

Finally, the second-order neurones from the gate to the thalamus are another level where modulation may occur. These neurones may transmit data concerning the nature of the noxious stimulus resulting in activation of both motor and sensory cortices, i.e. leading to both reactionary and sensory responses to noxious stimulation. These will again be modulated by past experience and emotional states, etc. The role of the cerebral cortex in either sensory perception in general or pain perception in particular is, however, still uncertain. Undoubtedly the cortex and other parts of the forebrain, e.g. the limbic system, are implicated in motivation, emotion, and pain memory, although their exact involvement in pain mechanisms has yet to be defined.

In 1975, two of the five endorphins (morphine receptors in the central nervous system) were noted to be associated with antinociceptive mechanisms.[24] These polypeptides behave like morphine by binding to morphine receptors to obtund pain. Encephalin and β-endorphin may therefore act as chemical neuromodulators, influencing both pain threshold and pain tolerance,[25,26] further compounding the complexity of the mechanics of pain.

Orofacial pain

Orofacial pain may be carried by myelinated or unmyelinated afferents from a receptive field, with:

(1) High-threshold mechanoreceptive (A) afferent fibres activated only by intense mechanical stimuli.
(2) Heat nociceptive (A) afferents that respond to intense heat.
(3) Strong mechanical stimuli and polymodal nociceptive (C) afferents that are responsive to intense mechanical, thermal and chemical stimuli.

These afferents are conveyed to the trigeminal (gasserian) ganglion where their primary afferent cell bodies are located. They then enter the brain stem to traverse the trigeminal spinal tract before entering the trigeminal nuclear complex (primarily the nucleus caudalis). Within this nucleus caudalis there appear to be three general types of nociceptive neurones:

(1) Nociceptive-specific neurones that respond exclusively to noxious mechanical and thermal stimuli.
(2) Wide-dynamic range neurones that respond to non-noxious as well as noxious stimuli.
(3) Low-threshold mechanoreceptive neurones that respond to light touch, pressure or facial hair movement, rather than noxious mechanical or heat stimuli.

Some of the neurones project to the thalamus via a pathway that may cross in the brain stem to the contralateral side. Others traverse to the reticular formation, cranial nerve motor nuclei (e.g. subnucleus oralis and the main trigeminal sensory nucleus) or other subnuclei. Obviously, the somatosensory cerebral cortex is involved in both general sensory perception as well as pain perception, although the role of other cortical regions, e.g. limbic system, has yet to be defined.

Secondary effects of pain

There is generally a close segmental relationship between the primary initiating pain and secondary effects of the noxious stimulus. Most secondary symptoms occur in structures innervated by the same major nerve that mediates the primary pain. These secondary effects may include:

(1) Sensory effects resulting in referred pains and secondary hyperalgesias, e.g. angina pectoris radiates to the top of the left shoulder, left arm and left side of the neck. The exact mechanism of referred pain is unclear but appears to depend on convergence of afferent inputs to central neurones from both the source and the referral sites, in addition to central summation. For instance, afferent inputs from facial, tooth pulp, pharyngeal and laryngeal sites may converge on the trigeminal brain stem complex and underlie certain types of referred pain in the orofacial region.

(2) Autonomic effects resulting in vasomotor and glandular symptoms, e.g. facial flushing with a dental abscess.

(3) Motor effects resulting in trigger point and myospastic activity in segmentally related skeletal muscles, e.g. masseter muscle pain with temporomandibular joint malfunction. For instance, local occlusal interferences may trigger increased muscular activity, changes in jaw position, muscle fatigue and pain. Interestingly, there appear to be no significant differences between the occlusions of patients affected by this disorder and those without it, thereby throwing into question the over-reliance on occlusal rehabilitation as a treatment order of this condition.

Pain aetiology (causes)

No single noxious stimulus results specifically in pain. Pain is therefore stated to have a multimodal aetiology. Nevertheless, there are some specific pathological processes that are commonly associated with pain. A few are mentioned here, primarily to illustrate the complexity of pain. Much more information concerning these aetiologies may be found in standard textbooks of pathology.

Inflammation

Tissue injury initiates an inflammatory response. Such a response characteristically includes pain. Inflammatory pain is actually a reaction to the chemical inflammatory mediators of bradykinin and prostaglandins. These chemical mediators not only result in vasodilatation and increased capillary permeability but also alter local receptor sensitivity and receptivity.[27–30] The pain threshold is lowered as a result of such mediator activity, the net result including increased nociceptor sensitivity to stimulation. Higher-threshold mechanoreceptors may also become sensitized to a wider variety of stimuli. As a result, spontaneous primary pain and stimulation-evoked primary hyperalgesia may occur. A prostaglandin-like substance may also be released in the central nervous system that sensitizes nociceptive interneurones to mechanical and chemical stimuli. The net result is that the neural pathways related to inflammatory pain become more sensitive to the action of opiates.[31]

Pain of inflammatory origin may involve different kinds of tissue innervated by receptors with different reactive responses. Superficial pain may be inflammatory in origin (e.g. gingivitis), whereas visceral inflammatory pain may result from inflammatory changes in the adjacent tissues, e.g. arteritis or lymphadenitis. Inflammatory pain is therefore but a component of a symptom complex.

Muscle pain

Most muscle pain is noninflammatory in origin. Sometimes it results from muscle spasm, sometimes it is reactive, and sometimes it is protective. For example, muscle splinting is a temporary protective mechanism resulting in muscle pain and weakness. As a consequence, such muscle splinting serves to rest the muscle until the symptoms have disappeared.

Vascular pain

Patients with vascular pain (e.g. migraine) frequently display a characteristic emotional overlay with personality features of insecurity and tension. Four possible conditions have been associated with vascular pain discomfort:[32]

(1) Vasodilatation and increased vascular permeability.
(2) Tissue oedema at the painful site.
(3) Oedema of the vessel wall and perivascular tissues.
(4) Associated muscle pain.

Thus, whereas vascular spasm and associated ischaemia contribute to the aetiology of vascular pain, other features may also occur.

Neural pain

Cutting or crushing a peripheral nerve induces anaesthesia due to afferent impulse interruption. Other symptoms may also occur, including paraesthesia, hyperaesthesia, hyperanalgesia or spontaneous pain. These symptoms may characterize the local area supplied by the nerve or may radiate to a much larger area.

Short term neural compression is usually painless, and/or results in anaesthesia. Chronic neural compression, however, ultimately leads to myelin nerve sheath degeneration. Loss of the myelin sheath may result in impulses travelling through the demyelinated region passing (shorting) to adjacent nerve fibres in a random manner, often reflected as pain, e.g. trigeminal neuralgia.[33]

Trauma, bacterial infection and inflammation may result in inflammatory changes of the nerve fibre itself.[1] As a result the threshold of C fibres may be lowered, thus making them more sensitive to nociceptive stimuli and there may be partial or complete abolition of the reactivity of the Aδ fibres.[34] Thus the peripheral inhibitory mechanisms of pain modulation may be reduced, leading to the net neural activity being perceived as pain.[21]

Other causes of pain

Pain may result from a variety of pathological events, including:

(1) Spontaneous events, without obvious cause.
(2) Elevation of body temperature, e.g. fever.
(3) A general response to abnormal allergic, emotional, endocrine, metabolic or toxic conditions.
(4) Direct noxious chemical, mechanical or thermal insults.

Categories of facial pain

Pain from the face or oral cavity may be classified into three general categories: somatic, neurogenous or psychogenic.

Somatic pain

Somatic pain may result from stimulation of neural receptors or peripheral nerves. If superficial in origin, the clinical characteristics include:

(1) Bright pain with a stimulating quality.
(2) Accurate pain localization.
(3) Accurate correlation between lesional site and pain source.
(4) Temporary pain abolition by topical anaesthetic application to the site.

If deep in origin, the clinical characteristics include:

(1) Dull pain, depressing in quality.
(2) Variable localization of diffuse pain.
(3) Site of pain may/may not correlate with lesional site.
(4) Frequent display of secondary central excitatory effects.

Neurogenous pain

As neurogenous pains are generated within the nervous system itself, nerve receptor or fibre stimulation is unnecessary. The clinical characteristics of such neurogenous pains include:

(1) Bright, burning pains with a stimulating quality.
(2) Good localization.
(3) Close correlation between site of pain and lesion.
(4) Possible accompaniment by other sensory, motor and/or autonomic symptoms.

Psychogenic pain

Psychogenic pain may reflect somatic or neurogenous pain intensification, or may be a psychoneurotic manifestation. The characteristics of psychogenic pain include:

(1) The site of pain often has no correlation with a possible cause.
(2) The clinical behaviour and/or response to therapy may be non-physiological, unexpected or unusual.

Odontogenic pain (toothache)

A tooth is primarily innervated from the maxillary or mandibular division of the trigeminal nerve that pass essentially through the apical foramen. These nerve fibres are evident at the cap stage of odontogenesis.[35] Whereas in the fully developed tooth, some nerves terminate in the pulp proper, the majority pass towards the coronal pulpal walls and roof to form the subodontoblastic nerve plexus. Nerve fibres from this plexus then pass into the overlying odontoblastic layer, and comprise both myelinated and unmyelinated nerve fibres (some of which may be autonomic in origin). Thermal, osmotic, electrical, therapeutic and pharmacolgical stimuli result in pulpal nerve excitation,[36] although the degree of specificity remains obscure. In fact both myelinated (A) and unmyelinated (C) fibres pass through the apical foramen into the root canal and generally branch infrequently until the coronal aspect where they fan out towards the pulpal dentine border as Rashkow's plexus. The density of this plexus varies, tending to be greater at the tips of the coronal pulp horns. From this subodontoblastic nerve plexus, nerve fibres are distributed in the pulpodentinal border zone, with terminals showing a characteristic head-like structure.

Some of the small (<1 μm diameter) nerve fibres in the odontoblastic zone are closely applied to the odontoblasts, and others enter the predentine to pass in the dentinal tubules for variable distances.[37-39] Some of these nerve fibres may, however, have an autonomic efferent rather than nociceptive afferent function. Also, there is little evidence that these fibres pass to the amelocemental junction (clinically the most sensitive region of the tooth). Thus, although these nerve fibres may be associated with tooth-ache, other mechanisms may also be responsible.

The odontoblastic transduction theory contends that a dental stimulus excites either an odontoblast or its process which then transmits the excitation to adjacent nerve fibres. Such a view is supported by the close association between odontoblasts and subodontoblastic nerve plexus, in addition to the neural crest origin of the odontoblasts themselves. The hydrodynamic theory contends that enamel or dentinal stimulation causes an outward or inward flow of dentinal tubular contents, the resultant disturbances being translated as pulpal nerve excitation.[40] Conceivably, more than one mechanism may be involved.

The innervation of the pulp includes both afferent neurones that conduct sensory impulses and efferent autonomic neurones that principally provide neurogenic modulation of the blood flow in the pulp. Myelinated axons appear mostly associated with pain sensory function and have the following properties:

(1) Relatively fast conduction velocity.
(2) Relatively slow stimulation threshold.
(3) Considered to convey impulses conceived as sharp and penetrating.

The pain sensory unmyelinated nerve fibres passing into the pulp tissue are generally considered to exhibit the following properties:

(1) Relatively slow conduction velocity.
(2) Relatively high stimulation threshold.
(3) Considered to convey impulses conceived as dull and lingering.

Pulpal (including nociceptive) stimuli result in neuronal activity in widely dispersed CNS regions, including:

(1) Trigeminal brain stem sensory nuclei.
(2) Cranial nerve motor nuclei.
(3) Cerebellum.
(4) Reticular formation.
(5) Ventrobasal thalamus.
(6) Hypothalamus.
(7) Somatosensory cerebral cortex.
(8) Orbital cerebral cortex.

Pulpal stimulation thereby produces emotional, motivational and other behavioural changes, in addition to the appropriate reflex responses. The innervation of tooth pulps exhibits marked variability, with an increase in the number of myelinated axons from the time of first eruption to some time after eruption. This correlates with newly erupted healthy teeth being less sensitive than older healthy teeth. With aging, however, the number of axons entering a tooth generally decreases. This again correlates well with clinical findings of a reduction in pulpal sensitivity with increasing age.

Pain control

Many procedures are available for the control of pain. These include:

(1) Pharmacological agents: local and general anaesthetic agents, analgesic drugs, e.g. morphine.
(2) Therapeutic procedures: acupuncture, transcutaneous electrical stimulation, audioanalgesia, hypnosis.
(3) Psychiatric counselling.
(4) Neurosurgery.

All these methods are directed toward blocking pain transmission either at the periphery before the impulses enter the brain or within the brain.

The reader is referred to more clinically oriented textbooks for a more detailed exposition of these topics.

Conclusions

Pain is a multidimensional experience involving both the sensation evoked by a noxious stimulus but also the reaction to it. The sensation of pain therefore depends in part on the patient's past experience, personality and level of anxiety. The neural basis for pain is, however, poorly understood, with the gate theory emphasizing some of the polymodal interactions involved. These complex interactions have yet to be fully evaluated.

Review questions

1. Describe the various types of pain receptors found in the body.
2. What are the possible causes of pain?
3. Describe the possible mechanisms for pain from a grossly carious tooth using the gate theory.
4. Compare tooth-ache with somatic facial pain.
5. How can pain be controlled?

References

1. DALESSIO, D.J. (1972) *Wolff's Headache and Other Head Pain*. New York: Oxford University Press
2. DUBRUL, E.L. (1980) *Sicher's Oral Anatomy*, 7th ed. St. Louis: C.V. Mosby
3. WIESENDANGER, M., HAMMER, B. and HEPP-REYMOND, M.C. (1970) Corticofugal control mechanisms of somatosensory transmission in the spinal trigeminal nucleus of the cat. In *Trigeminal Neuralgia*, edited by R. Hassler and A.E. Walker. Stuttgart: Georg Thieme
4. YAKSH, T.L. and HAMMOND, D.L. (1982) Peripheral and central substrates involved in the rostral transmission of nociceptive information. *Pain*, **13**, 1–85
5. CLARK, D., HUGHES, J. and GASSER, H.S. (1935) Afferent function in the group of nerves of slowest conduction velocity. *Am. J. Physiol.*, **114**, 69
6. BISHOP, G.H. (1966) Fibre size and myelination in afferent systems. In *Pain*, edited by R.S. Knighton and P.R. Dumke. Boston: Little Brown
7. COLLINS, W.F., NULSEN, F.E. and SHEALY, C.N. (1966) Electrophysiological studies of peripheral and central pathways conducting pain. In *Pain*, edited by R.S. Knighton and P.R. Dumke. Boston: Little Brown
8. WALL, P.D. (1984) Mechanisms of acute and chronic pain. In *Advances in Pain Research and Therapy*, edited by L. Kruger and J.C. Liebeskind. New York: Raven Press
9. MENSE, S. and MEYER, H. (1981) Bradykinin-induced sensitization of high-threshold muscle receptors with slowly conducting afferent fibres. *Pain (Suppl.)*, **1**, s204
10. CHAHL, L.A. and IGGO, A. (1977) The effects of bradykinin and prostaglandin E1 on rat cutaneous afferent nerve activity. *Br. J. Pharmacol.*, **59**, 343–347
11. HIGGS, G.H. and MONCADA, S. (1983) Interactions of arachidonate products with other pain mediators. In *Advances in Pain Research and Therapy*, edited by J.J. Bonica, U. Lindblom and A. Iggo, Vol 5, pp. 617–626. New York: Raven Press
12. GREENBERG, S. and PALMER, G.C. (1978) Biochemical basis of analgesia: metabolism, storage, regulation and actions. *Dent. Clin. North. Am.*, **22**, 31–46
13. PATEROMICHELAKIS, S. and ROOD, J.P. (1981) Effects of prostaglandin E on A-beta and A-delta mechanoreceptor responses. *Pain (Suppl.)*, **1**, s203
14. BECK, P.W. and HANDWERKER, H.O. (1974) Bradykinin and serotonin effects on various types of cutaneous nerve fibres. *Pflügers Arch. Ges. Physiol.*, **347**, 209–222
15. MESSING, R.B. and LYTTLE, L.D. (1977) Serotonin-containing neurons: their possible role in pain and analgesia. *Pain*, **4**, 1–21
16. ZIMMERMANN, M. (1979) Peripheral and central nervous mechanisms of nociception, pain, and pain therapy. In *Advances in Pain Research and Therapy*, edited by J.J. Bonica, J.C. Liebeskind and D.G. Albe-Fessard, Vol 3, pp. 3–32. New York: Raven Press
17. LEMBECK, F., DONNERER, J. and COLPAERT, F.C. (1981) Increase in substance P in primary afferent nerves during chronic pain. *Neuropeptides*, **1**, 175
18. YASPHAL, K., WRIGHT, D.M. and HENRY, J.L. (1982) Substance P reduces tail-flick latency: implications for chronic pain syndromes. *Pain*, **14**, 155–167
19. KEELE, K.D. (1975) A physician looks at pain. In *Pain: Clinical and Experimental Perspectives*, edited by M. Weisenberg. St Louis: C.V. Mosby
20. CHAHL, L.A. and KIRK, E.J. (1975) Toxins which produce pain. *Pain*, **1**, 3–49
21. MELZACK, R. and WALL, P.D. (1965) Pain mechanisms: a new theory. *Science*, **150**, 971–979
22. CASEY, K.L. and MELZACK, R. (1967) Neural mechanisms of pain: a conceptual model. In *New Concepts of Pain*, edited by E.L. Way. Philadelphia: F.A. Davis
23. WALL, P.D. (1978) The gate control theory of pain mechanisms: a re-examination and restatement. *Brain*, **101**, 1–18
24. BASBAUM, A.T. (1981) Brainstem control of nociiception: the contribution of the monoamines. *Pain (Suppl.)*, **1**, s231
25. WATKINS, L.R. and MAYER, D.J. (1982) Organization of endogenous opiate and non-opiate pain control systems. *Science*, **216**, 1185–1192
26. VON KNORRING, L., ALMAY, B.G. and JOHANSSON, F. (1978) Pain perception and endorphin levels in cerebrospinal fluid. *Pain*, **5**, 359–365
27. BURGESS, P.R. and PERL, E.R. (1973) Cutaneous mechanoreceptors and nociception. In *Handbook of Sensory Physiology*, edited by A. Iggo, Vol 2, pp. 29–78. Heidelberg: Springer Verlag
28. BEITEL, R.E. and DUBNER, R. (1976) The response of unmyelinated (C) polymodal nociceptors to thermal stimuli applied to a monkey's face. *J. Neurophysiol.*, **35**, 1160
29. LIM, R.J.S. (1970) Pain. *Ann. Rev. Physiol.*, **32**, 269
30. HANDWERKER, H.O. (1976) Influences of algogenic substances and prostaglandins on the discharges of unmyelinated cutaneous nerve fibres identified as nociceptors. In *Advances in Pain Research and Therapy*, edited by J.J. Bonica and D.G. Albe-Fessard, Vol 1, pp. 41–45. New York: Raven Press
31. FERREIRA, S.H. (1983) Prostaglandins: peripheral and central analgesia. In *Advances in Pain Research and Therapy*, edited by J.J. Bonica, U. Lindblom and A. Iggo, Vol 5, pp. 627–634. New York: Raven Press
32. WOLFF, H.G. (1963) *Headache and Other Head Pain*. New York: Oxford University Press
33. SWEET, W.H. (1977) Trigeminal neuralgia. In *Facial Pain*, edited by C.G. Alling and P.E. Mahan. Philadelphia: Lea & Febiger
34. BIGELOW, N., HARRISON, I. and GOODELL, H. (1945) Studies on pain: quantitative measurements of two pain sensations of the skin with reference to the nature of the 'hyperalgesia of peripheral neuritis'. *J. Clin. Invest.*, **23**, 503
35. PEARSON, A.A. (1977) The early innervation of the developing deciduous teeth. *J. Anat.*, **123**, 563–577
36. MATTHEWS, B. (1977) Responses of intradental nerves

to electrical and thermal stimulation of teeth in dogs. *J. Physiol. (Lond.)*, **264**, 641–664

37. FEARNHEAD, R.W. (1963) The histological demonstration of nerve fibres in human dentine. In *Sensory Mechanisms in Dentine*, edited by D.J. Anderson. Oxford: Pergamon Press
38. CORPRON, R.E. and AVERY, J.K. (1973) The ultrastructure of intradental nerves in developing mouse molars. *Anat. Rec.*, **175**, 585–606
39. ANDERSON, S.A. (1979) Pain control by sensory stimulation. In *Advances in Pain Research and Therapy*, edited by J.J. Bonica, J.C. Liebskind and D.G. Albe-Fessard, Vol 3, pp. 569–585. New York: Raven Press
40. BRANNSTROM, M. and ASTROM, A. (1972) The hydrodynamics of the dentine: its possible relationship to dentinal pain. *Int. J. Dent.*, **22**, 219–227

2

Mastication

Introduction

Masticatory movements comprise exceedingly complex and co-ordinated neuromuscular events. They include not only mandibular elevation and depression but also opposing tooth alignment and accurate regulation of masticatory forces. However, whether mastication utilizes some of the neuromuscular pathways and mechanisms used in the programmed rhythmic motor behaviour of suckling, or whether the maturing nervous system develops new mechanisms triggered by tooth eruption, remains enigmatic.

These masticatory activities require the co-ordinated activity of several groups of muscles attached primarily to the mandible. These muscles appear to have shorter contraction times than most other body muscles. They also incorporate muscle spindles to monitor their activity, especially the elevator muscles. The masticatory muscles appear to have no Golgi tendon organs to monitor tension, although periodontal ligament and oral mucosal mechanoreceptors conceivably provide sufficient motor neurone feedback. Masticatory muscle control and co-ordination are partly a function of brain stem centres. These are not only capable of generating oscillatory activity patterns, independent of feedback from the periphery, but may also initiate rhythmic chewing movements. In this respect, mastication is a rhythmical activity with many similarities to respiration, locomotion and other innate rhythms. There is, however, scant information concerning the roles for the brain stem centres, basal ganglia, cerebellum or cerebral cortex in masticatory control. The existence of jaw reflexes (jaw jerk, jaw-opening and jaw-closing) suggest that neural connections could provide the following:

(1) Length servomechanisms for jaw movement control.
(2) Positive feedback mechanisms to reinforce elevator muscular contraction forces when the teeth contact a bolus.
(3) Protective mechanisms which limit the maximum forces developed on the teeth and mucous membranes.

Masticatory mandibular movements

Subjects with good dentitions usually have greater masticatory efficiency than partially dentate or edentulous individuals.[1] These last two types of patient do not compensate for lack of masticatory efficiency by increased numbers of chews, however, but tend to swallow rather larger food boluses.

The range of mandibular masticatory movements were first described by Ulrich[2] and Bennett[3] at the turn of the century. They showed that there was no fixed axis of mandibular rotation. Normal movements always involve simultaneous hinge and sliding condylar movements. Even the small mandibular movements from rest to occlusion always involve some posterior condylar movement, in addition to rotation. Some individuals are capable of producing pure hinge movements on occlusal opening, but only for the initial opening phases. With maximum opening, the condyles move forward, beyond the lowest part of the articular eminence. This forward condylar movement is even greater when the mandible is protruded with the teeth in contact. When the mandible is moved to one side, the condyle on that side moves downward. A posterior condylar movement is also possible from centric occlusion. Such posterior mandibular movements from a centric relationship occur during swallowing, but not during masticatory movements.[4] Thus the condyle may rotate and translate to allow the jaw to open and close during masticatory mandibular movements.[5] The condylar head does not abut directly on the temporal bone, however, as there is a joint cavity. There is also an intervening meniscus that divides the joint cavity into upper and lower compartments. It is generally considered that hinge movements occur in the lower compartment and translational movements in the upper compartment, although both movements may occur in each compartment to a variable extent.

During mastication, there is an opening phase, during which there may be some lateral deviation, and a closing phase which begins with a lateral component towards the working side. There is also a lateral component back towards centric occlusion in the final closing phase, which is often guided by gliding tooth contacts.[6,7] In fact, the chewing cycle can be considered to comprise three phases:

(1) An opening phase.
(2) A closing phase.
(3) An occlusal phase.

During both the opening and beginning of the closing phases, the masticatory muscles undergo isotonic contraction or relaxation. In the latter part of the closing and occlusal phases, however, tension builds up in the elevator muscles. Elevator muscular contraction is strictly isometric only when the teeth are in contact or when there is a hard unyielding object in between them. During chewing, the change from isotonic to isometric contraction is usually not abrupt but rather a gradual change during the latter part of the closing phase. The opening movement appears to be only just sufficient for the teeth to clear the bolus; tooth contact with the bolus occurs soon after the beginning of the closing phase.[7] Mastication is characterized not only by a simple straight opening and closing of the jaw but also retrusive, protrusive and lateral jaw movements. Bilateral chewing is far less common than unilateral chewing since one side of the jaw is usually favoured in mastication. Each chewing cycle lasts approximately 0.8–1.0 s.[8]

During the closing phase of mastication, the temporalis muscle on the working side is the first to become active, followed by both masseters and the temporalis of the balancing (non-working) side.[6,9] The masseter and medial pterygoids are the first to become active during an incisive movement.[10] The lateral pterygoid muscle is active during both mandibular protrusion and opening,[11] although it is not strictly a mandibular depressor. The suprahyoid muscles (digastric, geniohyoid and mylohyoid muscles) become active during jaw opening, although hyoid stabilization through infrahyoid and stylohyoid muscle contraction is a necessary prerequisite.[12] During the initial phase of isotonic closing from an open position, the depressor muscles are first activated.[6] The depressor muscles then gradually relax to allow the mouth to be closed by the passive tension in the elevator muscles and ligaments.

During opening, there is usually a lateral mandibular shift to the working (functional) side. The mandible then swings back during closure into the intercuspal position. Tooth contact glides (or slides) may occur as the opposing teeth contact one another during the initial phases of opening or terminal phases of closing. Thus both the condylar head and mandibular body move during mastication. The working-side condyle moves laterally during the opening phase, whereas the opposing condyle on the balancing side moves medially downwards and forwards. The working-side condyle rapidly resumes its position within its fossa early in the closing phase, whereas the balancing-side condyle moves back into its fossa in the later phase of closing. Such mandibular movement patterns are not fixed, however, but may be affected by a number of factors, including food bolus consistency, individual masticatory habits and the state of the dentition.

Tooth contact

A maximum force of about 50 kg can be developed between the molar teeth of a dentate patient, although forces of up to 150 kg have been recorded between the molar teeth in Eskimos.[13] This maximum force can be increased by exercise and practice.[14] The maximum force occurs between the first molars, and falls off by about 10 kg in the incisor region.[15] It is not known whether this maximum biting force is limited by protective reflexes centring on periodontal membrane receptor excitation and elevator muscle inhibition, or the physical properties of the masticatory muscles themselves coupled with tooth depression within their periodontal membranes. In fact, both mechanisms may be involved. Since the maximum force developed by a muscle depends in part on its length, the biting force is maximal when the teeth are separated by a few millimetres.[16,17] In a small proportion of cases, the maximum biting force is limited by pain from the teeth[18], especially in patients with advanced chronic periodontal disease. During normal function, however, a force of 7–15 kg occurs during swallowing and chewing.[19–21] If the bite is raised on one tooth, that tooth, and the opposing tooth in the opposite jaw, will be subjected to increased masticatory stress. In such instances, the total tension developed by the elevator muscles may be reduced, presumably due to increased periodontal mechanoreceptor stimulation.[22]

Thus a number of factors may influence the biting force including:

(1) The particular tooth (greater forces occur between the molars than incisors).
(2) Dietary consistency.
(3) Degree of chronic periodontal disease.
(4) Jaw separation.
(3) Tooth-cusp configuration.
(6) Natural or artificial teeth.
(7) Biting practice.

The masticatory system is relatively unique compared with other bodily movements in that it is often terminated by abrupt contact between hard tissues. The periodontal supporting tissues provide only limited cushioning.[23] Such a situation places a significant role on the neural regulating mechanisms of the muscles of mastication. The original claims that only negligible contacts occur between the teeth during mastication are not true.[24] In fact, the closing movements during chewing are all directed towards the position of maximal intercuspal contact, with tooth contact occurring in up to 100% of the strokes in a chewing sequence.[6,25–27] The number of tooth contacts may vary with food type and increases towards the end of a chewing cycle; this is associated with reduced food-particle size towards the end of the masticatory cycle.[26] In some instances, the teeth contact on only one side of the jaws, due to displacement of the loaded teeth in their sockets[28] and mandibular bending.[29] Often there appears to be a gliding movement between the opposing tooth cusps as they pass into and out of maximal contact.[6] During such gliding movements, eccentric tooth contacts may occur.[30] In some patients, such gliding contacts cannot be detected, as vertical chopping movements predominate.[6] In such instances, there is no mechanical guide to the final path of mandibular closure, so that mandibular movements must be dependent on neural mechanisms. During swallowing, tooth contacts occur both in the position of maximal intercuspation[26] and with the mandible in a more retruded position,[27] although such retrusive mandibular movements do not occur during mastication.[27]

Abnormal tooth contacts have been implicated in the aetiology of periodontal tissue pathogenesis, in addition to temporomandibular joint and masticatory muscle malfunction. Such abnormal tooth contacts may result in a dentist performing tooth reshaping in the form of extensive crown and bridge therapy or changing the normal occlusal relationship between the upper and lower teeth. There is, however, no conclusive evidence that a traumatic occlusion develops physiologically in the absence of chronic periodontal disease or that abnormal tooth contacts or particular jaw relationship patterns ever provide the primary causes of periodontal disease, temporomandibular joint disease or masticatory muscle malfunction.[31–33]

The normal mechanisms which determine the position of a tooth in the dental arch would be expected to prevent the development of a traumatic occlusion. Also a tooth would be expected to maintain this position during function, since abnormal forces would result in a change of tooth position until a new equilbrium position was achieved. Thus an occlusion which had developed physiologically would already be in optimal equilibrium; such an optimal equilibrium could not be improved by orthodontic or occlusal rehabilitative therapy. If the occlusion were to be changed for aesthetic or food stagnation reasons, then an alternative position of non-traumatic equilibrium would have to be achieved. If the functional forces were greater than normal, reflex changes in masticatory muscle activity might occur as a result of increased periodontal membrane mechanoreceptor activity. Altered tooth contacts might also lead to abnormal masticatory muscle activity if the normal synaptic events forming part of the control mechanisms regulating masticatory muscle activity were disturbed.

Neural masticatory receptors

The various co-ordinated masticatory activities of the mandible are reflected by the appropriate muscle function. Each mandibular skeletal muscle comprises an active contractile portion, comprising large numbers of extrafusal striated muscle fibres, and a passive elastic component comprising fascia, ligaments and tendons. Both elements contribute to muscle tone at rest or in contraction, although the relative contribution of each appears to be a function of muscle length. Each muscle is innervated by α-efferent motor neurones that supply the extrafusal muscle fibres, whereas γ-efferents supply the intrafusal fibres of the muscle spindles. As with other skeletal muscles, the masticatory muscles may undergo isotonic contraction (shorten to produce jaw movement against constant load) or isometric contraction (produce contractile tension with no change in length). Each muscle comprises fibres that exhibit rapid twitch contraction (fast or white fibres that are quickly fatigable) or slow twitch contraction (fatigue-resistant and atuned to the maintenance of mandibular posture). There are also muscle fibres with intermediate properties.

Contraction of individual muscle fibres is a function of a muscle unit. The latter comprises a single α motor neurones, its α-efferent nerve fibre and a number of muscle fibres. The size of a motor unit reflects the number of individual muscle fibres supplied. An increase in muscle tension involves the following:

(1) An increase in individual motor unit discharge frequency.
(2) An increase in the number of motor units discharging (recruitment)–the smaller motor units become activated first, with the larger units becoming activated at higher tensions.
(3) Increased motor unit discharge synchrony.

Sensory receptors in skeletal muscles generally comprise two basic groups: free and encapsulated nerve endings. Free nerve endings are generally believed to be primarily associated with pain perception, although some may be sensitive to non-noxious stimuli, e.g. muscle stretch.

Muscle spindles

Muscle spindles of the orofacial muscles are similar to those elsewhere in the body.[34] They comprise stretch-sensitive, slowly-adapting specialized (intrafusal) mucscle fibres that are contained within a capsule lying parallel to the extrafusal muscle fibres. The spindle generally has a double afferent innervation:

(1) Large (12–20 μm diameter) group Ia mylinated afferent fibres terminate as annulo-spiral (primary) endings in the central region of each intrafusal fibre.
(2) Smaller (4–12 μm diameter) group II myelinated afferent fibres ending on either side of the central region as spray (secondary) endings.

The efferent (motor) supply to the intrafusal fibres is derived from γ motor neurones located within the central nervous system. Some muscles, e.g. mandibular elevators (masseter, medical pterygoid and temporalis) have large numbers of spindles,[36] whereas the digastric, facial and lateral pterygoid muscles contain few, if any, muscle spindles.[37–39] This suggests that these latter muscles have either alternative means of proprioceptive control, e.g. free nerve-endings, and/or depend on other stretch-sensitive afferents, e.g. receptors in the temporomandibular joint. The masseter, temporalis and medial pterygoid muscles contain numerous spindles that relay information to the brain about muscle length.[35] In fact, the number of spindles/g muscle is much greater in the muscles of mastication than in the upper limb muscles,[40] although only about 50% compared with the muscles that move the fingers.[41–42]

The spindle afferents from the masseter, temporalis and medial pterygoid muscles appear unique, in that their cell bodies reside within the central nervous system. In fact, the axons bypass the trigeminal ganglion and enter the pons in the motor rather than the sensory root of the trigeminal nerve. The cell bodies of these large unipolar cells reside in the trigeminal mesencephalic nucleus. Collaterals form monosynaptic connections with elevator muscle α motor neurones in the trigeminal motor nucleus.[43] Destruction of the trigeminal ganglion or the trigeminal root between the ganglion and the pons is not followed by degeneration of synaptic terminals in the trigeminal motor nucleus.[44] This confirms that the cell bodies of the spindle afferents are within the CNS. The mesencephalic nucleus contains cells of fibres which innervate muscles on the same side of the body,[43] although input may also be received from nerves supplying contralateral muscles.[45,46] Lesions in the trigeminal mesencephalic tract produce no detectable degeneration of fibres in the nerves to the anterior belly of the digastric or mylohyoid muscles,[44,47,48] and there do not appear to be afferents responding to passive stretch of the depressor muscles from either the mesencephalic nucleus[47] or the trigeminal ganglion.[49]

There is a concept that the muscle spindles may be involved in correcting small errors between the intended and actual mandibular movements and maintaining a constant posture against the effects of gravity. Originally, the γ motor neurones were considered to provide the command signal for a movement, with the muscle spindles acting as an error detector in a follow-up length servomechanism. The spindles are still considered as providing length feedback but in a system whereby muscle contraction is servo-assisted rather than being totally dependent on a follow-up length servomechanism.[42] This is because muscle movement results from central coactivation of both α and γ motor neurones, rather than α motor neurones alone. Thus, if a nut is cracked between the teeth, the unloading reflex results in a sudden switching off of the powerful elevator muscle contraction as soon as the nut cracks. The sudden shortening of the elevator muscles will cause a decrease in the spindle discharge with a consequent reduction in α neurone activity. Throughout the bite and crack, the masticatory system behaves as though it were attempting to move the mandible so the distance between the teeth was slightly less than the diameter of the nut. Forces of up to 100 kg can be developed between the teeth under such conditions, but rarely do they crash together when the resistance suddenly disappears. Thus the spindles of the mandibular elevators may monitor individual spindle output without interrupting their connections with other neurones.

Golgi tendon organs

The Golgi tendon organs are receptors primarily located at muscle-tendon junctions (or temporomandibular joint capsule). They are innervated by Ib myelinated afferent (8–12 μm diameter) fibres. There is no evidence of such units within the masticatory muscles, or tension receptor afferents in the trigeminal ganglion.[49]

Periodontal mechanoreceptors

The periodontal ligament contains mechanoreceptors that respond to forces applied to the teeth.[50] These mechanoreceptors have a wide range of properties:

(1) Some are excited by just a few microns of tooth displacement.[51]
(2) Some are less sensitive and respond only to much larger forces.
(3) Some exhibit directional sensitivity, with nerve fibres responding maximally to forces in one particular direction.[52]
(4) Some are slowly adapting and produce continuous discharge when a constant stimulus is applied.
(5) Some adapt more rapidly, producing only a few impulses immediately when stimulated.[53]
(6) Some are very rapidly adapting units and do not respond unless a very rapid stimulus is applied.
(7) Some are very slowly adapting units and provide a constant discharge that can be increased or decreased by applying forces in specific directions.[54]

The actual location of these various units has yet to be defined, however, although conceivably some may be associated with the surrounding soft tissues, rather than in the periodontal membrane itself, e.g. palatal mucosa[51] and tongue.[55]

Most single fibres respond to mechanical stimulation of just one tooth, although some also respond to stimulation of up to three adjacent teeth.[56] Whether this results from nerve branching with a single nerve supplying the receptors of more than one tooth, or mechanical coupling between the teeth, remains obscure. Fibres which respond to mechanical stimulation of a tooth can often also be excited by pressure on the adjacent mucous membrane or gingiva. This again may reflect indirect periodontal membrane receptor stimulation.

The conduction velocities of the periodontal membrane mechanoreceptor fibres range from 25 to 80 m/s, with the majority between 40–50 s.[53,57] The cell bodies of some of these fibres are located in the trigeminal (gasserian) ganglion, with others in the trigeminal mesencephalic nucleus.[43,58] Responses to mechanical stimulation of the teeth have also been reported from interneurones in the supratrigeminal,[59] main sensory and rostral part of the spinal trigeminal nuclei.[60,61]

Mucous membrane receptors

There are some cells in the mesencephalic nucleus, main sensory and spinal trigeminal nuclei[61] that respond to pressure in the palate, particularly in the region just distal to the central incisors.[43] There is no evidence of specialized nerve endings in the oral mucosa.

Joint receptors

Free nerve fibres comprise the predominant receptor in the temporomandibular joint capsule.[62] In addition, a few complex receptors have been recorded, including Ruffini, Pacinian and Golgi receptors. These last appear to be confined to the lateral aspect of the joint capsule and lateral ligament and supplied by a branch of the auriculotemporal nerve. The majority of myelinated nerve fibres innervating the temporomandibular joint are small in diameter (up to 2 μm) There are some up to 12 μm, however, which presumably innervate the more complex receptors. These receptors appear to be associated with joint location preception.[62]

Central neural connections

Muscle spindle afferents from the mandibular elevators (masseter, medial pterygoid and temporalis) enter the mandibular division of the trigeminal. The cell bodies of these nerves reside in the trigeminal mesencephalic nucleus (not the trigeminal ganglion), along with some of the primary afferents responding to tactile stimulation of one or more teeth, the palatal mucosa and cutaneous regions of the face. Most afferent fibres responding to tactile stimuli, including those from the temporomandibular joint and muscle nociceptive afferents, have their cell bodies within the trigeminal ganglion. The unipolar, bipolar and multipolar cells form clusters within the mesencephalic nucleus. Conceivably the associated tight junctional contacts and synapses between these cells facilitate afferent signal amplification, thereby regulating the signals before passing to the trigeminal motor nucleus or higher centres of the brain. The central axonal processes of the masticatory muscle spindle afferents leave their cell bodies in the trigeminal mesencephalic nucleus to pass to the trigeminal motor nucleus. This forms the jaw-jerk reflex arc. In addition, these muscle afferents pass to other regions of the central nervous system including the cerebellum and cerebrum. Such muscle afferent input to the cerebral cortex may contribute to jaw motility control or jaw position sense. Interestingly, other cranial nerves, e.g. VII, XII, may also comprise muscle afferent fibres, possibly facilitating mandibular movement control.

The muscle, cutaneous, temporomandibular joint and intraoral afferents serve as the afferent limbs of the many reflex activities associated with the oral cavity. The afferent fibres pass much of their sensory input via one or more synapses to the cranial nerve motor nuclei, which then supply the α-efferent motor neurones that effect muscle contraction. Most of these are simple reflexes. More complex reflex functions are required for masticatory and swallowing mandibular movements. There is therefore a hierarchy of reflex complexity:

(1) Simplex reflexes, e.g. mandibular depression.
(2) Complex reflexes, e.g. masticatory activities.

Many of the interneurones involved in these various reflex activities are located within the sensory cranial nuclei, in the supratrigeminal nucleus or the diffuse reticular formation interposed between the sensory and motor nuclei.

Jaw reflexes

Jaw reflexes are roughly comparable to spinal reflexes although there are some fundamental differences.

(1) Some primary afferent cell bodies are located within the trigeminal mesencephalic nucleus.
(2) Many orofacial muscles lack Golgi tendon organs or muscle spindles.
(3) The γ-efferent (fusimotor) control system is incomplete, due to the lack of muscle spindles in many muscles.
(4) Reciprocal innervation is limited, due to the sparsity of muscle spindle and tendon afferent fibres. This may be compensated for by afferent inputs from receptors in the periodontal membrane and temporomandibular joint.
(5) The conduction velocity of orofacial efferent fibres may be slower than their spinal counterparts.

The motor neurones involved in these reflexes lie predominantly within the trigeminal motor nucleus, except for those supplying the posterior belly of the digastric muscle which are derived from the motor neurones of the accessory facial nucleus.

Jaw-closing reflex

The simple jaw-closing (jaw-jerk) reflex has a 6 ms latency period between stimulus and movement. This monosynaptic reflex involves stretch-induced masseter or temporalis muscle spindle activation, with the afferents passing to the trigeminal motor nucleus via the trigeminal mesencephalic nucleus. Efferents then effect appropriate muscle contraction.

Tapping on the chin initiates a jaw-jerk reflex analogous to the knee jerk. After a brief depression of the mandible, there is a reflex response in the masseter and temporalis muscles, following an 8 ms latency delay. If the jaw jerk is repeated with the subject voluntarily biting on a hard object, there is a marked increase in reflex masseter muscular activity. After this initial response, the masseter does not return immediately to the previous level of activity, but passes through a period of decreased activity, during which the masseter is totally inactive. This is termed the silent period. It is not possible to establish the exact duration and latency of such silent periods as they depend on many factors, including the amount of activity at the time the stimulus was applied and the degree of mouth opening.

Activation of the elevator muscles in the jaw jerk involves a monosynaptic reflex with Ia spindle afferents.[63] An increase in response during voluntary contraction of the elevator muscles[64] indicates that the contraction is accompanied by an increase in γ motor neurone activity to increase elevator muscle spindle sensitivity. If the voluntary contraction were solely due to α motor neurone activation, then the chin tap would have produced less spindle-stretch, resulting in a smaller monosynaptic reflex. If the teeth are clenched together with nothing between them, the jaw jerk is depressed, although the silent period is still present.[65] Indeed, there is evidence that the peridontal ligament mechanoreceptors produce monosynaptic reflex inhibition on the same side.[66]

There is no detectable response in either the elevator or depressor muscles of a relaxed subject if the chin is tapped from underneath, i.e. there is no reverse jaw jerk. There is also no response if the stimulus is applied while the subject contracts his depressor muscles against resistance. These data suggest that there are few muscle spindles and no stretch reflex in the digastric muscle.[67]

By contrast, rapid jaw closing by mandibular elevator muscle contraction results in an unloading reflex.[68] The effects in the jaw muscles are those which would be expected if the elevator muscle spindles suddenly stopped firing. This would cause a decrease in elevator α motor neurone excitation and removal of some inhibition from the depressor α motor neurones, assuming that there is reciprocal innervation. The spindles in the mandibular depressors, therefore, exhibit an insignificant role.

Jaw-opening reflex

The jaw-opening reflex is a response to orofacial stimuli and involves two or more synapses and excitation of the motor neurones that supply the digastric and inferior head of the lateral pterygoid muscles. The interneurones, relaying the sensory afferents from the orofacial region to the digastric motor neurones, are located in the trigeminal spinal tract nucleus and adjacent reticular formation. The trigeminal spinal tract nucleus also relays afferent inputs from the face, oral mucosa, teeth and temporomandibular joints to the motor neurones.

Electrical oral mucosal stimulation of a subject whose elevator and depressor muscles are relaxed results in now jaw muscle activity.[69] When the elevator muscles are voluntarily contracted, however, there is masseteric inhibition, with two periods of inhibition with latencies of 15 and 45 ms and a brief interim of normal reactivity. Similar responses have been reported following electrical stimulation from several intraoral sites.[70–72] With reduction in stimulus intensity, however, only one latent period occurs,[70] and no response at all if the intensity is only just above the sensory threshold.[73] Electrical stimulation of the face, palate, gingiva, periodontium, tooth pulp, laryngopharyngeal mucosa, temporomandibular joint or lips produces similar effects.[70,74]

After stimulation, a slight opening movement occurs[71] presumably reflecting elevator muscular inhibition. This opening could evoke a stretch reflex in the elevator muscles and provide a contribution to the overall response, including the synchronization of activity between and after the two inhibitory phases.[71]

Mechanical stimulation of the teeth causes similar effects to those produced by electrical stimulation. When the elevators of depressors are relaxed, there is no detectable muscular response as the teeth are tapped. When the elevators are contracted, however, and the tooth is tapped, then there is elevator muscular inhibition, although no response occurs in the digastric muscle.[75–77] The latency and duration of this response depends on many factors, with the minimum latency of inhibition being about 13 ms. This inhibition of elevator activity may be entirely the result of periodontal mechanoreceptor activity, although some activity remains after neutralization of afferent activity by local anaesthesia.[84] This latter may reflect the presence of a jar reflex, in which bone vibration causes excitation of the elevator spindles and transitory synchronization of elevator motor units. This could present as increased and decreased motor activity, with the decreased period presenting as a silent period. There is general agreement that stimulation of the periodontal mechanoreceptors causes elevator muscular inhibition, although there is no comparable change in digastric muscle activity when the depressors are relaxed or contracted.[75]

Just prior to the silent period produced by tapping a tooth, there is transient activation of the elevator muscles with a latency of 7 ms.[77,78] This elevator activation has been compared in latency to the monosynaptic jaw jerk. Mechanical stimulation of the mucous membranes and lips[70] also causes a short latency of elevator muscle activity.

Tooth contact reflexes

When the upper and lower teeth are snapped together, reflex changes occur in the elevator muscles, similar to those produced by mechanical single tooth stimulation. This transient activation is followed by a silent period associated with later phases of increased and decreased activity. There are no comparable effects on the depressor muscles. A silent period may comprise a frequent occurrence in normal masticatory tooth contacts[79,80] reflecting periodontal mechanoreceptor activity, although muscle spindles may also be involved. If elevator muscle contraction resulted from co-activation of α and γ efferents, intrafusal fibre contraction in the elevator spindles would result in increased spindle discharge when movement was suddenly arrested. As a result, there would be elevator muscle activation by the monosynaptic reflex pathway and a silent period.

Jaw-unloading reflex

When the jaw is suddenly unloaded, a protective reflex immediately limits further jaw-closing muscular activity. This sudden reduction or complete cessation of elevator muscle activity is associated with reflex excitement of the jaw-depressor muscles. The receptors responsible for this reflex have yet to be discerned.

Horizontal jaw reflexes

Lateral, protrusive and retrusive reflex mandibular reflexes are important in finely controlled mastica-

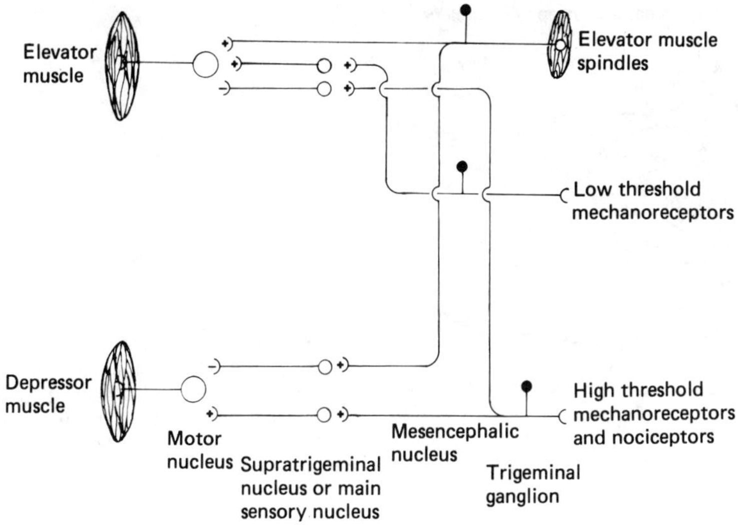

Figure 2.1 Summary of reflex arcs by which intra-oral stimuli result in changes to depressor and elevator muscle activity.

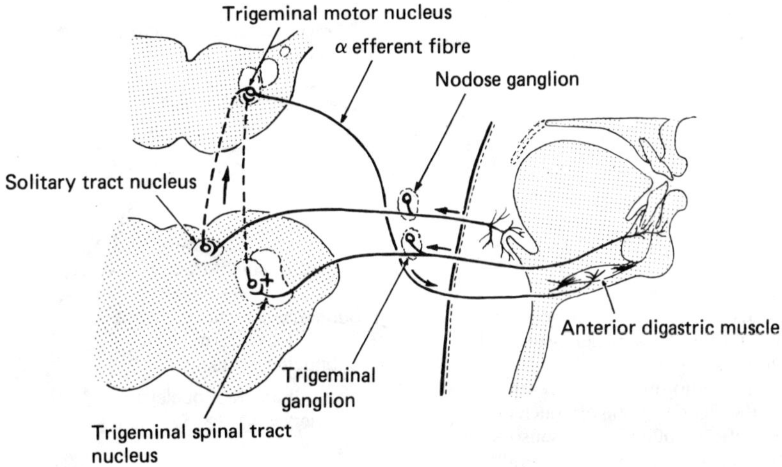

Figure 2.2 Jaw-opening reflex in the anterior digastric muscle evoked from intra-oral or pharyngolaryngeal stimulation.

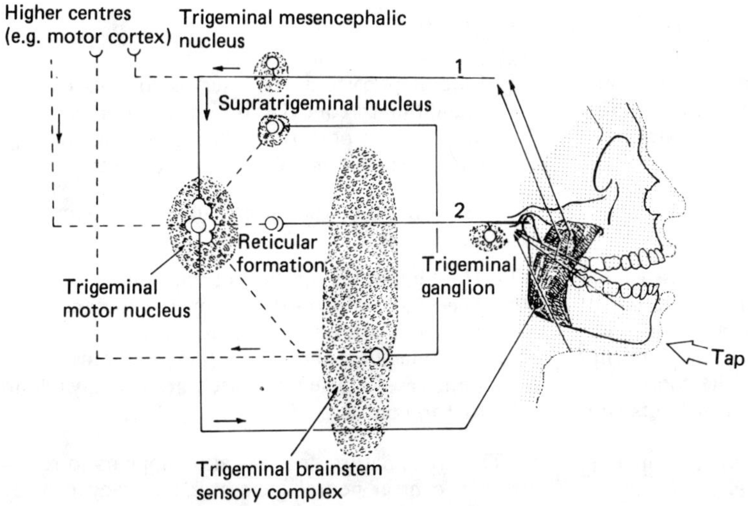

Figure 2.3 Probable central reflex pathways from lower tooth or chin tap. Pathway 1 mainly excites jaw-closing motor neurones involving trigeminal motor nucleus. Pathway 2 mainly inhibits these motor neurones via one or more synapses in the supratrigeminal nucleus, trigeminal brain stem nuclei or reticular formation. Some information in both pathways also passes to higher brain centres, where it may modulate descending motor neurones in the motor nucleus. Peripheral receptors of these pathways are located in skin, periodontal ligament, mucous membrane, periosteum, temporomandibular joint and muscles.

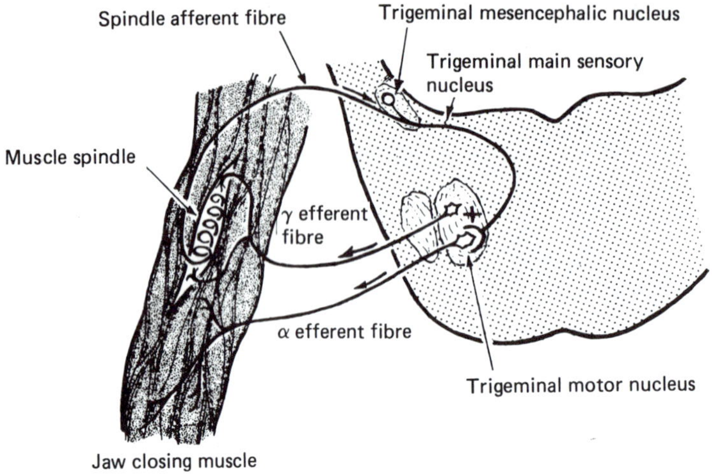

Figure 2.4 Jaw-changing reflex where muscle spindle afferent stimulation leads to trigeminal motor nucleus activation (+) relaying efferent data to the intrafusal fibre of the spindle *and* the jaw-closing muscle.

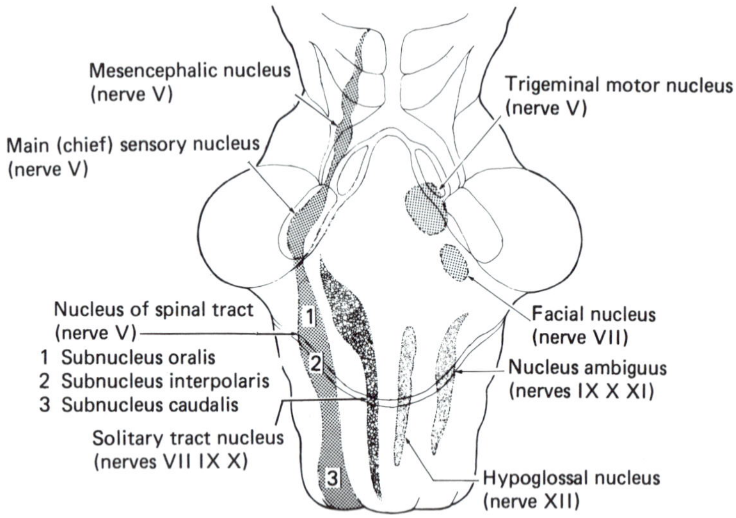

Figure 2.5 Principal sensory and motor brain stem nuclei associated with cranial nerves V–XII. For clarity, motor nuclei are presented on the right and sensory nuclei on the left, although in fact sensory and motor nuclei occur bilaterally.

tory mandibular movements. Although lateral mandibular movement reflexes, resulting from lateral pterygoid contraction, can be elicited from tactile tooth or oral mucosal stimulation,[81] these reflex pathways have been subjected to scant enquiry.

Mastication

The mandibular and condylar movements associated with mastication are the co-ordinated result of sequenced mandibular muscle contraction (*Figures 2.1–2.5*). The muscles of the tongue, face and lips are also important for maintaining the food bolus between the teeth,[82,83] as evidence in patients with Bell's (facial nerve) palsy.

The muscles responsible for mandibular opening may be placed in the following order of activity:

(1) Mylohyoid.
(2) Digastric.
(3) Lateral pterygoid. This serves to stabilize the mandibular condyle or move the condyle anteriorly or posteriorly during opening, closing and protrusive mandibular movements.[81]

The primary muscles responsible for mandibular closing include:

(1) The temporalis on the working side.
(2) The temporalis on the balancing side and both masseters after a 50–100 ms delay.
(3) Both masseter and medial pterygoid muscles; in some cases, these two muscle groups may be the first to contract.

The cyclic nature of mastication appears to result from a central neural generator (chewing centre) located in the brain stem reticular formation.[79] The interval between masticatory strokes is often remarkably regular during a chewing sequence, suggestive of some overall regulatory mechanism. Conceivably, such a centre generates the basic cyclic pattern of masticatory muscle activity, although this may be influenced by peripheral afferents from other regions including the face and mouth, in addition to central influences from other parts of the brain, e.g. emotion, stress and volition. Mastication is therefore not a peripherally triggered event, although a voluntary effort is not required for the continued masticatory activity once started. Volition may, however, be associated with masticatory initiation or cessation, reflecting overall cerebral cortical influences. Mastication can occur, however, in decerebrate animals and anencephalic patients, although the movements may be disturbed due to lack of higher control. Although mandibular movements are not peripherally evoked, sensory inputs can facilitate or suppress centrally induced mandibular movements. Such sensory afferents may reflexly influence brain stem motor neurone activity or affect higher cortical centres whose descending pathways may also affect the chewing centre. Conceivably, the basic opening and closing mandibular movements are primarily chewing-centre dependent, whereas more refined muscle activities are probably under peripheral and central control.

Maxillomandibular relations

Mandibular rest position

In the rest (postural) position, the mandible is generally assumed to be maintained in a fairly constant position relative to the maxilla, when a patient is relaxed with the anterior teeth being separated by a few millimetres. The maintenance of such a position is assumed to be a function of some postural control mechanism whereby a low level of elevator muscle activity opposes the effects of gravity.[84]

This rest position has important denture construction connotations. However, experimental data have repeatedly shown that there is no single constant position of the mandible when the patient is at rest.[85,86] Low levels of activity occur in the mandibular elevator and depressor muscles when a subject is in the rest position.[87–90] Changes in this activity level may occur with gravitational changes, e.g. following tilting of the patient's head.[90] Such an equilibrium position may result from passive forces of the muscles, ligaments and joint capsules,[91] with muscle activity being required to accomodate mandibular positional deviations, i.e. in an manner analogous to erect posture maintenance by trunk muscle activity.

Conclusions

It is the main function of the dentist to ensure that patients can bite and masticate their food in an efficient manner. The problem is that there is still a dearth of information concerning the 'proper' method for the opposing teeth to meet together during chewing. As a result, great care has to be taken to ensure that the patient's masticatory ability is improved, rather than worsened, by dental treatment.

Review questions

1. Describe the events when you suddenly crack the shell of a hazel-nut between your teeth.
2. How could 'premature' tooth contact interfere with normal masticatory movements?
3. Discuss the physiological role of periodontal mechanoreceptors.
4. What is the significance of the mandibular rest position?
5. What central influences can affect masticatory movements?

References

1. GUNNE, H.S. (1985) Masticatory efficiency and dental state. A comparison between two methods. *Acta Odontol. Scand.*, **43**, 139–146
2. ULRICH, J. (1959) The human temporomandibular joint. *J. Prosthet. Dent.*, **9**, 399–406, translated by U. Posselt from the original text dated 1896
3. BENNETT, N.G. (1908) A contribution to the study of the movement of the mandible. *Proc. R. Soc. Med.*, **1**, 79–95
4. KIDD, W.L. and SANDER, A. (1961) A study of posterior mandibular movements from intercuspal occlusal position. *J. Dent. Res.*, **40**, 419–425
5. NEVARKI, K. (1976) An analysis of the mandibular movement from rest to occlusal position. *Acta Odontol. Scand. (Suppl.)*, **129**, 19
6. AHLGREN, J. (1966) Mechanism of mastication. *Acta Odontol. Scand. (Suppl.)*, **24**, 44
7. MURPHY, T.R. (1965) Timing and mechanism of human masticatory stroke. *Arch. Oral Biol.*, **10**, 981–993
8. GILL, H.I. (1971) Neuromuscular spindles in human lateral pterygoid muscles. *J. Anat.*, **109**, 157–167
9. MOLLER, E. (1967) The chewing apparatus. *Acta Physiol. Scand. (Suppl.)*, **69**, 280
10. CARLSOO, S. (1956) An electromyographic study of the activity of certain suprahyoid muscles (mainly the anterior belly of the digastric muscle) and of the reciprocal innervation of the elevator and depressor muscles of the mandible. *Acta Anat.*, **26**, 81–93
11. CARLSOO, S. (1956) An electromyographic study of the

activity and anatomic analysis of the mechanics of the lateral pterygoid muscle. *Acta Anat.*, **26**, 339–351

12. LEHR, R.P., BLARTON, P.L. and BIGGS, N.L. (1971) An electromyographic study of the mylohyoid muscle. *Anat. Rec.*, **169**, 651–660
13. WAUGH, L.M. (1939) Dental observations among Eskimo. *J. Dent. Res.*, **15**, 355–366
14. BREKUS, P.J., ARMSTRONG, W.D. and SIMON, W.J. (1941) Stimulation of the muscles of mastication. *J. Dent. Res.*, **20**, 87–92
15. WORNER, H.K. and ANDERSON, M.N. (1944) Biting force measurements on children. *Aust. Dent. J.*, **48**, 1–12
16. BOOS, R.H. (1940) Intermaxillary relation established by biting power. *J. Am. Dent. Assoc.*, **27**, 1192–1199
17. TUELLER, V.M. (1969) The relationship between the vertical dimension of occlusion and forces generated by closing muscles of mastication. *J. Prosthet. Dent.*, **22**, 284–288
18. BLACK, G.V. (1895) An investigation of the physical characters of the human teeth in relation to their diseases and to practical dental operations, together with the physical characteristics of filling materials. *Dent. Cosmos*, **37**, 469–484
19. ANDERSON, D.J. (1956) Measurement of stress in mastication. *J. Dent. Res.*, **35**, 671–673
20. NYQUIST, C. and OWALL, B. (1968) Masticatory load registrations during function. *Odontal. Revy*, **19**, 45–54
21. ATKINSON, H.F. and SHEPHERD, R.W. (1967) Masticatory movements and the resulting force. *Arch. Oral Biol.*, **12**, 195–202
22. ANDERSON, D.J. and PICTON, D.C.A. (1958) Masticatory stresses in normal and modified occlusion. *J. Dent. Res.*, **37**, 312–317
23. JERGE, C.R. (1964) The neurologic mechanism underlying cyclic jaw movements. *J. Prosthet. Dent.*, **14**, 667–681
24. JANKELSON, B., HOFMAN, G.M. and HENDRON, J.A. (1953) The physiology of the stomatognathic system. *J. Am. Dent. Assoc.*, **46**, 375–386
25. ADAMS, S.H. and ZANDER, H.A. (1964) Functional tooth contacts in lateral and centric occlusion. *J. Am. Dent. Assoc.*, **69**, 465–473
26. ANDERSON, D.J. and PICTON, D.C.A. (1957) Tooth contact during chewing. *J. Dent. Res.*, **36**, 21–26
27. PALMEIJER, J.H.N., GLICKMAN, I. and ROEBER, F.W. (1968) Intra-oral telemetry. *J. Prosthet. Dent.*, **19**, 151–159
28. PICTON, D.C.A. (1963) The effect on normal vertical tooth mobility on the rate of thrust and time interval between thrusts. *Arch. Oral. Biol.*, **81**, 291–299
29. PICTON, D.C.A. (1962) Distortion of jaws during biting. *Arch. Oral Biol.*, **7**, 575–580
30. GRAF, H. and ZANDAR, H.A. (1963) Tooth contact pattern in mastication. *J. Prosthet. Dent.*, **13**, 1055–1066
31. RAMFJORD, S.P. (1961) Bruxism: a clinical and electromyographic study. *J. Am. Dent. Assoc.*, **62**, 21–44
32. SCHAERER, P. and STALLARD, R.F. (1966) Effect of occlusal interference on tooth contact during mastication. *Helv. Odontol. Acta*, **10**, 49–56
33. SCHAERER, P., STALLARD, R.E. and ZANDER, H.A. (1967) Occlusal interferences and mastication: an electromyographic study. *J. Prosthet. Dent.*, **17**, 438–449
34. CODY, F.W.J., LEE, R.W.H. and TAYLOR, A. (1971) Classification of jaw muscle spindle afferents in the cat. *J. Physiol.*, **222**, 82–83P
35. FREIMANN, R. (1954) Untersuchungen über Zahl und Anordnung der Muskelspindeln un den Kaumuskeln des Menschen. *Anat. Anz.*, **100**, 258–264
36. FRANKS, A.T. (1965) The control of movements in the temporomandibular joints. *Ned. Tijdschr. Tandheelkd.*, **72**, 605–619
37. BOSSY, J. (1958) A propos de l'innervation proprioceptive du muscle stylohyoiden et du ventre proterieux du muscle gastric. *Arch. Anat. Histol. Embryol.*, **41**, 37–50
38. VOSS, H. (1956) Zahl und Anordnung der Muskelspindeln in den oberen Zungenbeinmuskeln, im M. trapezius und M. latissimus dorsi. *Anat. Anz.*, **103**, 443–446
39. WINKLER, G. (1957) L'innervation proprioceptive des muscles sanshyoidieus et génio-hyoidien chez l'homme. *Arch. Anat. Histol. Embryol.*, **40**, 169–178
40. DELLOW, P.G. and LUND, J.P. (1971) Evidence for central timing of rhythmical mastication. *J. Physiol.*, **215**, 1–13
41. COOPER, S. (1960) Muscle spindles and other muscle receptors. In *Structure and Function of Muscle*, edited by G.H. Bourne. New York: Academic Press
42. MATTHEWS, P.B.C. (1972) *Mammalian Muscle Receptors and their Central Connections*. London: Arnold
43. CORBIN, K.B. (1940) Observations on the peripheral distribution of fibres arising in the mesencephalic nucleus of the fifth cranial nerve. *J. Comp. Neurol.*, **73**, 153–177
44. SZENTAGOTHAI, J. (1948) Anatomic considerations of monosynaptic reflex arcs. *J. Neurophysiol.*, **11**, 445–454
45. SMITH, R.D., MARGARIAN, H.Q. and NIEMER, W.T. (1967) Bilateral relationships of the trigeminal mesencephalic nuclei and mastication. *J. Comp. Neurol.*, **131**, 79–91
46. SMITH, R.D., MARCARIAN, H.Q. and NIEMER, W.T. (1968) Direct projections from the masseteric nerve to the mesencephalic nucleus. *J. Comp. Neurol.*, **133**, 495–502
47. CORBIN, K.B. and HARRISON, F. (1940) Function of the mesencephalic root of the fifth cranial nerve. *J. Neurophysiol.*, **3**, 423–435
48. THELANDER, H.E. (1924) The course and distribution of the radix mesencephalica trigemini in the cat. *J. Comp. Neurol.*, **37**, 207–220
49. BEAUDREAU, D.E. and JERGE, C.R. (1968) Somatotrophic representation in the Gasserian ganglion of tactile peripheral fields in the cat. *Arch. Oral Biol.*, **13**, 247–256
50. ANDERSON, D.J., HANNAM, A.G. and MATTHEWS, B.

(1970) Sensory mechanisms in mammalian teeth and their supporting structures. *Physiol. Rev.*, **50**, 171–195

51. YAMADA, M. (1967) Interactions between the tactile sense and the mobility of the tooth. *J. Dent. Res.*, **46**, 1256
52. NESS, A.R. (1954) The mechanoreceptors of the rabbit mandibular incisor. *J. Physiol.*, **126**, 475–493
53. PFAFFMANN, C. (1939) Afferent impulses from the teeth due to pressure and noxious stimulation. *J. Physiol.*, **97**, 207–219
54. HANNAM, A.G. (1969) Spontaneous activity in dental mechanosensitive units in the dog. *Arch. Oral Biol.*, **14**, 793–801
55. SMITH, R.D. and MARCARIAN, H.Q. (1968) Centripetal localisation of tooth and tongue tension receptors. *J. Dent. Res.*, **47**, 616–621
56. HANNAM, A.G. (1970) Receptor fields of periodontal mechanosensitive units in the dog. *Arch. Oral Biol.*, **15**, 971–978
57. HANNAM, A.G. (1968) The conduction velocity of nerve impulses from dental mechanoreceptors in the dog. *Arch. Oral Biol.*, **13**, 1377–1383
58. JERGE, C.R. (1963) Organisation and function of the trigeminal mesencephalic nucleus. *J. Neurophysiol.*, **26**, 379–392
59. JERGE, C.R. (1963) Function of the nucleus supratrigeminalis. *J. Neurophysiol.*, **26**, 393–402
60. EISENMAN, J., LANDGREN, S. and NOVIN, D. (1963) Functional organisation in the main sensory trigeminal nucleus and in the rostral subdivision of the nucleus of the spinal trigeminal tract in the cat. *Acta Physiol. Scand. (Suppl.)*, **59**, 214
61. KRUGER, L. and MICHEL, F. (1962) A single neuron analysis of buccal cavity representation in the sensory trigeminal complex of the cat. *Arch. Oral Biol.*, **71**, 491–503
62. THILANDER, B. (1961) Innervation of the temporomandibular joint capsule in man. *Trans. R. Sch. Dent. Stockh.*, Umea, No. 7
63. MCINTYRE, A.K. and ROBINSON, R.G. (1959) Pathway for the jaw-jerk in man. *Brain*, **82**, 468–474
64. HANNAM, A.G. (1972) Effect of voluntary contraction of the masseter and other muscles upon the masseteric reflex in man. *J. Neurol. Neurosurg. Psychiatry*, **35**, 66–71
65. HUFSCHMIDT, H.J. and SPULER, H. (1962) Mono- and polysynaptic reflexes in trigeminal muscles in man. *J. Neurol. Neurosurg. Psychiatry*, **25**, 332–335
66. GOLDBERG, L.J. (1972) The effect of jaw position on the excitability of two reflexes involving the masseter muscle in man. *Arch. Oral Biol.*, **17**, 565–576
67. BLOM, S. (1960) Afferent influences on tongue muscle activity. *Acta Physiol. Scand. (Suppl.)*, **49**, 170
68. HANNAM, A.G., MATTHEWS, B. and YEMM, R. (1968) The unloading reflex in masticatory muscles of man. *Arch. Oral Biol.*, **13**, 361–364
69. GOLDBERG, L.J. (1971) Masseter muscle excitation induced by stimulation of periodontal and gingival receptors in man. *Brain Res.*, **32**, 369–381
70. BRATZLAVASKY, M. (1972) Pauses in activity of human jaw closing muscles. *Exp. Neurol.*, **36**, 160–165
71. YEMM, R. (1972) Reflex jaw opening following electrical stimulation of oral mucous membrane in man. *Arch. Oral Biol.*, **17**, 513–523
72. YU, S.K., SCHMITT, A. and SESSLE, J.B. (1973) Inhibitory effects on jaw muscle activity of innocuous and noxious stimulation of facial and intraoral sites in man. *Arch. Oral Biol.*, **18**, 861–870
73. YEMM, R. (1972) The response of the masseter and temporal muscles following electrical stimulation of the oral mucous membrane in man. *Arch. Oral Biol.*, **17**, 23–33
74. HOFFMAN, P. and TONNIES, J.F. (1948) Nachweis des völlig konstanten Vorkrommens des Zunger-Kieferreflexes. *Pflügers Arch. Ges. Physiol.*, **250**, 103–108
75. BEAUDREAU, D.E., DAUGHERTY, W.F. and MASLAND, W.S. (1969) Two types of motor pause in masticatory muscles. *Am. J. Physiol.*, **216**, 16–21
76. HANNAM, A.G., MATTHEWS, B. and YEMM, R. (1969) Changes in the activity of the masseter muscle following tooth contact in man. *Arch. Oral Biol.*, **14**, 1401–1406
77. SESSLE, B.J. and SCHMITT, A. (1972) Effects of controlled tooth stimulation on jaw muscle activity in man. *Arch. Oral Biol.*, **17**, 1597–1608
78. HANNAM, A.G., MATTHEWS, B. and YEMM, R. (1970) Receptors involved in the response of the masseter muscle to tooth contact in man. *Arch. Oral Biol.*, **15**, 17–24
79. AHLGREN, J. (1967) Kinesiology of the mandible. *Acta Odontol. Scand.*, **25**, 593–611
80. AHLGREN, J. (1969) The silent period in the EMG of the jaw muscles during mastication and its relationship to tooth contact. *Acta Odontol. Scand.*, **27**, 219–227
81. SESSLE, B.J. and GURZA, S.C. (1981) Jaw movement-related activity and reflexly induced changes in the lateral pterygoid muscle of the macaque monkey. *Arch. Oral Biol.*, **27**, 167–173
82. AHLGREN, J. (1966) Mechanisms of mastication. *Acta Odontol. Scand.*, **24**, 1–109
83. MOLLER, E. (1966) The chewing apparatus. *Acta Physiol. Scand.*, **69**, 1–229
84. POSSELT, U. (1963) *The Physiology of Occlusion and Rehabilitation*. Oxford: Blackwell
85. BANDO, E., FUKUSHIMA, S., KAWABATA, H. and KOHNO, S. (1972) Continuous observations of mandibular positions by telemetry. *J. Prosthet. Dent.*, **28**, 485–490
86. GRIFFITHS, M.J. and DIBDIN, G.H. (1974) Telemetry of mandibular posture. *J. Dent.*, **3**, 261–266
87. CARLSOO, S. (1952) Nervous coordination and mechanical function of the mandibular elevators. *Acta Odontol. Scand. (Suppl.)*, **10**, 11
88. KAWAMURA, Y., KATO, I. and TAKATA, M. (1967) Jaw closing muscle activities with the mandible in the rest position. *J. Dent. Res.*, **46**, 1356–1362

89. LEHR, R.P., BLARTON, P.L. and BIGGS, N.L. (1971) An electromyographic study of the mylohyoid muscle. *Anat. Rec.*, **169**, 651–660
90. LUND, P., NISHIYAMA, T. and MOLLER, E. (1970) Postural activity in the muscles of mastication with the subject upright, inclined and supine. *Scand. J. Dent. Res.*, **78**, 417–424
91. YEMM, R. and BERRY, D.C. (1969) Passive control in mandibular rest position. *J. Prosthet. Dent.*, **22**, 30–36

3

Taste

Introduction

The general sensory nerve fibres innervating the orofacial tissues provide a wealth of information on the tactile features, pressure, temperature and potentially harmful qualities of objects coming into contact with the oral tissues. While the total experience of taste represents the integration of information derived from olfactory qualities, as well as other sensory features, of the stimulus (e.g. temperature of soup affects the assessment of its saltiness), the sensation of taste is the dentist's primary concern. Taste receptors are localized on the tongue and palatal oral mucosa, where they are especially vulnerable to the effects of a wide variety of oral or systemic disorders and treatments. Indeed, over two million North Americans probably have taste problems, although the subjective nature of taste prohibits the collection of accurate data. This is partly the result of the variety of terms that are used to describe taste anomalies:

1. Hypogeusia (ageusia)–reduced or total lack of taste.
2. Dysgeusia (cacogeusia)–unpleasant or bad tastes.

Disorders of taste can be physically upsetting and induce mental stress and worry. Indeed, symptoms of depression are frequently associated with taste dysfunctions. Disorders of taste may also be associated with a wide range of neurological and musculoskeletal disorders, including intracranial trauma, stroke and 'multiple sclerosis. Salivary gland function can also affect the sensation of taste, e.g. following localized injury, radiation and the side-effects of drugs and medications. Abnormal taste responses have also been associated with patients with diabetes mellitus, disseminated (widespread) cancer, cystic fibrosis and renal dysfunction. Unfortunately there have been all too few investigations on this important oral sensory input.

Taste

Taste may be defined as the detection and recognition of liquid phase stimuli. Taste (or gustation) is a sensation that is developed well before birth. Initially, therefore, it may comprise part of the monitoring system of the amniotic environment. After birth, the complex process of taste may be subdivided into a number of component aspects.[1]

Preneural taste events

There is really very little data concerning the events immediately preceding the stimulation (depolarization) of the component taste buds. It is, however, assumed to be influenced by a variety of factors, including:

(1) Stimulus characteristics.
(2) Taste support systems.
(3) General taste bud characteristics.
(4) Specific taste bud receptor characteristics.
(5) Mechanisms of stimulus–receptor binding.

Neural taste events

Similarly, the neural events following taste bud stimulation have been subjected to scant neurological investigation. It is again assumed that such neurogenic transmission is influenced by a variety of factors, including:

(1) Transduction of the chemical binding energy to an electrically recognizable generator potential.
(2) Neural transmission of the generator potential.
(3) Formation of the action potential and its axonal conduction.
(4) Transmission of the action potential to those brain centres involved with taste detection and recognition.
(5) Central nervous system integration of the received signals.

Taste stimuli

Present-day dogma contends that taste stimuli represent four primary qualities, salt, sweet, sour and bitter;[2] this is in fact a condensation of previous views that there were ten primary qualities. The characteristics of taste stimuli, which are essential for their detection and recognition at a molecular level, have yet to be defined for any taste stimulus.

The sweet taste

The sweet taste is not caused by any single class of chemicals, but several, including:

sugars	esters
glycols	amino acids
alcohols	sulphonic acids
aldehydes	halogenated acids
ketones	inorganic salts of lead and beryllium
amides	

Most of the substances that cause a sweet taste are therefore organic chemicals, and a slight molecular change can cause a change in taste from sweet to bitter, e.g. the addition of a simple radical. Thus the stimuli that produce a sweet response are diverse, so that the simple view that carbohydrates are equivalent to sweet cannot hold.[4] There is a theory that all stimuli that are sweet have a specific molecular structure, with two component functional groups equivalent to a strong acid and a strong base. Some form of complementarity may then exist with the taste receptor, such that hydrogen bonding or some other form of energy-requiring process takes place at a specific molecular distance of 0.3 nm between these two component functional groups.[4] This latter proposition remains theoretical.

The sour taste

The best correlation between taste stimulus and taste response concerns the sour taste for the hydrogen ion concentration and/or the degree of dissociation of the acid.[3] There are, however, exceptions to this general rule, in that all acids are not sour (e.g. amino acids are sweet).

The bitter taste

Like the sweet taste, the bitter taste is not caused by any single type of chemical. Bitter substances, represented by alkaloids (including many of the drugs used in medicine, e.g. quinine, caffeine, strychnine and nicotine), ureas, and other long-chain organic substances containing nitrogen, represent a diversity of sensory stimuli, although many anomalies exist. For instance, saccharin tastes sweet at low concentrations but bitter at high concentrations, and even at low concentrations there is a bitter after-taste. Some substances have a sweet taste on the front of the tongue, where taste buds with special sensitivity to the sweet taste are principally located, and a bitter taste on the back of the tongue, where taste buds more sensitive to the bitter taste are located.

The bitter taste, when it occurs in high intensity, usually results in a patient rejecting a particular food or medication. This is undoubtedly an important function of the bitter taste sensation, since many of the deadly toxins found in poisonous plants are alkaloids, and these all cause intensely bitter tastes.

The salt taste

The salty taste is elicited by ionized salts. The quality of the taste varies between one salt and another because the salts also elicit other taste sensations besides saltiness. In general, salts are detected and recognized by their cation, although the counter ion, the molecular species of the cation and other factors may also be involved.[3]

Obviously, considerably more work is required to define taste stimulus characteristics. There are, however, certain thresholds for stimulation of various taste sensations:

(1) The sour taste for hydrochloric acid averages 0.9 mmol/litre.
(2) The salty taste for sodium chloride averages 10 mmol/litre.
(3) The sweet taste for sucrose averages 10 mmol/litre.
(4) The bitter taste for quinine averages 8 μmol/litre.

This illustrates how much more sensitive is the bitter taste compared with the other taste sensations: an important protective function. Many patients are, however, taste blind for certain substances, especially for different types of thiourea compounds.

Taste support systems

The major taste support systems (*Figure 3.1*) include:

(1) Secretions of glands of the oral cavity which come into direct contact with the taste system.
(2) Physical structures that house the taste buds.

The salivary secretions are derived from both major and minor salivary glands and, with the diminution of their function, resulting either from radiotherapy[5] or Sjögren's syndrome,[6] taste acuity for all stimuli is either destroyed or markedly attentuated. Moreover, attempts to use artificial saliva substitutes have been universally unsuccessful in rectifying the abnormal taste function.[7] Conceivably, therefore, saliva contains some taste bud stimulatory factor(s).

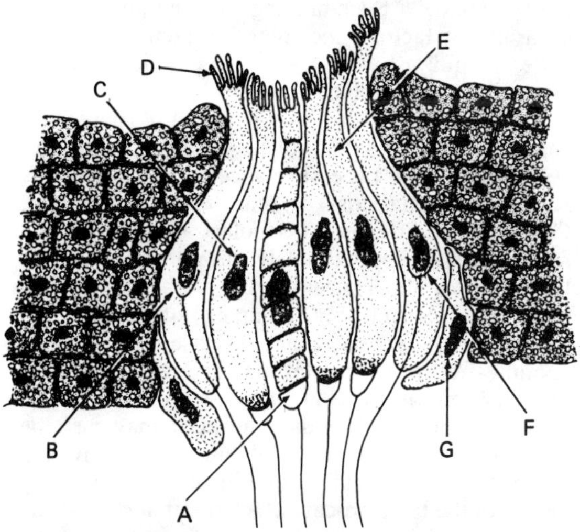

Figure 3.1 Diagrammatic representation of taste bud. A, type II cell with nerve fibres coiled around cell body; B and F, type I cells with nerve fibre invaginated into cell bodies; C and E, type III cells with synaptic nerve contacts; G, type IV (basal) cells.

Taste bud locations

The taste bud is composed of about 40 modified epithelial cells:

(1) Taste cells.
(2) Sustentacular (supporting) cells.

The taste cells are continually being replaced by mitotic division from the surrounding epithelial cells. The life span of each taste cell is limited and a taste bud actually comprises taste cells at various levels of maturity. The outer tips of the taste cells are arranged around a minute taste pore. From the tip of each cell several microvilli (taste hairs) protrude outwards into the taste pore towards the oral cavity. Interwoven among the taste cells is a branched terminal network of several taste nerve fibres, some of which invaginate into folds of the taste cell membranes. There is therefore an extremely intimate contact between the taste cells and the nerves.

Interestingly, the taste buds degenerate when the taste nerve fibres are destroyed. If, subsequently, the taste fibres regrow to the epithelial surface of the mouth, the local epithelial cells reform to a new taste bud. Presumably, this trophic function of a taste nerve fibre reflects the action of some protein trophic factor secreted by the nerve endings.

Taste buds in the oral cavity are present in papillae, e.g. the fungiform papillae. These papillae and buds are innervated by the chorda tympani branch of the lingual nerve. The papillae are red, circular and small, varying from 1 to 4 mm in diameter. These papillae are slightly elevated above the lingual surface, and are surrounded by smaller, more numerous, spiny-like papillae, the filiform papillae, which do not contain taste buds. The taste buds in the fungiform papillae are usually multiple, varying between one and eight, and may also contain specialized pressure, tactile and temperature receptors. They also contain both myelinated and unmyelinated nerve fibres unrelated to the taste buds.[8]

Over the posterior one-third of the tongue are the circumvallate papillae arranged in the V-shaped groove. These papillae are circular and 2–15 mm in diameter. These papillae are commonly elevated from the lingual surface, with the taste buds lying in the papillary and contra-papillary crypt surfaces. They and their buds are innervated by the glossopharyngeal (IXth) nerve. In addition to the taste buds, these papillae also contain specialized pressure, tactile and temperature receptors, as well as myelinated and unmyelinated nerves unrelated to the taste buds.[8]

Over the palate there are palatal papillae which house taste buds opening directly into the oral cavity. These 5–20 papillae are mainly centred at the hard/soft palate junction. They are innervated by both the glossopharyngeal and vagus nerves. The taste buds in these papillae are mainly single and surrounded by small salivary glands.

Papillae and taste buds may occur in other oral and pharyngeal locations, including the lips, inner surface of the lingual mucosa, epiglottis, various pharyngeal regions and the upper one-third of the oesophagus as well as the pharynx.[9]

Taste buds

Although all the taste buds are capable of responding to each taste quality, their response characteristics are concentration dependent. Thus, differentiation of sensory discrimination may be observed. Taste buds in fungiform papillae appear to respond in a rather more uniform manner to low concentrations of both sweet and salt taste substances,[10] whereas the taste buds in the vallate papillae appear to respond in a rather uniform manner to low concentrations of sweet substances and only to higher concentrations of salt, sour and bitter stimuli.[11] Taste buds in the palatal papillae respond in a uniform manner to both sour and bitter substances, although they respond to salt and sweet at relatively high concentrations.[10] Thus the greatest number of taste buds in the oral cavity are involved with the response to sweet, and fewest to sour or bitter substances. Thus, in taste loss secondary to metabolic or trace metal abnormalities,[12] secondary to irradiation or depressed salivary flow,[7] the sensation of sweet is least affected. By contrast, the bitter taste quality is usually the first taste sensation to be affected in pathological disturbances.

Taste buds comprise 20–50 cells. The taste buds from the fungiform and palatal papillae are relatively long and slender, whereas those from the vallate papillae are more globular. The component cells all comprise cell processes that extend to the pore region of the bud, and all the cells have desmosomal junctions one with another. No blood or lymphatic vessels are associated with any portion of the taste bud. Conceivably, epithelial cells adjacent to the outer membrane of the taste bud migrate into the bud and under the influence of neural and possibly salivary stimuli differentiate into the specialized cell types that comprise the taste bud. The nerve fibres enter and leave the taste bud at its base and these unmyelinated fibres generally extend only halfway into the bulk of the bud. Both adrenergic and cholinergic nerve fibres have been found in the taste buds.

Within the bud, three major cell types have been described.[13]

Type I cells (80%)

These contain neural synapses, the direction of which suggests an afferent transmission from nerve to bud. The cells are regarded as serving a neurotransmitter function.

Type II cells (15%)

These contain neural synapses, the direction of which suggests an afferent transmission from nerve to bud, as in type I cells. They also contain intracellular helical bundles extending over the cell length and are regarded as serving a neurotransmitter function, with some contractile properties.

Type III cells (5%)

These contain neural synapses, the direction of which suggests an afferent transmission from bud to nerve. The cells are regarded as receptor cells in the taste bud.

Mechanics of taste

The initial event in the process of taste presumably involves the binding of the taste stimulus to the taste bud receptor on the exposed receptor membrane of the taste bud.[1,14] Such binding may be influenced by a variety of factors, including interaction between taste stimuli, hormones,[15] ganglionic blocking agents[11] and proteolytic enzymes.

The membrane of the taste cell is negatively charged on the inside with respect to the outside. Application of a taste substance to the taste hairs results in partial loss of this negative potential. Generally, the degree of depolarization of the cell membrane is approximately proportional to the logarithm of the concentration of the stimulating substance. Conceivably, complex interactions between adenyl cyclase, guanyl cyclase and the taste stimulus–receptor complex may be important to the transduction of the binding energy to form the generator potential, although there may also be initiators, integrators and inhibitors. Conceivably, acetylcholine may play a role in some of the early events of the taste process which occur at or near the pore of the taste bud[1]. The function of the adrenergic fibres of the taste bud remain obscure.

Once the generator potential is formed, it is conducted by neural or modified neural elements to the synapse where true depolarization occurs.[16]

Subsequently, these signals are translated along the VIIth, IXth and Xth cranial nerve branches to the ipsilateral nucleus of the tractus solitarius, with second-order neurones subsequently translating the information to the parietal and anterior opercular–insular cortex via the ventral posterior thalamus.[17] This cursory description is necessarily simplified, since the detailed neuronal interactions have yet to be defined. Generally, the taste pathways closely parallel those of the somatic pathways from the tongue.

From the tractus solitarius, a large number of impulses are transmitted directly to the superior and inferior salivary nuclei. These, in turn, transmit impulses to the major salivary glands to help to control the secretion of saliva during the ingestion of food.

Taste preferences

The phenomenon of taste preference almost certainly results from some mechanism located in the central nervous system, although taste buds may become sensitized to the needed nutrient.[18] Thus previous experience with unpleasant or pleasant tastes plays a major role in determining a patient's taste likes and dislikes. Such previous experience influences suggest that taste preference reflects a central rather than local (peripheral) mechanism.

Pathological taste afflictions[22–24]

Pathological processes can affect taste at most stages of the taste process. For instance, miraculin produces attenuation or blocking of sour and bitter tastes.[18] This glycoprotein binds tightly to the taste bud receptor.

Abnormalities in taste support systems usually produce decreased taste acuity. For instance, xerostomia accompanying Sjögren's syndrome,[7] salivary gland tumours or irradiation[19] result in both degenerative changes in the taste buds, as well as taste abnormalities. Taste abnormalities have also been described in cyanocobalamin and retinol deficiencies, and a return to normality with restitution of the vitamin deficiency. In addition to surgical interruption of the nerves supplying the taste buds,[20] taste changes may also be associated with a host of systemic and local diseases, including:

(1) Influenza and various other infectious diseases.
(2) Post-partum or post-general or local anaesthesia.
(3) Hypothyroidism.
(4) Cirrhosis.
(5) Cushing's syndrome.
(6) Zinc deficiency.
(7) Collagen diseases.
(8) Leukaemia.

A number of drugs result in taste abnormalities, especially antibiotics, tranquillizing agents, steroids and anticancer drugs.

Untreated adrenocortical insufficiency and pancreatic cystic fibrosis have been associated with taste disturbances, whereas some untreated hypertensive patients have a craving for sodium chloride. Phenylthiourea is appreciated by about 80% of the population as extremely bitter but has no taste at all for the remaining 20% of the population. This distribution follows a simple Mendelian pattern, with non-tasters exhibiting an increased prevalence to glaucoma.[21]

Patients with craniofacial hypoplasia exhibit normal taste detection whereas taste recognition is grossly deficient. Although patients with congenital and genetic abnormalities commonly exhibit taste loss, taste and olfaction sensitivity are intimately intertwined.

Abnormalities of olfaction may be either qualitative or quantitative. These symptoms may be caused by local lesions in the nose, e.g. vasomotor rhinitis, or intracranial diseases, e.g. tumours. In both situations, disturbances in olfaction may be associated with taste dysfunction.

Conclusions

There is still much to be learned about how information on taste is transduced and coded in the nervous system. It is generally believed that cells in a taste bud or single peripheral taste fibre do not react exclusively to a single stimulus but rather to selected qualities of the stimulus. It is likely that branches of the facial, glossopharyngeal and vagus nerves receive input from the receptor cells in the taste buds, which then pass to the rostral part of the solitary tract, where there is a second relay to the parabrachial nucleus of the pons, and a third relay to the ventrobasal complex of the thalamus. From this area, sensory input then passes to the cortical taste area in the rhinal sulcus in addition to the lateral hypothalamus, amygdala and red nucleus of the stria terminalis.

Review questions

1. What disease entities are known to be associated with taste disturbances?
2. Why is saliva crucial to the sensation of taste?
3. Describe the functional morphology of a taste bud.
4. What are the probable neurological pathways for the sensation of taste from the tongue tip to the central nervous system?

References

1. HENKIN, R.I. and BRADLEY, D.F. (1971) *Steroids, Hormones and Brain Function*. Los Angeles: University of California Press
2. OHRWALL, H. (1901) Die Modalitäts und Qualitätsbegriffe im der Sinnesphysiologie und deren Bedeutung. *Arch. Physiol. Scand.*, **11**, 245–272
3. SKRAMLIK, E. (1926) *Handbook der Physiologie der niederen Sinne*. Bdl. Leipzig: Georg Thieme
4. SHALLENBERGER, R.S. and ACREE, T.E. (1971) *Handbook of Physiology, Chemical Senses II*. Berlin: Springer
5. HENKIN, R.I. (1972) Disorders of taste and smell. *JAMA*, **220**, 870–871
6. CATALANOTTO, F.A. and SWEENEY, E. (1973) The effects of surgical desalivation of the rat upon taste acuity. *Arch. Oral Biol.*, **18**, 941–951
7. HENKIN, R.I., TALAL, N., LARSON, A. and MATTERN, C.F.T. (1972) Abnormalities of taste and smell in Sjögren's syndrome. *Ann. Int. Med.*, **76**, 375–383
8. HENKIN, R.I. (1967) *Symposium on Oral Sensation and Perception*. Springfield: C.C. Thomas
9. LALONDE, E.R. and EGLITIS, J.A. (1961) Number and distribution of taste buds on the epiglottis, pharynx, larynx, soft palate and uvula in a human newborn. *Anat. Rec.*, **140**, 91–95
10. BURKL, W. (1954) Uber das Vorkommen von Geschmacksknopsen im mittleren Drittle des Osophagus. *Anat. Anz.*, **100**, 320–321
11. MATTERN, C.F.T., DANIEL, F.T., WENDELL, A. and HENKIN, R.I. (1970) The ulltrastructure of the human circumvallate papilla. *Anat. Rec.*, **167**, 175–182
12. HENKIN, R.I., SCHECHTER, P.J., RAFF, M.S., BRONZERT, D.A. and FRIEDEWALD, W.T. (1974) *Clinical Applications of Zinc Metabolism*. Springfield: C.C. Thomas
13. MURRAY, R.G. and MURRAY, A. (1970) *Ciba Foundation Symposium on Mechanism of Taste and Smell in Vertebrates*. London: Churchill
14. MERTZ, W. and CORNATZER, W.E. (1971) *Newer Trace Metals and Nutrition*. New York: Dekker
15. HENKIN, R.I. (1974) *Handbook of Physiology*. New York: American Physiological Association
16. MORITA, H. (1959) Initiation of spike potentials in contact chemosensory hairs of insects. *J. Cell Comp. Physiol.*, **54**, 189–204
17. BURTON, H. and BENJAMIN, R.M. (1971) *Handbook of Sensory Physiology*. Berlin: Springer
18. KARAHARA, K. and BEIDLER, L.M. (1968) Taste modifying protein from miracle fruit. *Science*, **161**, 1241–11243
19. MACCARTHY-LEVINTHAL, E.M. (1959) Post radiation mouth blindness. *Lancet*, **ii**, 1138–1139
20. GUTH, L. (1958) Taste buds on the cat's circumvallate papilla after reinnervation by glossopharyngeal, vagus and hypoglossal nerves. *Anat. Rec.*, **130**, 25–37
21. KOLKER, A.E. and HETHERINGTON, J. (1970) *Becker-Schaffer's Diagnosis and Therapy of the Glaucomas*. St Louis: C.V. Mosby
22. SCHIFFMAN, S.S. (1983) Taste and smell in diseases. *N. Engl. J. Med.*, **308**, 1337–1343
23. MATTES, R.D. (1984) Salt taste and hypertension: a critical review of the literature. *J. Chronic Dis.*, **37**, 195–208
24. YAMAMOTO, T. (1984) Taste responses of cortical neurones. *Prog. Neurobiol.*, **23**, 273–315

4

Deglutition

Introduction

To survive, we must meet the nutritional requirements of the physiological system by obtaining food and assimilating it within the body. The digestive system transports food internally from the environment to a tissue interface for nutrients to reach cellular components of the biological system. The passage of the bolus from the mouth to the oesophagus requires the interaction of both the respiratory and digestive tracts, with deglutition (swallowing) providing for the propulsion of the food from the oral cavity into the stomach, as well as providing a protective reflex for the digestive and upper respiratory tracts.[1,2] As a protective reflex, deglutition has been evoked to assist in:

(1) Removal of aspirated particles that have entered the larynx and lower respiratory tract to be propelled by a cough, or other clearing gesture, back into the pharynx.
(2) Removal of particles originally trapped in the nasopharynx.
(3) Returning material influxed from the stomach into the oesophagus and pharynx.

Despite the fact that the processes of deglutition have been subjected to intense investigation,[3–8] there remain considerable voids in our present understanding of this complex system.

Swallowing dynamics

The simple constrictor arrangement of the pharynx is enclosed within a vertical set of muscles descending to the pharynx from the styloid process and basicranium.[3] The superior constrictor is external to salpingopharyngeus, palatopharyngeus and palatolaryngeus, and the inferior constrictor is external to stylopharyngeus. The tongue, hyoid bone and larynx comprise an intrinsically mobile column controlled by muscles joining it to the basicranium, mandible and pterygoid regions of the face. In man, the upper 2 cm portion of the oesophagus is striated muscle[9] and continues the muscular pattern of the pharynx as it is held in position by its continuity with the pharynx. In contrast, the lower two-thirds of the oesophagus is stabilized by its fascia and penetration through the diaphragm; its musculature is non-striated. A transition zone therefore exists between the cervical and thoracic levels of the oesophagus in which striated and smooth muscle fibres intermingle.[10]

Cinefluorographic studies have defined three basic phases in deglutition.[11–13]

(1) There is the voluntary transfer of material from the mouth to the pharynx.
(2) This is followed by an involuntary (reflex-dependent) phase, comprising the highly co-ordinated transport of material away from the mouth or buccal cavity by a contraction wave of the pharyngeal constrictor muscles, past a relaxed cricopharyngeus muscle into the upper oesophagus.
(3) There is an involuntary transport phase whereby the food passes along the oesophagus through a relaxed lower oesophageal sphincter into the gastric cardia.

The oral phase

The swallowing co-ordination begins with withdrawal of the soft palate from its position against the pharyngeal portion of the tongue. After oral mastication of a solid food mass, or with the intake of a liquid, the dorsal portion of the tongue forms a spoon-shaped depression in the anterior midline: the food mass is contained anteriorly and laterally by the tip of the tongue interacting with the labial muscles. In this collection phase, the containment is developed anteriorly by the tip of the tongue positioned against the palatal mucosa adjacent to the maxillary teeth. Laterally, the tongue seals against the buccal teeth and palatal mucosa. Posteriorly, the pharyngeal portion of the tongue arches to meet the posterior portion of the palate.[14] At this time, the lips are apart and maxillary and mandibular incisors are not in contact.

After the bolus is formed and is on the dorsal surface of the tongue, the tip of the tongue is placed on the anterior alveolar ridge just in front of the maxillary central incisors. During this anterior alveolar phase, the voluntary opening of the peripheral seal begins with the depression of the posterior tongue and elevation of the soft palate. Concurrently, the lips are closed and the maxillary and mandibular incisors come together. The anterior half of the tongue is then pressed against the maxillary alveolar ridge and the anterior half of the hard palate in rapid sequence, moving the bolus posteriorly on the dorsum and root of the tongue towards the pillars of the fauces – the midpalatal phase. This movement, particularly of a liquid, is probably assisted by gravity. The soft palate is elevated to allow the bolus to pass through the faucial isthmus and, in its final elevation, becomes triangular in shape and contacts the adjacent pharyngeal wall to prevent penetration of the bolus into the nasopharynx. The posterior pharyngeal wall contributes to closure of the palatopharyngeal isthmus by a general inwards and forwards constriction. Glossectomy, with or without replacement by a prosthetic device, destroys this propulsion action, so that the subject must tilt the head back for deglutition.[15]

The pharyngeal phase

As the bolus reaches the soft palate immediately prior to the pharyngeal component of deglutition, the hyoid bone is brought to a preparatory position by moderate elevation. Intra-oral manipulation and respiration are arrested for the duration of the pharyngeal phase.[3] The pharyngeal phase begins as the bolus is carried between the tongue, the approximated soft palate, the constrictor wall and the epiglottis: the posterior compression phase. It has been suggested that partial leakage of the bolus to the receptive field innervated by the superior laryngeal nerve occurs prior to the main movement of the bolus and this accounts for the initiation of the pharngeal reflex.[16] The tongue is the principal carrier of the bolus: its posterior mass is rolled back on the hyoid bone, while maintaining the bolus within the indentation of its dorsal surface.[3] The posterior part of the tongue moves in a posterior and superior direction to convey the well-contained bolus into the pharynx.

The pharynx then demonstrates two basic movements: the elevation of the whole pharyngeal tube, followed by a descending peristaltic wave.[13]

The pharyngeal constrictors move upwards and forwards and begin propelling the bolus through the pharynx with a sequential contraction. This engulfing action of deglutition takes approximately 100 ms. The pharynx develops considerable force as it ejects the food bolus into the oesophagus, with a velocity of 100 cm/s being reached, about half of the velocity at which blood is ejected into the aorta from the heart.[17] Simultaneously, the larynx rises and is pulled under the root of the tongue; the epiglottis folds down over the laryngeal opening. During this phase of pharyngeal constriction, the epiglottis tips inferoposteriorly and the true and false vocal cords protect the laryngeal vestibule by constricting the laryngeal aperture. Thus the epiglottis facilitates passage of the bolus through the piriform fossae and into the oesophagus. This pharyngeal phase is completed when the soft palate returns to its original position and the larynx is reopened for respiration.

The oral phase of deglutition is subjected to

marked individual variability, whereas the pharyngeal swallowing movements are generally consistent. For instance, the maxillary and mandibular teeth usually make contact during swallowing, when the bolus passes from the oral cavity into the pharynx and while the bolus is in the pharynx. This tooth contact is considered to stabilize the mandible while the hyoid and larynx execute supero-anterior movements. Tooth contact, lip and tongue movements, however, vary considerably between patients.[11] For instance, in glossopharyngeal breathing, the tongue, palate and upper pharynx move normally, whereas the inferior constrictor closes the lower pharynx, while the larynx opens to admit the bolus of air.

The oesophageal phase

The final stage of deglutition, the oesophageal phase, begins 600–900 ms after initiation of the pharyngeal phase, and as the food passes the pharyngo-oesophageal sphincter.[18] The peristaltic contractions begin in the cervical level of the oesophagus and take on average 8 s to reach the oesophagogastric junction. This peristaltic sequence of the oesophagus during deglutition, termed primary peristalsis, is distinct from secondary peristalsis, which is initiated by distension as a bolus is placed directly within the oesophagus.[19]

Muscular co-ordination

The importance of deglutition in transport and protection is illustrated by the frequency: 2400 swallows per day increasing to 300/h during eating.[20] Such activity is aided by contraction of craniofacial muscles in addition to those of the oesophagus and pharynx. For instance, swallowing involves contraction of the medial pterygoid, masseter and temporalis muscles, along with the mylohyoid and anterior belly of the digastric. Electromyographic studies have shown that the suprahyoid suspensory muscles (affecting the position of the posterior region of the tongue), the muscles around the posterior pillars of the fauces and the muscles involved in closure of the palatopharyngeal isthmus are primarily involved in the initial swallowing stages, whereas the lower pharyngeal muscles, beginning with the middle pharyngeal constrictor, constrict within 125–135 ms later. The primary peristalsis of the oesophagus begins as the bolus enters the oesophagus in a continuation of the motion begun by the pharynx.

Requirements for swallowing

The essential physiological requirements for deglutition thus comprise the following:

(1) Development of a bolus.
(2) Prevention of disbursal of the bolus during deglutition.

Table 4.1 Muscles of the face

Muscle	*Origin*	*Insertion*	*Nerve*	*Action*
Orbicularis oris	Neighbouring muscles, mostly buccinator	Skin around lips and angles of the mouth	Facial	Closes, opens, protrudes, inverts, and twists lips
Zygomaticus minor	Zygomatic bone	Orbicularis oris in upper lip	Facial	Draws upper lip upwards and outwards
Levator labii superioris	Below infra-orbital foramen in maxilla	Orbicularis oris in upper lip	Facial	Pulls up or elevates upper lip
Levator labii superioris alaeque nasi	Process of maxilla	Skin at mouth angle, orbicularis oris	Facial	Raises angle of mouth
Zygomaticus major	Zygomatic bone	Fibres of the orbicularis oris, angle of the mouth	Facial	Draws upper lip upwards, draws angle of the mouth upwards and backwards: the smiling muscle
Levator anguli oris (caninus)	Canine fossa of maxilla	Lower lip near angle of the mouth	Facial	Raises corners of mouth
Depressor anguli oris	Outer surface and above lower border of mandible	Skin of cheek, corner of mouth, lower border of mandible	Facial	Draws lower lip down, draws angle of mouth downwards and inwards
Depressor labii inferioris	Lower border of the mandible	Skin of lower lip, orbicularis oris	Facial	Depresses lower lip
Mentalis	Incisive fossa of mandible	Skin of chin	Facial	Pushes up lower lip, raises chin
Risorius	Platysma, fascia over the masseter	Angle of mouth, orbicularis oris	Facial	Draws corners or angle of mouth outwards, causes dimples, gives expression of strain to face
Buccinator	Alveolar process of maxilla, buccinator ridge of mandible	Angle of mouth, orbicularis oris	Facial	Flattens cheek, holds food in contact with teeth, retracts angles of the mouth

(3) Development of differential pressures facilitating bolus propulsion.
(4) Prevention of food or fluid entering the nasopharynx or larynx.
(5) Rapid transit of the bolus through the pharynx, minimizing the suspension of respiration.
(6) Prevention of gastric reflux during oesophageal emptying.
(7) Clearing of residual material from the pharyngo-oesophageal tract.

This is therefore a very complex process, which can be illustrated by consideration of some of the component muscles (*Tables 4.1–4.5*).[25,26]

(1) The tongue movements that initiate deglutition require the concomitant contraction of the

Table 4.2 Muscles of mastication

Muscle	*Origin*	*Insertion*	*Nerve*	*Action*
Temporalis	Temporal fossa of skull	Ramus and coronoid process	Trigeminal	Elevates or closes mandible, retracts mandible
Masseter	Zygomatic arch	Ramus	Trigeminal	Elevates or closes mandible
Medial pterygoid	Palatine bone, lateral pterygoid plate, tuberosity of maxilla	Ramus	Trigeminal	Elevates or closes mandible
Lateral pterygoid	Greater wing of sphenoid and lateral pterygoid plate	Neck of condyle	Trigeminal	Depressor or opener of mandible, protrudes mandible, permits side-to-side movement

Table 4.3 Muscles of the soft palate

Muscle	*Origin*	*Insertion*	*Nerve*	*Action*
Levator veli palatini	Apex of temporal bone	Palatine aponeurosis of soft palate	Vagus, accessory	Raises soft palate
Tensor veli palatini	Fossa of sphenoid bone	Palatine aponeurosis of soft palate	Trigeminal	Stretches soft palate
Palatoglossus	Undersurface of soft palate	Side of tongue	Vagus, accessory	Raises back of tongue during first stage of swallowing
Palatopharyngeus	Soft palate	Pharyngeal wall	Vagus, accessory	Shuts off nasopharynx during second stage of swallowing
Uvulae	Posterior nasal spine, palatine aponeurosis	Into uvula to form its chief bulk or content	Vagus, accessory	Shortens and raises uvula

Table 4.4 Muscles of the pharynx

Muscle	*Origin*	*Insertion*	*Nerve*	*Action*
Palatopharyngeus	Extends from soft palate to pharyngeal wall	Posterior border of thyroid cartilage, pharyngeal aponeurosis	Pharyngeal plexus, accessory	Narrows oropharynx, elevates pharynx, shuts off nasopharynx
Stylopharyngeus	Medial side of root of styloid process	Superior and inferior borders of thyroid cartilage	Glossopharyngeal	Raises and dilates pharynx
Salpingopharyngeus	Pharyngeal end of auditory tube	Blends with palatopharyngeus	Pharyngeal plexus, accessory	Raises nasopharynx, draws lateral pharyngeal walls up

Table 4.5 Suprahyoid muscles

Muscle	*Origin*	*Insertion*	*Nerve*	*Action*
Mylohyoid	Inner surface of mandible	Upper border of hyoid bone	Trigeminal	Elevates tongue and floor of mouth, depresses jaw when hyoid bone is in fixed position
Digastric (anterior belly)	Intermediate tendon by loop of fascia to hyoid bone	Lower border of mandible	Trigeminal	Raises hyoid bone if jaw is in fixed position, depresses jaw if hyoid bone is in fixed position
Geniohyoid	Mental spine of mandible	Hyoid bone	Cervical (C1 and C2) through hypoglossal	Draws hyoid bone forward, depresses mandible when hyoid bone is in fixed position
Stylohyoid	Styloid process of temporal bone	Body of hyoid at greater cornu	Facial	Elevates hyoid and tongue base
Hyoglossus	Greater cornu of hyoid	Into tongue sides	Hypoglossal	Tongue depression
Genioglossus	Upper genial tubercle of mandible	Hyoid, inferior tongue, tip	Hypoglossal	Protrusion, depression
Styloglossus	Anterior border of styloid process	Into side of tongue	Hypoglossal	Elevates up and back
Palatoglossus	Anterior surface of soft palate	Dorsum and side of tongue	Glossopharyngeal, vagus, accessory	Narrows fauces, elevates posterior tongue

mylohyoid, geniohyoid and digastric muscles in the floor of the mouth.

(2) The styloglossus and hyoglossus muscles force the root of the tongue against the soft palate and posterior pharyngeal wall.

(3) The levator and tensor veli palatini muscles elevate the soft palate, with additional shortening and dorsal thickening until approximation against the posterior pharyngeal muscle prevents nasopharyngeal regurgitation.

(4) The middle and inferior pharyngeal constrictor muscles narrow the hypopharynx and contribute to the peristaltic movements involving the posterior pharyngeal wall, generally between Passavant's ridge and the cricopharyngeal sphincter.

(5) The dorsal and downward tilting of the epiglottis, resulting from muscular elevation of the larynx, contraction of the floor of the mouth, along with elevation and posterior movement of the hyoid bone.

Bolus motion

The bolus is then sucked into the laryngopharynx by the production of a zone of negative pressure, resulting from the upward movement of the hyoid and larynx along with the forward and posterior motion of the latter. This creates a pulling force and increases the anteroposterior diameter of the laryngopharynx. Contraction of the intrinsic laryngeal muscles then shortens and widens the aryepiglottic, vocal and vestibular folds, producing an airtight soft stopper for the subepiglottic region. This eliminates the loss of air from the respiratory tract, which would oppose the sucking effect. Epiglottic depression does not completely close the laryngeal aditus, however, resulting in the frequent insertion of small particles of the bolus into that opening for a short distance.

A liquid bolus is usually split by the epiglottis, travelling on each side of the larynx through the piriform recesses to rejoin behind the cricoid cartilage. The epiglottis acts as a ledge, checking the descent of the bolus and obviating early closure of the larynx. Protection of the larynx during deglutition is effected in part by contraction of the sphincteric muscle girdle that surrounds it. This occurs without elevation of the larynx. In fact, the larynx may be closed at any stage during deglutition, but is always closed when the last of the bolus leaves the pharynx, at which point material entering the laryngeal vestibule is squeezed out. The cover provided by the epiglottis bending over the laryngeal entrance prevents the deposition of residue, and reinflation of the airway carries any residue up into the vallecula. In the absence of epiglottic function, repeated swallowing removes food from the laryngeal entrance prior to airway reinflation.

Passage of the bolus through the oesophagus requires the co-ordinated activity of the oesophageal inlet, the oesophageal outlet and the body of the oesophagus. The inlet comprises visceral striated muscle that maintains the lumen in a closed position and is integrated with the tongue and hypopharynx. The high-pressure zone, which is equivalent to the upper oesophageal sphincter, relaxes promptly on swallowing to coincide with pharyngeal contraction and movement of the bolus into the upper end of the oesophagus. Only in the act of deglutition does the pressure in the oesophagus fall, although a pressure gradient between the oesophagus and stomach is maintained, so the lumen does not open too widely. Deglutition initiates a moving, ring-like contraction that sweeps rapidly through the upper striated portion and less rapidly through the lower smooth muscle portion. The terminal outlet is located 1–2 cm above the diaphragm, and is termed the gastro-oesophageal vestibule. Evacuation of this vestibule filled from above inhibits reflux of the stomach's content into the oesophagus, and it thus functions as a valve. Proximal to this vestibule, there is a functional ampulla that serves as a collecting area where pressure is built by the peristaltic wave moving towards it.

Nervous control of swallowing *(Tables 4.6, 4.7)*

Deglutition is usually initiated by sensory impulses transmitted as a result of stimulation of receptors on the fauces, tonsils, soft palate, base of the tongue and posterior pharyngeal wall. These sensory impulses reach the brain stem primarily through the VIIth, IXth and Xth cranial nerves, while the efferent function is mediated through the IXth, Xth, and XIIth cranial nerves. The cricopharyngeal sphincter opening is reflexive, relaxation occurring at the time when the bolus reaches the posterior pharyngeal wall prior to reaching this sphincter.

Table 4.6 Afferent controls in swallowing

Sensory function	*Innervation*
General sensation, anterior two-thirds of tongue	Lingual, trigeminal (V)
Taste, anterior two-thirds of tongue	Chorda tympani, facial (VII)
Taste and general sensation, posterior one-third of tongue	Glossopharyngeal (IX)
Mucosa of vallecula	Internal branch of superior laryngeal, vagus (X)
Primary afferent	Glossopharyngeal (IX)
Secondary afferent	Pharyngeal branch of vagus (X)
Tonsils, pharynx, soft palate	Glossopharyngeal (IX)
Pharynx, larynx, viscera	Vagus (X)

Table 4.7 Efferent controls in swallowing

Efferent stage	*Innervation*
Oral	
Masticatory, buccinator, floor of mouth	Trigeminal (V)
Lip sphincter	Facial (VII)
Tongue	Hypoglossal (XII)
Pharyngeal	
Constrictors and stylopharyngeus	Glossopharyngeal (IX)
Palate, pharynx, larynx	Vagus (X)
Tongue	Hypoglossal (XII)
Oesophageal	
Oesophagus	Vagus (X)

Control of swallowing involves three phases:

(1) The voluntary control of the oral preparatory phase.
(2) The voluntary and involuntary control of the pharyngeal phase.
(3) The involuntary control of the oesophageal phase.

In the preparatory phase, the basic purpose of mastication and intraoral manipulation is to create a bolus of proper size and consistency for transport to the pharynx and oesophagus. The second and third phases of swallowing demonstrate involuntary reflexive central nervous system control, which may be based on a swallowing centre.

Initiation of swallowing

Although reference is often made to the 'swallowing centre', this is probably an oversimplification. It is likely that modulation of the processes of deglutition results from impulse activity in cranial nerves other than those intermittently associated with swallowing itself. For instance, salivatory preparation of the bolus cannot occur in the absence of cholinergic activity mediated through the peripheral and autonomic nervous systems. Also, the striated muscle mediating deglutition in the pharynx, cricopharyngeal sphincter and upper one-third of the oesophagus, are under the control of impulses originating in motor neurones of the corresponding cranial nerve nuclei, whereas the smooth musculatures associated with deglutition are innervated by cholinergic vagal preganglionic fibres that synapse with a plexus in the muscle itself, resulting in postganglionic release of acetylcholine. The upper oesophageal sphincter adjacent to the cricopharyngeus is under control of the nucleus ambiguus and the dorsal motor nucleus of the vagus nerve (X), whereas the lower oesophageal sphincter is partially under vagal control. The extrinsic oesophageal musculature is under influence of the vagus nerve and the sympathetic nervous system (cervical and thoracic ganglia) with intrinsic neuro-ramifications by way of Auerbach and Meissner plexuses (parasympathetic postganglionic neurones in the gastrointestinal submucosal layer).

Continuation of swallowing

The sequence of movements comprising deglutition stems from a time-related (temporal) sequence of excitation and inhibition that occurs bilaterally in approximately 30 different muscles, including orbicularis oris, temporalis, masseter, mylohyoid, geniohyoid, palatopharyngeus and superior constrictor. Many of these muscles are termed obligate deglutition muscles, in that they always participate in swallowing activity in a rigid temporal pattern relative to one another and are relatively insensitive to sensory feedback and modulation once the process of deglutition has been initiated. There are also facultative deglutition muscles, which may or may not participate and are sensitive to sensory modulation. These latter muscles are primarily involved in stabilizing the tongue and effecting an anterior oral seal. There are also maturational changes in the muscles of deglutition since, prior to the eruption of the teeth in infants, the facial muscles act as facultative muscles, whereas in the adult the masticatory muscles are more dominant. The infantile (or tooth apart) swallow is also characterized by an active tongue thrust. Retention of this immature mode of deglutition may comprise an aetiologic factor of anterior malocclusions, especially the anterior open bite. Tooth apart swallows are, however, normal in adults when fluids or soft foods are consumed. Thus during the process of deglutition the consistency of the food bolus determines whether the teeth will come into occlusion.

Central control

Although deglutition is reflexly triggered from the periphery, the sequence and timing of the component movements is controlled by the central nervous system. In common with masticatory movements, deglutition is dependent upon the activity of the swallowing centre. In response to a peripheral stimulus, or central command to swallow, the neuronal programme of this centre exerts a sequential all-or-none pattern of excitatory and inhibitory effects on the various motor neurones supplying the muscles of deglutition. Although much of the detailed descriptions of the component central elements remain obscure, the neurones of the solitary tract nucleus appear to be intimately involved in selecting the incoming sensory inputs, along the Vth, Xth and XIth cranial nerves from the larynx or pharynx, that are appropriate for triggering the process of deglutition. It is unclear how this centre can distinguish between sensory inputs resulting in gagging, cough or deglutition as all emanate from the larynx or pharynx. This deglutition centre also receives input from central descending pathways from a number of cerebral cortical and subcortical sites, including the cerebral cortex, amygdala and midbrain. Such inputs can initiate or modify the pattern of deglutition through interaction with the peripheral inputs to the brain stem. Thus, although not generally susceptible to central control, the patterned sequence of events associated with deglutition can be modified by learning, e.g. following surgery for carcinoma of the larynx. The deglutition centre can also function without sensory feedback, i.e. it only needs sensory input to trigger the sequence. Deglutition is therefore not very sensitive to sensory inputs and, once triggered, will proceed to completion in most instances. A small degree of sensory modification is, however, possible. For instance, the patterning of facultative muscle activities appears dependent on the type and consistency of the bolus being swallowed. In addition, silent periods can be produced in both obligate and facultative muscle activities by stimuli that may be related to the production of other protective reflexes of the alimentary tract or respiratory tract, i.e. these latter may take precedence over the process of deglutition. Finally, the motor control of the processes of deglutition passes from the trigeminal (e.g. to the digastric, masseter, mylohyoid muscles), facial (e.g. to the orbicularis oris), glossopharyngeal, vagus and accessory (e.g. to the pharyngeal constrictors, and thyroarytenoid muscles, via the nucleus ambiguus) and hypoglossal cranial nerves (e.g. to the genioglossus and geniohyoid muscles).

Thus a functional deglutition centre appears to exist, having selective mechanisms for activation by appropriate stimuli. These have a defined spatio-temporal code, with interconnection of component cells resulting in a virtually invariable sequence of excitation and inhibition so that swallowing is the same regardless of its manner of initiation and with precision of organization resulting in control over relevant motor neurones. Corollaries of these features are that feedback regulation is not necessary for swallowing to proceed, that the output of the centre is highly stable, and that activity in the centre exerts inhibition upon possibly competing centres. The specific motor neurone pools involved in deglutition appear independent of the action of others in terms of the pattern of response. The deglutition centre, as defined by numerous studies, reveals that its location is in the reticular substance between the posterior pole of the seventh nucleus and the anterior pole of the inferior olive. It is of interest to note that unilateral destruction of this area by disease abolishes swallowing unilaterally.

The immature swallow

In the neonate, the soft palate occupies much of the volume of the upper pharyngeal region[21] which is much more compact than that of the adult. The mouth then acts as a piston within a cylinder during the suckling movement.[22] In the premature or small infant, short suckling bursts are followed by deglutition, whereas the normal mature infant swallows during prolonged suckling.[22] Thus, as the infant develops, the pharynx elongates and enlarges, with the soft palate becoming more mobile. The facial skeleton elongates and the oral chamber enlarges as the tongue increases in length. The epiglottis descends and alters the obligate nasal respiration, so that the older child can use either oral or nasal respiration.[23]

The infant swallows differently from the adult.[24] The alveolar ridges are apart (because the tongue protrudes between them) and the mandible is stabilized by the tongue and facial muscles. As the diet changes towards more compact, high-density foods, and the deciduous teeth erupt, the teeth come together during deglutition and the tongue does not protrude. Thus the tip of the tongue assumes a position near the incisive foramen of the palate and the mandible is increasingly stabilized by the elevator and depressor masticatory muscles. The labial and buccinator muscles are used less as the mandibular muscles become more important to deglutition. Infantile deglutition can, however, persist or recur and can be demonstrated well into adolescence. For instance, premature loss of the deciduous teeth may result in the tongue adapting to the surrounding space, leading to recurrence of the infantile swallow. Usually, the tongue retracts to the normal space following permanent incisor tooth eruption, followed by the return to a mature pattern of deglutition.

Neuromuscular control of swallowing

The highly integrated activities of deglutition depend on a combination of voluntary and involuntary control of the position of lips, teeth, jaws, cheeks and tongue, all partly mediated by the trigeminal (Vth) nerve innervated muscles that control the mandible and the masseter. Both of these muscle groups are involved in the control of leverage, stabilization and centring of the movable parts of the oral cavity. Therefore, mastication depends primarily on the Vth nerve, whereas the muscles of the lips and cheeks depend on motor functions of the VIIth nerve. All of the extrinsic muscles of the tongue depend on the motor function of the XIIth nerve, except for the palatoglossus (elevator of the tongue root) which is innervated by the vagus. All of the intrinsic muscles of the tongue are innervated by the XIIth nerve. All of the soft palate muscles are innervated by the vagus, except the tensor veli palatini, which is innervated by the Vth nerve. The stylopharyngeus is innervated by the IXth nerve and functions to widen the pharynx, whereas the palatopharyngeus is innervated by the Xth nerve. The maxillary and mandibular sensory divisions of the Vth nerve are primarily involved in providing sensation pertaining to the lips, palate, teeth, inner mouth and proprioceptive aspects of the muscles of mastication. The gag reflex, as well as nasal regurgitation, depends on the function or dysfunction of the IXth and Xth nerves.

The voluntary components of deglutition probably have their origin in higher cerebral centres, which operate on striated muscles, but involve the development of 'automatisms' that still may be subject to voluntary monitoring and control, although they appear involuntary. These include the habits of mouth control and chewing. Many of the neuromechanisms dependent upon the combination of the pathways referred to above combine in complex reflexes other than deglutition, e.g. cough and gag, and others that have variable expression at different stages of life, e.g. suckling of infancy and the biting reflexes dependent on masseteric stretch.

At the cortical level, the inferior portion of the precentral gyrus of the insula produces the movements of deglutition on electrical stimulation and these may result from efferent connections to the hypothalamus and then to the medulla, where the swallowing centre has been identified (in the region of the fourth ventricle and the Xth cranial nerve nucleus).

The swallowing centre co-ordinates efferent impulse flow by the following:

(1) Vth and Xth nerves to the levators (soft palate).
(2) Xth nerve to the pharyngeal constrictors, through the cervical and thoracic spinal nerves to the diaphragm and intercostals.
(3) Vth and XIIth nerves to the extrinsic muscles of the larynx.
(4) Xth nerve to the intrinsic muscles of the larynx and oesophagus.

The cervical oesophagus may receive two efferent supplies, one from the recurrent laryngeal and another from the pharyngo-oesophageal nerve arising from proximal to the nodose ganglion or from an oesophageal branch of the external laryngeal portion of the superior laryngeal nerve.

Sequentially timed discharges from the medullary centre mediate the movement of the bolus through successive levels of the oesophageal musculature. Oesophageal distension is signalled on visceral efferent nerves passing in the upper five or six thoracic sympathetic roots, presumably to the thalamus and inferior postcentral gyrus where they give rise to symptoms of pressure, burning, gas, and aching. Because of the widespread ramifications and functional significance of the vagus nerve, lesions in the vagal system may have far-reaching deleterious effects on coughing, swallowing, breathing and phonation. Deglutition is a lower-level response, yet its afferent side can be stimulated by voluntary movements of the tongue and larynx. This is subserved by separation of corticobulbar fibres, with some remaining ipsilateral and others providing contralateral innervation to the nucleus ambiguus (motor nucleus of IX and X). The latter forms the brain stem locus from which special visceral efferent fibres arise.

Fibres originating in the nucleus ambiguus innervate the pharyngeal, laryngeal and upper oesophageal striated muscles. The vagus is formed from dorsal efferent and inferior salivary nuclei. It also innervates the heart, lungs and gastrointestinal smooth muscle, in addition to carrying afferents for taste and pharyngeal sensation. Above the nodose ganglion, the vagus sends branches to the pharyngeal plexus, which supplies the mucosa and musculature of the pharynx, larynx and upper oesophagus, where it is accompanied by branches from the neighbouring sympathetic ganglia.

The superior laryngeal nerve is sensory to the laryngeal mucosa and motor to the cricothyroid muscle. The vagus terminates as the recurrent laryngeal nerve that supplies muscles intrinsic to the larynx, but not the cricopharyngeal muscle (which is supplied by a branch from the pharyngeal plexus).

Disordered swallowing

Disorders of deglutition (frequently termed dysphagia) primarily result from either neurological or mechanical factors.[27–32] They are briefly considered here as they shed a clinical light on to the mechanisms of the various processes involved.

Neurological disorders

The intimate relationship of the last four cranial nerves (IX–XII) results in the possibility of many combinations of nerve lesions that have similar common pathways in terms of symptomatology, including loss of strength of the voice, hoarseness, nasal speech, difficulty in swallowing and nasal regurgitation or aspiration. Referred or directly mediated painful sensations in the region of the external ear and scalp may draw attention to the IXth and Xth cranial nerves, while weakness and wasting of the sternomastoids, trapezei and tongue may implicate the XIth and XIIth nerves. A neurological cause of dysphagia is more likely if the anatomy is normal without deformity, although symmetry may be misleading since it may represent bilateral lesions. Since the larynx is innervated by the Xth nerve, paralysis of one or both vocal cords may be completely separate from neurological involvement of the palatopharyngeal apparatus. Neurological involvement of the orobuccal phase of deglutition is related to its volitional nature. Involvement of the reflexly controlled pharynx and the mixed functions of the larynx affect not only swallowing but speaking and breathing. Thus dysarthria, dysphagia and dysphonia may all coexist, as in Parkinsonism. Disorders of the basal ganglia, cerebellum and sensory feedback mechanisms may be associated with dysphagia. Pathology of the brain stem affecting swallowing frequently takes the form of bulbar palsy, poliomyelitis, trauma, vascular anomalies and brain stem tumours. The brain stem may also be involved in many congenital degenerative disorders, e.g. amyotrophic lateral sclerosis. A key finding associated with brain stem involvement is failure of the cricopharyngeal muscle to relax during swallowing, with accompanying pharyngeal retention, stasis and nasal regurgitation. Neurological causes of dysphagia are generally identified through such factors as the duration of the deglutition process, difficulties with liquids and solids, nasal regurgitation, and the presence or absence of heartburn. Hoarseness may indicate intrinsic laryngeal disease or relate to carcinoma, or it may be accompanied by recurrent laryngeal nerve paralysis complicating such diseases as poliomyelitis.

Oropharyngeal dysphagia is frequently accompanied by a decreased gag reflex, weakness of cervical or facial muscles and often a speech disorder. It is a common cause of dysphagia and, if it progresses to pharyngeal paralysis, it may cause sensory changes secondary to painful lesions of the mouth and tongue. Such diseases include scarlet fever, mumps, viral infections, monilia, peritonsillar abscess, carcinoma and syphilis. Pharyngeal paralysis often results from poliomyelitis, multiple sclerosis, cerebrovascular accident (stroke) involving the brain stem or diphtheria affecting the IXth and Xth nerves. Muscle weakness leading to pharyngeal involvement is found in myasthenia gravis, myotonic dystrophies and scleroderma.

Movement of the bolus from the mouth to the stomach occurs in an organized fashion only if the necessary neuromuscular and neuroregulatory controls are intact. The inherent complexity of the processes of deglutition probably predisposes its delicately balanced neural control to potential failure from a myriad of disease enitities. Most disorders of deglutition are not without cause, however, and a few examples are considered below to illustrate the scope of the complex nature of deglutition.

The neurogenic causes of dysphagia include:

Acquired central disorders

(1) Stroke syndromes and vascular disorders:
  infarction of the internal capsule;
  infarction of the brain stem;
  vasculitis.
(2) Movement disorders:
  Parkinson's disease;
  Huntington's disease.
(3) Poliomyelitis and other systemic infections:
  diphtheria;
  rabies;
  tetanus.
(4) Amyotrophic lateral sclerosis.
(5) Other causes:
  multiple sclerosis;
  tuberculosis;
  syphilis;
  neoplasms;
  degenerative disorders.

Acquired peripheral disorders

(1) Recurrent laryngeal neuropathy.
(2) Cranial neuropathies:
  diabetes;
  leukaemia;
  lymphoma;
  carcinoma.
(3) Other neuropathies.

Neurodevelopmental disorders

(1) Syringomyelia.
(2) Cerebral palsy.

Mechanical disorders

Patients with mechanical disorders of deglutition evidence difficulty secondary to the loss of sensory guidance of the structures necessary to complete a normal swallow. The central, and most of the peripheral, neurological controls for deglutition are intact, although the structures needed to complete the act are not. Even though causes and mechanisms of the neurological and mechanical disorders of deglutition are different, some of the problems are shared: for example, excessive expectoration of fluid resembling saliva (sialorrhoea), masticatory difficulties, oral and pharyngeal pooling, lengthened swallowing transit times, difficulty in channelling food into the oesophagus, and aspiration. (Aspiration is defined as the residual unswallowed pharyngeal content that is drawn into the larynx and trachea by inspiration following an attempt at a normal swallow.)

Most of the patients with mechanical dysphagia have had oral, pharyngeal or laryngeal structures removed or reconstructed during surgery for cancer, although there may be other causes:

(1) Acute inflammations:
  acute pharyngitis;
  lingual tonsilitis;
  herpes simplex;
  chemical inflammation due to corrosive fluid swallowing.
(2) Trauma:
  tooth brush abrasion;
  loose-dentures.

Macroglossia (tongue enlargement)

Secondary to radiotherapy or surgery of the tongue. Hypothyroidism.

Surgery

Especially surgical resection for carcinoma of the tongue; laryngectomy; tracheotomy tubes.

Mechanical dysfunction of deglutition is usually the result of oral and/or pharyngeal structures being surgically removed or altered, thereby impairing the displacement of food to the pharynx. Even though some patients have adequate sensory and motor components for oral and pharyngeal feeding post-operatively, most have significant dysphagia. Additionally, the majority have adequate cortical skills needed for the rehabilitation of feeding.

Conclusions

The physiological mechanisms responsible for deglutition are exceedingly complex, even without considering the protective gag and cough reflexes. Much more information is, however, required before the mechanisms underlying disturbed swallowing reflexes can be understood.

Review questions

1. Describe the actions of the soft palate during swallowing.
2. How is the musculature of the mouth co-ordinated during swallowing?
3. How might the central nervous system influence the mechanism of swallowing?
4. Why may the immature swallow persist into adolescence?
5. Discuss the mechanical disorders of swallowing.

References

1. HENDERSON, R.D.C., WOOLF, C. and MARRYATT, G. (1976) Pharyngooesophageal dysplasia and gastrooesophageal reflux. *Laryngoscope*, **86**, 1531–1539
2. STOREY, A.T. (1976) Interactions of alimentary and upper respiratory tract reflexes. In *Mastication and Swallowing: Biological and Clinical Correlates*, edited by B.J. Sessle and A.J. Hannam. Toronto: University of Toronto Press
3. BOSMA, J.F. (1957) Deglutition: pharyngeal stage. *Physiol. Rev.*, **37**, 275–300
4. DOTY, R.W. (1968) Neural organization of deglutition. In *Handbook of Physiology, Alimentary Canal*, edited by C.F. Code, 4, pp. 1861–1902. Washington: American Physiological Society
5. DUBNER, R., SESSLE B.J. and STOREY, A.T. (1978) *The Neural Basis of Oral and Facial Function*. New York: Plenum
6. INGELFINGER, F.J. (1958) Esophageal motility. *Physiol. Rev.*, **38**, 533–584
7. CODE, C.F. and SCHLEGEL, J.F. (1968) Motor action of the oesophagus and its sphincters. In *Handbook of Physiology, Alimentary Canal*, edited by C.F. Code, 4, pp. 1821–1839. Washington: American Physiological Society
8. POPE, C.E. (1974) Esophageal physiology. *Med. Clin. North Am.*, **58**, 1181–1199
9. AREY, L.B. and TREMAINE, M.J. (1933) The muscle content of the lower esophagus. *Anat. Rec.*, **56**, 315–320
10. JANSSENS, J. (1978) The Peristaltic Mechanism of the Esophagus. *PhD Thesis*, University of Leuven, Belgium
11. CLEALL, J.F. (1965) Deglutition: a study of form and function. *Am. J. Orthod.*, **51**, 566–594
12. SAUNDERS, J.B., DAVIS, C. and MILLER, E.R. (1951) The mechanism of deglutition (second stage) as revealed by cineradiography. *Ann. Otol. Rhinol. Laryngol.*, **60**, 897–918
13. SHELTON, R.L., BOSMA, J.F. and SHEETS, B.V. (1960) Tongue, hyoid and larynx displacement in swallow and phonation. *J. Appl. Physiol.*, **15**, 283–288
14. NAGASHIMA, J. (1977) Studies on morphological changes of the soft palate during deglutition and phonation by x-ray TV cinematography. *Shika Gakuho*, **77**, 1–37
15. KOTHARY, P.M., PAYMASTER, J.C. and POTDAR, G.G. (1974) Radical total glossectomy. *Br. J. Surg.*, **61**, 209–212
16. STOREY, A.T. (1968) Laryngeal initiation of swallowing. *Exp. Neurol.*, **20**, 359–365
17. FISHER, M.A., HENDRIX, T.R., HUNT, J.M. and MURRILLS, A.J. (1978) Relation between volume swallowed and velocity of the bolus ejected from the pharynx into the esophagus. *Gastroenterology*, **74**, 1238–1240
18. CHRISTRUP, J. (1964) Normal swallowing of foodstuffs of pasty consistence. A cinefluorographic investigation of a normal material. *Dan. Med. Bull.* **11**, 79–91
19. ARIMORI, M., CODE, C.E., SCHLEGEL, J.F. and STURM, R.E. (1970) Electrical activity of the canine esophagus and gastroesophageal sphincter; its relation to intraluminal pressure and movement of material. *Am. J. Dig. Dis.*, **15**, 191–208
20. LEAR, C.S.C., FLANAGAN, J.B.J. and MOORREES, C.F.A. (1965) The frequency of deglutition in man. *Arch. Oral Biol.*, **10**, 83–100
21. BOSMA, J.F. (1973) Physiology of the mouth, pharynx and esophagus. In *Otolarngology*, edited by M.M. Pararella and D.A. Shumrick. Philadelphia: Saunders
22. GRYBOSKI, J.D. (1969) Suck and swallow in the premature infant. *Pediatrics*, **43**, 96–102
23. LAITMAN, J.T., CRELIN, E.S. and CONLOGUE, G.J. (1977) The function of the epiglottis in monkey and man. *Yale J. Biol. Med.*, **50**, 43–48
24. GARCIN, A. (1969) Embryologic concepts: physiologic and anatomic details of neonatal deglutition. *J. Fr. Otorhinolaryngol.*, **18**, 723–724
25. ARDRAN, G.M. and KEMP, F.H. (1951) The mechanism of swallowing. *Proc. R. Soc. Med.*, **44**, 1038–1040
26. ARDRAN, G.M. and KEMP, F.H. (1952) Protection of laryngeal airway during swallowing. *Br. J. Radiol.*, **25**, 406–415
27. DONNER, W.J. (1974) Swallowing mechanisms and neuromuscular disorders. *Semin. Roentgenol.*, **9**, 273–282
28. PALMER, E.D. (1976) Disorders of the cricopharyngeus muscle: a review. *Gastroenterology*, **71**, 510–519
29. POPE, C.E. (1977) Motor disorders of the oesophagus. *Postgrad. Med.*, **61**, 118–125
30. JEAN, A. (1984) Control of the central swallowing program by inputs from the peripheral receptors. A review. *J. Auton. Nerv. Syst.*, **10**, 225–233
31. LOGEMANN, J.A. (1983) *Evaluation and Treatment of Swallowing Disorders*. San Diego: College-Hill Press
32. GROHER, M.E. (1984) *Dysphagia–Diagnosis and Management*. Boston: Butterworths

5

The oral mucosa

Introduction

The oral cavity is lined by a stratified squamous epithelium, whose functions include:

(1) Forming a primary structural barrier between the internal and external environments.
(2) Protection against mechanical damage, entry of noxious substances or organisms, and loss of fluids.

The epithelium and the underlying connective tissue of the lamina propria exhibit functionally related regional variations in their structure, pattern of macromolecular synthesis and rate of regeneration. The oral mucosa therefore comprises a complex tissue so that it would be naïve to assign its function to be merely a simple lining function. In addition, the normal structure and function of the oral mucosa is frequently disturbed, either transitorily or permanently, as a result of infection, physical or chemical injury or other disease processes. Thus a knowledge of the normal oral mucosal metabolism is important in understanding the many oral soft tissue lesions that occur in the mouth.

The epithelial layer

Like the skin, the oral mucosa comprises a surface epithelium overlying a layer of connective tissue. This stratified squamous epithelium undergoes mitosis, synthetic activity and disintegration, leaving the underlying cells as a cohesive tissue. Although the stratified squamous epithelium has a basic function, this is modified in certain regions of the mouth. Thus, on the palatal and gingival regions (the masticatory mucosa), it is modified by the deposition of keratin for protection from masticatory forces, whereas the cheeks, lips, soft palate, floor of the mouth and ventral tongue surface exhibit a more simple, non-keratinized, lining mucosa. The oral mucosa is further modified by the presence or absence of a submucous layer, which largely determines the firmness or looseness of its attachment to the underlying bones or muscles. There are also regional variations in the oral mucosa. For instance, the thickness of the oral mucosa is greater in the cheek than in the floor of the mouth, with parallel differences in the rates of germinal cell layer mitosis. Regional differences also exist in the degree of keratinization, tonofibrils and size and shape of the intracellular keratohyaline granules, in addition to cell size. Thus the oral mucosa is both structurally and functionally a complex tissue.

There are conflicting opinions concerning the degree of interaction between the epithelial and connective tissue components of the oral mucosa. Some consider the epithelial phenotype to be an intrinsic property of the epithelial cells,[1] whereas others contend that the subepithelial connective tissue continuously modulates the overlying epithelium.[2] There is a general consensus that the interaction between the oral epithelium and underlying connective tissues are of clinical significance in relation to the processes such as the control of cell proliferation and migration in wound healing and the restoration of tissue morphology following various oral surgical procedures, e.g. grafting and wound healing. In a variety of diseases, epithelial changes may be secondary to changes in the subepithelial connective tissues, e.g. in lichen planus,[3] submucous fibrosis,[4] leukoplakia,[5] age and radiation therapy.[6]

Component cell layers

Generally, the oral mucosal epithelium can be considered to comprise several cell layers:

(1) *Stratum germinativum*: where cell division occurs.
(2) *Stratum spinosum*: where cells with long cytoplasmic processes are interspersed with an amorphous intercellular substance comprising predominantly chondroitin sulphate.
(3) *Stratum granulosum*: where there are flattened cells comprising keratohyaline granules.
(4) *Stratum corneum*: a relatively structureless cell layer due to progressive loss of individual cell outlines and nuclei. This layer is predominantly found in the masticatory, rather than lining, mucosa.

The oral mucosa, as with any other epithelial tissue, comprises multiple cell rows with no supporting stroma. In addition to the metabolic (housekeeping) activities common to most cells, epithelial cells undertake a number of specialized synthetic activities associated with the maintenance of a surface barrier, including:

(1) Synthesis of keratin.
(2) Degradation of other intracellular organelles.
(3) Synthesis of cell membrane and extracellular components associated with cell adhesion and barrier function.
(4) Basement membrane synthesis to provide attachment to the underlying connective tissues.
(5) Macromolecular synthesis associated with cell migration.

The relatively undifferentiated basal (or germinal) cells of the oral epithelium contain the range of organelles typical of most cell types (nucleus, mitochondria, Golgi apparatus, endoplasmic reticulum, ribosomes, etc). Such cells are already marked by the presence of epithelial-specific features, especially desmosomes and tonofilaments. With entry into the maturation pathway and emigration from the basal layer, a sequence of epithelial specific ultrastructural changes occurs including:

(1) Cell flattening.
(2) Increase in cell volume.
(3) Formation of keratohyalin.
(4) Appearance and discharge of membrane-coating granules into the distal extracellular space.
(5) Thickening of the plasma membrane.

At the base of the stratum corneum, an abrupt transition occurs, associated with loss of cell nuclei, mitochondria and other basic subcellular structures, and the uniform tight packing of tonofilaments which are embedded in a matrix to produce a uniform cell content.

The keratohyalin granules are irregular in shape, show a patchy variation in electron density and are intimately associated with free ribosomes.[7] In the masticatory mucosa, the transition phase of individual cells between the stratum granulosum and stratum corneum is a little less regularly sequenced than in the epidermis, and the keratin pattern of the resulting cell content differs in that it consists of a homogeneous electron-dense mass, often lacking the filament profiles typical of the epidermis and showing lipid droplet inclusions. Parakeratinization, marked by incomplete transition of cellular contents and only partial lysis of cell organelles, is common in gingival epithelium. The lining oral mucosa differ from epidermis and masticatory mucosae in that keratohyalin is rarely formed, nuclei are retained and condensation of the intracellular content comparable to that of keratinizing epithelia does not occur. In addition, glycogen storage granules are commonly found in the cells of the suprabasal strata. The functional activity of the majority of the intracellular organelles remains obscure but is presumably associated with intercellular cement, barrier substances and keratin matrix formation.

The formation of a mechanically resistant, relatively impermeable stratum corneum, comprising many layers of flattened anucleate cells, is common to many stratified squamous epithelia. The proteinaceous and highly cross-linked fibrous nature of the keratins provide the mechanical strength and resistance to chemical dissolution of the stratum corneum. The fibrous proteins of prekeratins and keratins form 8 nm filaments as a result of aggregation of triple-stranded helical monomers.[8] The fibrous proteins of keratins comprise a heterogenous class of polypeptide chains (MW 45 000–70 000 daltons) showing differences in individual polypeptides with site and pathological involvement.[8]

A wide range of antigenically distinct glycoproteins and glycolipids are present at the extracellular surface of the plasma membrane of epithelial cells, presumably associated with cell adhesion, cell recognition and cell contact phenomena. Evidence exists that dermal influence may be necessary for the appropriate epithelial synthesis of cell surface components,[9] and alterations in cell surface components have been reported in wound healing and diseases of the oral mucosa.[10]

Basement membrane zone

The epithelium of the oral mucosa is typically supported by a basement membrane zone, the papillary and reticular zones of the lamina propria, and beneath these the submucosa. Fibroblasts and fibrocytes form the principal cell population maintaining the fibres and ground substance of the subepithelial connective tissues. Resident cells of the macrophage/histiocyte and mast cell lineages are present in variable numbers. The vascular system, comprising endothelial cells, pericytes and specialized fibroblasts, is well developed and neural elements are present in regionally varying concentrations. Undifferentiated mesenchymal cells of uncertain lineage are also present and presumably form the stem cells for the replacement of lost or damaged tissues. The fibrous component of the lamina propria varies in terms of fibre density and type, predominantly comprising collagens Types I and III.[11] The turnover rate of oral mucosal collagen exhibits regional variations, and is generally faster than in skin.

The extracellular matrix of the basement membrane plays roles in epithelial attachment, cell differentiation and permeability. It often comprises the primary or secondary site of involvement in pathological conditions of the mucosa. The basal hemidesmosomal-bearing surface of epithelial cells lies adjacent to an electron-lucent zone, the lamina lucida. Beneath this is an electron-dense zone, the lamina densa, which is associated with fibres that anchor the basal lamina zone to the deeper structures. This region has been shown to comprise collagenous and non-collagenous glycoproteins and proteoglycans, whereas the lamina densa contains primarily Type IV (and Type V) collagen. Fibronectin is also reported to be present in the dermis, without accentuation in the basement membrane zone. The epithelial basement membrane appears to be synthesized by the basal epithelial cells, whereas the complete basement membrane complex requires a living and viable dermal substrate.

Epithelial–mesenchymal interactions

There is a considerable body of evidence to indicate the important role of epithelial–mesenchymal interactions in the development of epithelial structures.[12] Morphogenetic epithelial–mesenchymal interactions can be considered either directive or permissive in nature, with the final adult form of a tissue being the terminal result of a cascade of prior interactions.[13] There are indications that epithelial–mesenchymal interactions continue to play an important part in the maintenance of regionally specific differences in the structure of renewing epithelia during adult life.[11] Thus, the oral mucosa represents the terminal, and normally stable, state resulting from prior and continuing epithelial–mesenchymal interactions.

The underlying connective tissue is not essential for all aspects of growth and differentiation of adult oral mucosa, although human mucosal epithelium transplanted to deep connective tissue in mice fails to show normal maturation, unless combined with subepithelial connective tissue.[14] Tissue culture studies indicate potentially important roles of the subepithelial connective tissues in facilitating growth and permitting the expression of specific epithelial phenotypes. Other observations suggest that the epithelial phenotype may be an intrinsic property of epithelial cells,[15] although it is possible that the epithelial connective tissue continuously modulates the overlying epithelium.[16] In other words, the degree of interaction between the epithelial and underlying connective tissues has yet to be fully defined, although they may be significant in the control of oral mucosal renewal, particularly in surgical wound healing. In a variety of pathological conditions, epithelial changes may be observed secondary to changes in subepithelial connective tissues, e.g. in lichen planus, submucous fibrosis, leukoplakia, and following radiotherapy.[4] Thus the oral mucosa should be considered a functional unit comprising both epithelial and connective tissue components, rather than a mere epithelial structure.

Epithelial functions

In addition to the metabolic activities common to most cells, epithelial cells undertake a number of specialized synthetic activities associated with the maintenance of a surface barrier:

(1) Synthesis of keratin.
(2) Degradation of other intracellular organelles.
(3) Synthesis of cell surface and extracellular components related to cell adhesion and barrier function.
(4) Synthesis of the basement membrane complex which provides attachment of the epithelium to the underlying connective tissue.
(5) Synthesis of macromolecules associated with cell migration under certain circumstances, e.g. wound healing.

Epithelial renewal

The rate of epithelial replacement varies markedly between various regions of the oral mucosa. The functional significance of such differences is presumably related to rates of surface wear, which are affected both by the degree of surface trauma at any particular site and by the resistance of the epithelial surface to abrasion. The maintenance of regionally specific rates of cell proliferation when transplanted to distant sites indicates that the mitotic activity is not much affected by normal function and that mucosal proliferation is pre-adapted to its functional requirement.[14] Presumably this high rate of cell turnover provides a self-cleansing mechanism that prevents undue colonization or pentration of the epithelial surface by bacteria or fungi. The rate of surface replacement depends not only on the rate of cell proliferation per unit area of epithelial surface, but also on the area of the surface cells, i.e. the rate of oral mucosal replacement is approximately four times faster than that of the epidermis.[17]

As the lining mucosa is functionally elastic, the epithelium comprises large cells with pleated cell walls, large amounts of intercellular glycoprotein and elastic fibres within a less dense lamina propria. By contrast, the masticatory mucosa shows a more massive and inflexible stratum corneum, a greater area of epithelial–connective tissue interface and a dense collagenous lamina propria with large straight collagen fibres which serve to bind the epithelial–connective tissue structures together.

Mucosal permeability

The epithelial components of skin and oral mucosa form the primary barrier to permeability of water, electrolytes and larger molecules. No evidence exists for active transport of substances in relation to anatomical site, with passage apparently being confined to simple diffusion. The oral mucosa does not appear to be more permeable to water or ions than epidermis under comparable conditions of hydration. The effect of hydration of the oral mucosa, however, may be partially offset by components of saliva augmenting barrier function. Regional variation exists in permeability to water but not to ions or larger molecules. It has also been shown that the ability of a compound to cross oral epithelia is highly dependent upon its lipid solubility.[18] The role of the basement membrane in limiting oral mucosal permeability remains obscure, apart from limiting such larger molecules as immune complexes, inulin and dextran.

Epithelial cells other than keratinocytes

Melanocytes

Within the oral mucosal epithelium, melanocytes serve to protect the tissues from the effects of actinic radiation by the production and distribution of melanin pigment to the adjacent keratinocytes. Melanocytes are derived from the neural crest tissues after the eleventh week of fetal life and exist as typically basally positioned dendritic cells. Melanocytes lack desmosomes and tonofilaments and are locally self-replicating. They are found in many other internal sites of the body that are protected from actinic radiation. Thus their function in all sites remains obscure.

Langerhans' cells

Langerhans' cells comprise dendritic, aureophilic, intra-epithelial cells which are the peripheral arm of the immune system.[19] These cells have many functional and cell surface features in common with macrophages, including cell surface Fc-IgG and C3 receptors. The migration of Langerhans' cells across the basement membrane has been observed together with evidence for a bone marrow origin, in addition to being locally proliferative.[20] Langerhans' cells typically lie suprabasally within epithelia as regionally variable, regularly grouped cells. The exact role of Langerhans' cells in the immune system is obscure, although there is evidence for their role in contact sensitivity.

Merkel cells

Merkel cells are typically situated in the basal region of epithelia, predominantly associated with intra-epithelial nerves. They are generally assumed to function as touch receptors.

Other non-keratinocytes

Occasional leukocytic cells have been reported within the epithelium in addition to mast cells, polymorphonuclear leucocytes and lymphocytes. Conceivably these last cells may serve as precursors to Langerhans' cells.

Influences of oral mucosal renewal

In addition to comprising a renewing cellular population, the oral mucosa exhibits marked diurnal variation, albeit affected by a range of factors, including stress, adrenergic compounds, age, inflammation and trauma.

Little is currently known about the mechanisms by which epithelial proliferation is controlled. One of the earliest formulations of a general concept of growth regulation centred on a negative feedback mechanism in which diffusion of an inhibiting principle from differentiated cells acted on the general mass of the same tissue.[21] A wide range of factors have been formulated to suppress the rate of epithelial tissue proliferation, including adrenergic agents, prostaglandins, epidermal growth factors, mesenchymal factors, oestrogens and vitamin A.[22] In fact, this is currently an area of intense research activity, with the primary objective of determining the factors responsible for epithelial tumour formation.

Oral mucosal maturation

Stratified squamous epithelium can be considered to comprise:

(1) A progenitor cell compartment, located in the basal region.
(2) A differentiating compartment, which lies suprabasally.
(3) A functional compartment from which the cells are eventually shed.

In the normal steady state, the rate of cellular formation per unit area of epithelium is balanced by their rate of loss. This concept not only applies to the epithelium as a whole but also to the various component regions. Statistically, therefore, for every cell formed by division, one cell emigrates from the basal layer and one cell is shed. However, each division does not always produce one cell committed to mature and one to remain. Emigration from the basal cell layer continues in the absence of cell proliferation. Differential changes in cellular adhesion probably comprise the most important factor in determining the rate of cell migration.

The suprabasal strata of the epithelium have a highly ordered pattern of organization, with cells aligned to form a series of hexagonal units. Cells in the mitosis phase occur principally beneath the periphery of such units, with cell proliferation comprising a non-random event. Thus, continued renewal of the oral mucosa may be a function of only a small subpopulation of stem cells, which are the only cells capable of repeated division throughout life. The majority of proliferative cells are therefore committed to differentiation, maturation and death after a few divisions.[23] Thus the basal or germinative population of oral mucosal cells comprises a heterogeneous, rather than homogeneous, population. Stem cells are probably more slowly cycling than other proliferative cells and may have unusual patterns of division to reduce accumulation of errors associated with DNA replication. It is within this subpopulation that changes prior to carcinogenesis are thought to occur.[24]

The mechanism by which cells are lost from the surface epithelium remains obscure. The stratum corneum comprises essentially a mass of flattened inert keratinized cells, with programmed decomposition, or proteolytic breakdown of the extracellular cement, being the most likely cause of the loss of superficial cells.[25] In both normal and pathological states, the desquammation process may be influenced by surface environmental conditions, although the normal desquammation does not appear to depend on surface abrasion. Scanning electron microscopy has demonstrated that the surface of desquammating cells from various regions of the oral mucosa may be smooth, or folded into a honey-comb pattern of ridges.[26] These surface specializations may comprise a precise press-stud mechanism related to cellular adhesion.

The healing of oral mucosal wounds is similar to those of the skin. Mucosal wounds, however, heal more rapidly than those of other epidermal tissues.[27] The oral mucosa also responds similarly to skin to friction, ultraviolet light and inflammatory and carcinogenic factors, with a response including increased rates of cell proliferation and maturation leading to epithelial thickening.

Mucosal protection

Although there are general factors that influence host resistance to oral mucosal disease, e.g. heredity, race, sex, age, hormonal imbalance and nutrition, local factors are also involved. In addition to intrinsic factors, such as a continuous cellular desquammation and the keratin layer, saliva, due to mechanical lavage and antibacterial activity, determines the health of this tissue. Saliva may also contain specific protective factors, e.g. IgA, IgG and IgM immunoglobulins (antibodies). In addition, there is the normal battery of protective host defence mechanisms derived from the underlying connective tissue structures, e.g. macrophages, lymphocytes and polymorphonuclear leucocytes, in addition to a rich vascular and lymphatic network.

Keratinization

Keratins are a group of fibrous proteins resistant to autolysis and enzymic digestion. This property is probably the result of the disulphide (S–S) linkages between adjacent component polypeptide chains. These bonds are contained in the amino acid cystine, and it is the high content of cystine that is the most characteristic feature of the keratin molecule. The amount of cystine varies with the type of keratin, in addition to exhibiting regional and diurnal variation. Other types of cross-linkages are also important in joining the polypeptide chains of keratin. Hydrogen bonds provide links between two dipoles, one a hydrogen atom and the other either a nitrogen or oxygen atom: these hydrogen bonds are primarily responsible for the stability of the molecular configuration of keratin, with the polypeptide chains having a spiral configuration with the hydrogen bonds not only linking between adjacent chains, but also preventing extension. Salt linkages also form a number of cross-linkages between polypeptide chains, but are weaker than disulpide bonds.

Conclusions

This chapter focused on the epithelial component of the oral mucosa, although it is well to remember that the underlying mesodermal tissues also have a key role in mucosal metabolism. It is also important to realize that pathological lesions of the oral mucosa are frequently evident at the initial stages of development. In this regard, it is essential to know the structure and function of the normal mucosa in order to diagnose pathological anomalies at their earliest development stage.

Review questions

1. What is the function of the basement membrane?
2. List the functions of the non-keratinocytes in the oral epithelium.
3. What factors influence the rate of oral mucosal renewal?
4. How does the oral mucosa offer protection to the underlying tissues?
5. What metabolic functions occur in the component epithelial cell layers?

References

1. BILLINGHAM, R.E. and SILVERS, W.K. (1967) Studies on the conservation of epidermal specificities of skin and certain mucosas in adult mammals. *J. Exp. Med.*, **125**, 429–446
2. KARRING, T., LANG, B.P. and LOE, H. (1975) The role of the gingival epithelial tissue in determining epithelial proliferation. *J. Periodont. Res.*, **10**, 1–11
3. HOLMSTRUP, P. and DABELSTEEN, E. (979) Changes in carbohydrate expression of lichen planus-affected oral epithelial cell membranes. *J. Invest. Dermatol.*, **73**, 364–367
4. PINDBORG, J.J. (1980) Incidence and early forms of oral submucous fibrosis. *Oral Surg.*, **50**, 40–44
5. MACKENZIE, I.C., DABELSTEEN, E. and ROED-PETERSEN, B. (1979) A method for studying epithelial–mesenchymal interactions in human oral mucosal lesions. *Scand. J. Dent. Res.*, **87**, 234–243
6. HOPPS, R.M. and JOHNSON, N.W. (1974) Relationship between histological degree on inflammation and epithelial proliferation in macaque gingiva. *J. Periodont. Res.*, **9**, 273–283
7. MATOLTSY, A.G. and BALSAMO, C.A. (1975) A study of the components of the cornified epithelium of human skin. *J. Biophys. Biochem. Cytol.*, **1**, 339–360
8. BADEN, H.P. (1979) Keratinization in the epidermis. *Pharmacol. Ther.*, **7**, 393–411
9. KING, I.A. and TABIOWA, A. (1980) The dermis is required for the synthesis of extracellular glycosaminoglycans in cultured epidermis. *Biochim. Biophys. Acta*, **632**, 234–243
10. DABELSTEEN, E. and MACKENZIE, I.C. (1978) Expression of ricinus communis receptors on epithelial cells in oral carcinomas and oral wounds. *Cancer Res.*, **38**, 4676–4680
11. MINOR, R.R. (1980) Collagen metabolism. *Am. J. Pathol.*, **98**, 227–279
12. SENGEL, P. (1976) *Morphogenesis of Skin*. Cambridge: Cambridge University Press
13. SAXEN, L. (1977) Directive versus permissive induction: a working hypothesis. In *Cell and Tissue Interaction*, edited by J.W. Lash and M.M. Burger. New York: Raven Press
14. MACKENZIE, I.C. and HILL, M.W. (1981) Maintenance of regionally specific patterns of cell proliferation and differentiation in transplanted skin and oral mucosa. *Cell Tiss. Res.*, **219**, 597–607
15. BEER, A.E. and BILLINGHAM, R.E. (1970) Implantation, transplantation and epithelial–mesenchymal relationships in the rat uterus. *J. Exp. Med.*, **132**, 721–736
16. HEANEY, T.G. (1977) A histological investigation of the influence of adult porcine gingival connective tissues in determining epithelial specificity. *Arch. Oral Biol.*, **22**, 167–171
17. KVIDERA, E.J. and MACKENZIE, I.C. (1981) Surface clearance of oral mucosa and skin. *J. Dent. Res.*, **60A**, 939
18. SIEGEL, I.A. and IZUTSU, K.T. (1980) Permeability of oral mucosa to organic compounds. *J. Dent. Res.*, **59**, 1604–1605
19. STINGL, G. (1980) New aspects of Langerhans' cell function. *Int. J. Dermatol.*, **19**, 189
20. MACKENZIE, I.C. (1975) Labelling of murine epidermal Langerhans' cells with H3-thymidine. *Am. J. Anat.*, **144**, 127–136

21. WEISS, P. and KAVANAU, J.L. (1957) A model of growth and growth control in mathematical terms. *J. Gen. Physiol.*, **41**, 1–47
22. LAURENCE, E.B. (1980) The regulation of cell proliferation in normal epithelia. In *Oral Premalignancy*, edited by I.C. Mackenzie, E. Dabelsteen and C.A. Squier. Iowa City: University of Iowa Press
23. POTTEN, C.S. (1976) Identification of clonogenic cells in the epidermis and the structural arrangement of the epidermal proliferative unit. In *Stem Cells of Renewing Cell Populations*, edited by A.B. Carnie, P.K. Lala and D.G. Osmond. New York: Academic Press
24. LAJTHA, L.G. (1970) Stem cell kinetics. In *Regulation of Hematopoiesis*, edited by A.S. Gordon. New York: Appleton-Century-Crofts
25. BADEN, H.P., LEE, L.D. and KUBILUS, J. (1976) Intra- and extracellular cementing substances. *J. Cosmet. Chem.*, **27**, 433–441
26. MCMILLAN, M.D. (1979) The surface structure of the completely and incompletely orthokeratinized oral epithelium in the rat: a light, scanning and transmission electron microscope study. *Am. J. Anat.*, **156**, 337–352
27. SCIUBBA, J.J., WATERHOUSE, J.P. and MEYER, J. (1978) A fine structural comparison of the healing of incisional wounds of mucosa and skin. *J. Oral Pathol.*, **71**, 214–227

6

Immunology

Introduction

The scope of the subject of immunology is vast and primarily related to the host defence mechanisms (*Table 6.1*). Although the immune system is vital for survival, an immune reaction may cause fatal disease, e.g. an overwhelming hypersensitivity reaction to a bee sting. There are, in fact, a host of disorders affecting all organ systems that are clearly attributable to immunological reactions to exogenous agents, or to the abnormal development of immunity against the body's own tissues and cells. In this chapter, only the most important subject matter is considered, and the reader is encouraged to look further at the reviews listed in the reference section[1–22] to obtain a more comprehensive appreciation of immunology. Bear in mind also, that immunology is a subject with an intense investigative background: as such, the subject is in a constant state of flux and rapid change. Accordingly, only those aspects for which there is a firm basis are considered in this chapter.

What is immunology?

Immunology is the study of the processes by which the body defends and maintains the constancy of its internal milieu against invasion by foreign organisms, or the mutation or development of unwanted

Table 6.1 Defence systems

External	*Internal*
Normal flora	Secretions
Anatomical barriers	Complement system
Secretions	Chemotaxis
Acids	Opsonins
Mucus	Iron proteins
Sweat	Transferrin
	Lactoferrin
	Glycoproteins
	Lysozyme
	Polyamines
	Inflammatory responses
	Oedema
	Fever
	Phagocytic cells
	Neutrophils (PMNs)
	Monocytes
	Macrophages

cells or cell products within itself. The immune system comprises all the phenomena that result from the specific interaction between the cells of the immune system and antigens. If an antigen gains access into the body, two possible outcomes result.

Humoral response

This involves antibody synthesis and release within the blood and extracellular fluids. In this response, the humoral antibodies can combine with antigens (e.g. microbial toxins) to cause toxin neutralization, or they can coat the antigenic surfaces of micro-organisms and render them susceptible to lysis by complement, or phagocytosis by macrophages.

Cell-mediated response

This is manifested by sensitized lymphocytic production: the cells are then capable of interacting with antigen by means of specific cell surface receptors. In this response, the sensitized cells are responsible for such actions: a process that includes resistance against many intracellular micro-organisms (e.g. viruses, fungi, some bacteria) and foreign tissue graft rejection.

The lymphocyte is the principal cellular component in both types of response, so that the lymphoid tissues are the central structural components of the immune system (*Figure 6.1*). The two major types of lymphocytes involved are B cells and T cells. B cells (bursa-dependent lymphocytes) are progenitors of plasma cells that secrete antibodies. while T cells (thymus-dependent lymphocytes) are the mediators of cell-mediated immunity. Macrophages are also components of the immune system, although they do not give rise to sensitized cells themselves or produce antibodies (*Figure 6.2*).

Antibody production leads to:

(1) Activation (fixation) of complement components, leading to inflammatory response enhancement by the production of biologically

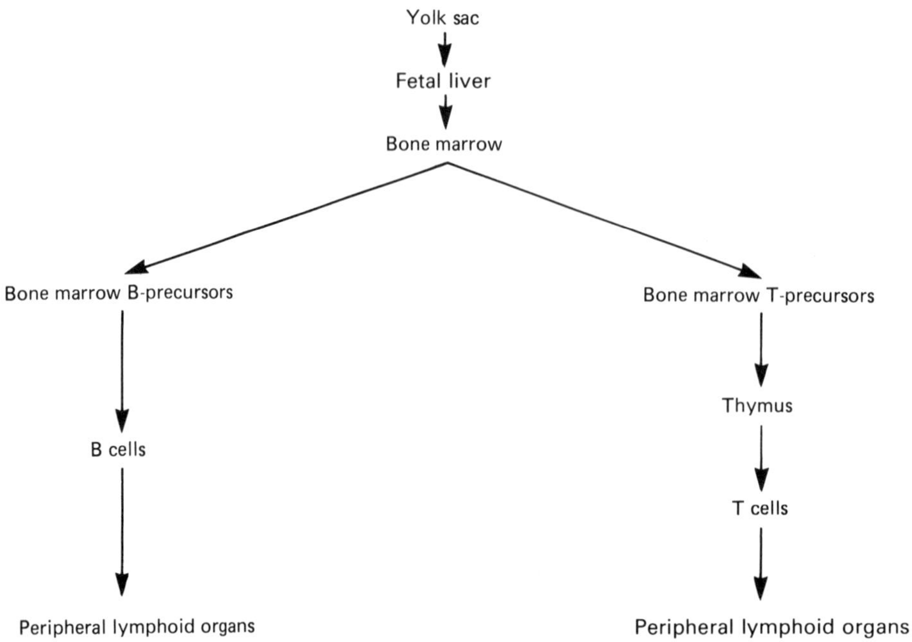

Figure 6.1 Origin of the immune system.

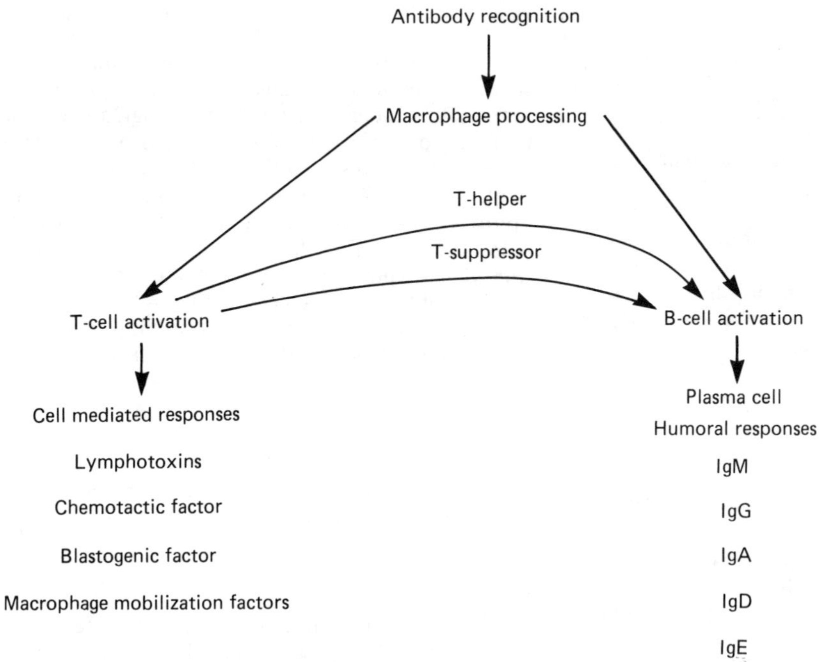

Figure 6.2 Major immune responses of T and B cells.

active molecules, and complement-induced opsonization which facilitates phagocytosis. In addition, antibodies lead to complement-mediated neutralization of certain viruses, as well as the lysis of cellular antigens.
(2) Direct neutralization of certain micro-organisms and viruses.
(3) Antibody-induced opsonization.
(4) Triggering of mast cell histamine release.
(5) Feedback regulation of antibody synthesis.

When T cells are stimulated by antigens, lymphokine secretion results in delayed-hypersensitivity reactions, secretion of antigen-specific helper factors which influence B cell differentiation and antigen-specific suppressor factor secretion to influence both B and T cell function. Antigen-stimulated T cells also secrete non-specific helper and suppressor factors that modulate lymphocyte function, in addition to the secretion of important growth factors, e.g. interleukin 2. Subsequent antigenic elimination depends upon the activation and amplification of non-specific effector cells or substances (e.g. complement activation or macrophage phagocytosis) following the interaction of specific products of the immune response with antigen.

Antigens

By definition, antigens induce immune responses. In most cases, antigenic ingestion by macrophages appears to be an essential prelude to antibody production. Antigens range from relatively simple macromolecules (e.g. serum albumin) to complex infectious micro-organisms. There are different categories of antigen, including:

(1) *Immunogen*: an antigen capable of inducing an immune response.
(2) *Tolerogen*: a molecule that induces a specific state of unresponsiveness or tolerance.
(3) *Haptens*: relatively small molecules that are not antigenic in themselves but can bind to a protein carrier to become antigenic.

There are also epitopes (antigenic determinants) which are specific sites on antigens that elicit a specific response, whereas an immunodominant determinant is an epitope that dominates in the induction of an immune response.

Antigens occur in a number of different chemical forms, including proteins and glycoproteins and polysaccharides, although nucleic acids and lipids are generally poor immunogens. In fact, the immunogenicity of an antigen depends upon its chemical nature, in addition to its foreignness, molecular size (the larger the molecule, the greater the immunogenicity), chemical complexity, accessibility of antigenic determinants, and host-related factors, including the health and nutritional status of the host. Thus antigens may induce immune system production of antigen-specific protein products which are collectively termed antibodies (immunoglobulins).

Antibodies

Antibodies (immunoglobulins) are glycoproteins that possess an antigen-binding region (Fab) and an Fc fragment that can attach to Fc receptors present on most lymphocytes, polymorphonuclear leucocytes and macrophages to provoke a variety of reactions, including complement activation. These biological properties depend on four distinct component heavy and light chain classes and subclasses,[2] which in turn depend on their amino acid sequences. Immunoglobulins are produced by B lymphocytes (B cells) and their fully differentiated cell form, plasma cells, having the same specificity for antigen in their cell surface receptors.

IgG

IgG is, in some ways, the most important, in that it forms up to 80% of circulating antibodies. It is produced in response to most infections and often provides persistent protection. IgG is, therefore, the characteristic serum immunoglobulin of a secondary immune response to antigen. There are four subclasses of IgG (IgG_1, IgG_2, IgG_3, IgG_4), with the heavy chain being responsible for the differences. Maternal IgG is the only immunoglobulin to cross the placenta. IgG binds to cell surface receptors of polymorphonuclear leucocytes, monocytes and some lymphocytes via the Fc region, in addition to complement fixation.

IgM

IgM is the first antibody to appear as the primary response to an antigenic stimulus, e.g. an infection. On further exposure, however, B cells switch to IgG production, since IgG is the most potent complement-fixing antibody. IgM is active in complement fixation and a potent agglutinator of particulate antigens and cellular antigens (e.g. bacteria). It also binds to surface receptors of T-helper cells.

IgA

This is the characteristic immunoglobulin of the secretory immune response and is also present in tears, saliva and colostrum. Being an agglutinator, it is often potent in neutralizing certain bacteria and viruses. It contains an additional (secretory) component that is added to polymeric IgA by certain epithelial cells as it is transported from the stromal side to the luminal side of an epithelial gland. This immunoglobulin provides protection of the mucosal surfaces of the body (including the oral cavity) from microbial colonization and penetration, primarily by replication of IgA-secreting plasma cells lining these sites.

IgD

IgD is a cell-surface receptor on immunocompetent B cells; its function remains controversial.

IgE

This reaginic antibody is generally associated with allergy. Most of the IgE is bound to the surface of basophils and mast cells, which when stimulated leads to the release of histamine, leukotrienes, and eosinophil chemotactic factors.

Cells of the immune system (*Table 6.2*)

T lymphocytes

T lymphocytes (T cells) are present in both the peripheral lymphoid tissues as well as in the circulating blood. In the lymph nodes they are located in the area between the follicles and in the deep cortex of the lymph nodes. T cells are also located in the periarteriolar sheaths of the spleen. In the peripheral blood, they constitute 60–70% of all lymphocytes. T cells are long-lived and form a large recirculating pool of cells. T cells have two main functions.

Table 6.2 Features of immunocompetent cells

Characteristics	*T cell*	*B cell*	*Macrophage*
Origin	Bone marrow	Bone marrow	Bone marrow
Differentiation	Thymus	Bone marrow	Bone marrow
Life-span	months/years	days/weeks	?
Lymphoid tissue localization	Perifollicular Periarteriolar	Germinal centres	Diffuse
Recirculation	Yes	Mainly static	Yes
Functions			
Cell-mediated immunity	Yes	No	Yes
Humoral immunity:			
Helper functions	Yes	No	Yes
Antibody synthesis	No	Yes	No
Memory	Yes	Yes	No

Cellular immune reactions

T cell functions include the following:

(1) Resistance against some viral and microbial infections.
(2) Delayed hypersensitivity reactions.
(3) Rejection of solid organ transplants.
(4) Resistance against new tumour formation.

Regulatory functions

T cells play important roles in modulating the immune response mediated by other T and B cells. In fact there are several subsets of T cells, each with specific facilitatory (T helper) or suppressive (T suppressor) roles.

B lymphocytes

B lymphocytes (B cells) are present in the blood and lymphoid tissue, including the bone marrow. They constitute 10–20% of the circulating lymphocytes together with the extra-oral lymph nodes and spleen.[24] There are, in fact, several intra-oral lymphoid aggregations that are important in this regard: the palatine tonsils; the lingual tonsils and the nasopharyngeal tonsils (adenoids).

B cells express surface immunoglobulin (Ig), in addition to two other receptors: a receptor for the Fc portion of the IgG (Fc receptor) and a receptor for the third component of complement (C3b receptor).

Proteins and polysaccharides are strong immunogens for B cells, whereas T cells recognize polysaccharides poorly, if at all. Lipids, nucleic acids and steroids are generally weak immunogens, unless conjugated to immunogenic carrier molecules. B cells may be stimulated directly by various soluble antigens, while most T cells can only recognize soluble antigens if they have been phagocytosed and presented by macrophages, i.e. they can only recognize foreign epitopes when they are on cell membranes. All immunocompetent lymphocytes derived from lymphoid stem cells undergo an antigen-independent proliferation and differentiation phase before they are released in the body as mature small lymphocytes.

K lymphocytes

These cells are characterized by the presence of an Fc receptor but they lack surface Ig and surface markers of T cells and are non-phagocytic. They therefore lack the typical markers for B cells, T cells or macrophages, although morphologically they resemble small or medium-sized lymphocytes and are sometimes termed 'null cells'. Due to their Fc receptors for IgG, these cells can lyse antibody-coated target cells by a process termed antibody-dependent cellular cytotoxicity.

NK lymphocytes

Natural killer (NK) cells are found in the peripheral blood and lymphoid tissues and are capable of lysing a variety of cells, including tumour cells, virus-infected cells and some normal cells, without previous sensitization. They may therefore provide important first-line defences against tumour formation and virus infection. Morphologically NK cells resemble small lymphocytes, although they possess Fc receptors and share some cell surface antigens with T cells and macrophages.

Langerhans' and dendritic cells

Langerhans' cells are found in the epithelium whereas dendritic cells are found in the lymphoid tissues. Both cells are extremely efficient in antigenic presentation. They therefore probably form a vital component of the immune system.

Macrophages (*Table 6.3*)

Macrophages are widely distributed in the lymphoid tissue as well as in circulating blood (monocytes). In the lymph nodes they are present in the walls of sinuses as well as the deep cortex. Macrophages are required to process and present the antigen to immunocompetent cells, in addition to acting as powerful effector cells in certain cell-mediated immune reactions resulting from the T cell secretion of lymphokines. Macrophages also produce a number of soluble factors that affect not only the growth and functioning of lymphocytes but also fibroblasts, endothelial and smooth muscle cells. The macrophage cell membrane also has two important receptors, one for the Fc portion of IgG and one for activated C3 (complement). Both these receptors facilitate phagocytosis of particulate matter. Thus macrophages not only play a crucial role in promoting recognition of an antigen by immunocompetent cells but are also closely associated with

Table 6.3 Macrophage functions

Lymphocyte proliferative regulation
Antigen uptake and processing
Antigen transfer to lymphocytes
Antigen-dependent T cell proliferative control
Cell-mediated response
Complement component production
Micro-organism phagocytosis
Enzyme/enzyme-inhibitor secretion
Promotion/inhibition of cellular replication, including lymphocytes
Polymorph (PMN) chemotactic factor secretion

lymphocytes in lymphoid organs. When an antigen is phagocytosed by a macrophage, most of it is digested and destroyed, although part is processed and presented to the lymphocytes in an immunogenic fashion. Thus, when an antigen is processed by macrophages, their epitopes are presented to lymphocytes in their native and digested forms. Macrophages also support many lymphoid cell interactions, including protection of the immune system from being flooded by excessive amounts of antigens in overwhelming infections. This prevents the development of immunological tolerance.

Antibody–antigen reactions

Antibody–antigen reactions may have a variety of results, including:

(1) Agglutinins, which cause microbial clumping to hamper their spread through the tissues.
(2) Opsonins, which render micro-organisms and other particulate matter more susceptible to phagocytosis.
(3) Precipitins, which precipitate soluble antigens out of solution, rendering them more susceptible to phagocytosis.
(4) Neutralizing antibodies, which inactivate and/or render viruses non-infective.
(5) Complement fixation (activation), that results from many antibody–antigen complexes, leading to lytic and bactericidal reactions. The other reactions mentioned above, however, are not complement-dependent.

Complement (*Figure 6.3*)

The complement system comprises at least 9 plasma proteins, most of which are produced by mac-

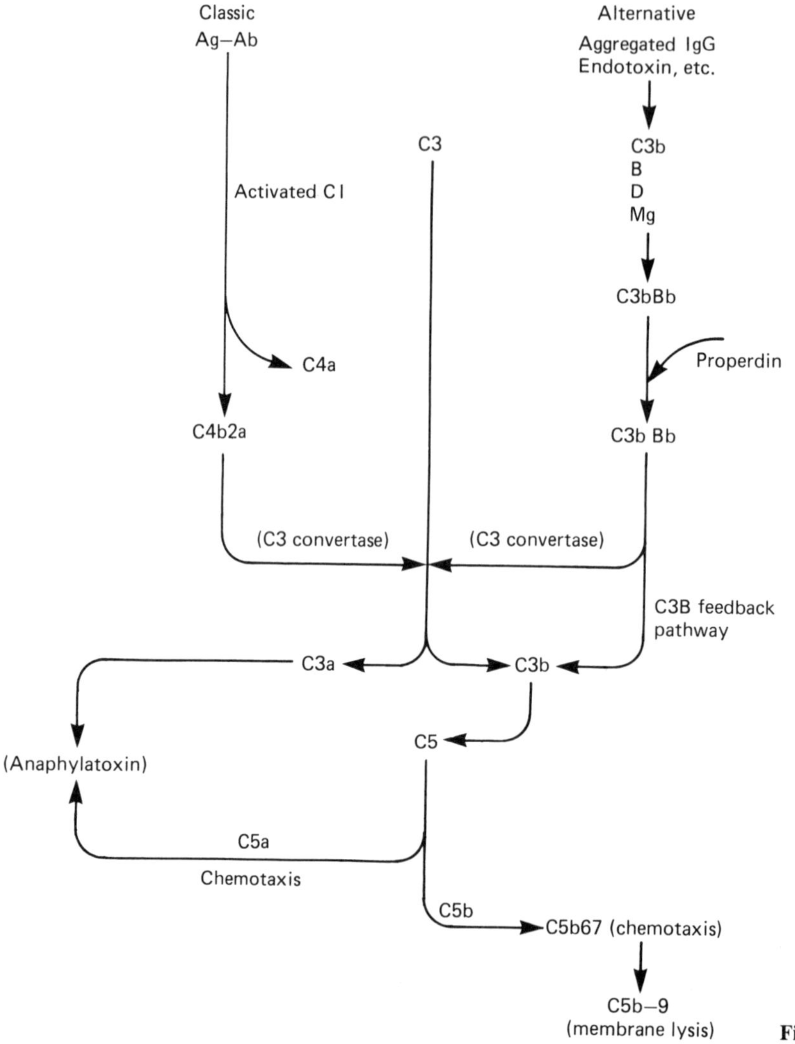

Figure 6.3 The complement system.

rophages (except C1). When this system is activated, a series of end-products and by-products are produced, most of which affect both the inflammatory and immunological reactions. This complement cascade may be triggered by a number of stimuli, including:

(1) Antibody–antigen complexes.
(2) Aggregated immunoglobulins.
(3) Antibody attachment to cell membranes.
(4) Some proteolytic enzymes, e.g. trypsin.

Classically, the complement cascade results in components in the following sequence, C142356789. There is also an alternative pathway that can be activated by aggregates of IgG, IgA or IgE, in addition to non-immunological mechanisms, e.g. endotoxin. These activators stimulate C3 convertase formation, causing cleavage of C3 and the remaining components, i.e. the remaining complement components react in the same sequence as in the classic pathway. The complement system, therefore, hinges on C3, the complement component present in highest concentration in the serum.

The effects of many of the components of complement include:

(1) *Chemotaxis*: C3a, C5a and C5b strongly attract polymorphonuclear leucocytes, thereby contributing to microbial phagocytosis in inflammatory reactions.
(2) *Cell lysis*: the culmination of the complete complement cascade results in microbial membrane damage and lysis.
(3) *Anaphylotoxis*: fragments of C3a and C5a (C3 and C5 fragments) lead to type 1 hypersensitivity reactions.
(4) *Kinin production*: this leads to increased vascular permeability associated with inflammation.

Types of immunity (*Figure 6.4*)

In order to understand this biological system, a few fundamental concepts are required.

Immunity is a term that refers to the resistance of a host organism to invasive pathogens or their toxic products. Immunity can be divided into two main types – non-specific and specific.

Natural resistance/non-specific immunity

This system does not involve specific recognition of a foreign agent and operates through various factors, including genetic control, physical and mechanical factors, biochemical, cellular and other factors. For instance:

(1) The oral mucosa provides a mechanical barrier that prevents irritation of the underlying connective tissues.
(2) The hydrochloric acid of gastric secretions, together with lysozyme in sweat, tears and saliva, exhibit antibacterial activity.
(3) Interferons comprise a family of glycoproteins that are produced within a few hours to every nucleated cell in response to a wide range of viral infections.
(4) A component of the blood, complement, comprises over 18 distinct serum protein factors that interact to contribute to the normal body defences potentiating phagocytosis of various microbes and parasites. Complement also

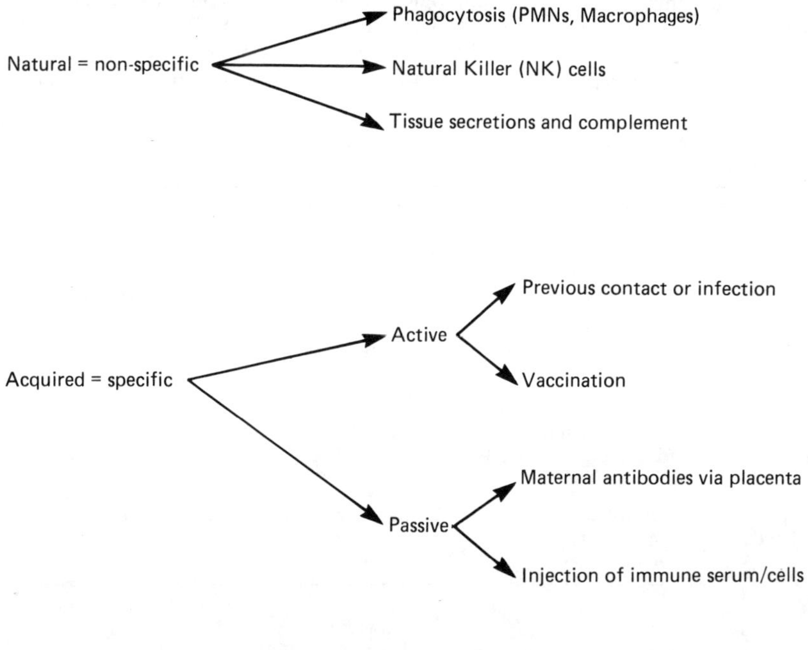

Figure 6.4 Types of immunity.

stimulates the inflammatory host defence mechanism.

Phagocytosis is a major component of the non-specific immune system. It is the process whereby a single phagocytic cell engulfs unwanted or mutated cells or invading infectious micro-organisms. Effective phagocytosis by polymorphonuclear leucocytes and monocytic macrophages early in the course of microbial invasion may readily render the invading organism non-pathogenic. Phagocytes also interact and co-operate with the complement and specific immune systems to potentiate their defensive action. Phagocytosis (a function of the reticulo-endothelial system) is a complex process that involves chemotaxis, attachment, ingestion, intracellular killing and digestion.

Intracellular killing is dependent upon powerful antimicrobial substances in the lysosomes – lysozyme, hydrogen peroxide and myeloperoxidase.

Macrophages also secrete lysozyme, complement factors and interferon, which all contribute to natural resistance (*see Figure 6.2*).

Specific immunity

This is a specific reaction of the body against non-self foreign agents, in which its immune products react specifically with the stimulating agent. Conventionally, specific immunity is divided into passive and active immunity.

Passive immunity involves either the transfer of antibodies or, in some diseases, of sensitized white blood cells from an immune to a non-immune person. Natural passive immunity is transferred across the placenta, whereas artificial transfer is the therapeutic use of various antitoxins or gammaglobulins, as in the treatment of tetanus or diphtheria. In certain diseases, e.g. tuberculosis, passive immunity can only be transferred by white blood cells from an immune person, not by antibodies. In both cases, passive immunity is short-lived, depending on the life-span of the antibody or the transferred cells in the recipient. Once they disappear, the host is again susceptible to the disease.

Active immunity occurs when a foreign (i.e. non-self) substance is encountered. An active immune response, with the production of specific antibodies and sensitized cells, may occur, although infrequently an antigen-specific unresponsiveness may result. This latter is termed immunological tolerance. An active immune response can follow natural clinical or subclinical infection, or be induced artificially by vaccination. Active immunity involves three essential characteristics – recognition, specificity and memory.

Hypersensitivity reactions (*Table 6.4*)

Contact with antigen not only results in the induction of protective immune responses but also reactions that may be damaging to the host. For instance, the immune reactions that occur in response to contact with exogenous antigens (e.g. drugs, foods, chemicals, dust, pollens and microbial agents) may result in a range of responses including skin itchiness (urticaria) to bronchial asthma. These reactions are termed hypersensitivity reactions, which may be initiated by either interaction with antigen and humoral antibody or cell-mediated immune mechanisms.

Type 1 (anaphylactic) hypersensitivity reactions

Anaphylaxis may be defined as a rapidly developing immunological reaction occurring within minutes after the combination of an antigen with antibody bound to mast cells or basophils in indfividuals previously sensitized to the antigen. The systemic

Table 6.4 Hypersensitivity states

Type	*Mediator*	*Mechanism*	*Disease example*	*Effect*
I Anaphylactic	IgE	IgE binds to mast cells releasing histamines, SHT, SRS-A	Anaphylactic reactions, atopic allergy	Bronchoconstriction, vasodilatation, increased vascular permeability
II Cytotoxic killer	Complement, killer lymphocytes	Lysis of cells with surface antigens	Haemolytic anaemia, thrombocytopenic purpura	Cell death
III Immune complex	Antibody/antigen/complement	Immune-complex formation, lysosomal enzyme release	Serum sickness	Blood vessel wall damage
IV Cell-mediated	Lymphokines, sensitized T cells	Cytotoxic action by lymphocytes or lymphokines	Contact dermatitis	Target cell death

response usually follows an intravenous injection of an antigen to which the host has already become sensitized, with a state of shock occurring within minutes. In the local reaction, localized skin responses, nasal and conjunctival discharge, hay fever, bronchial asthma or allergic gastrointestinal disturbances develop depending on the portal of entry of the allergen.

Type I reactions are mediated by IgE antibodies. An allergen stimulates IgE production by lymphocytes and plasma cells mainly in the tonsils, Peyer's patches and the lamina propria of the gastrointestinal and other mucosal surfaces, assisted by T-helper cells. Once the IgE antibodies are formed in response to the allergen, they have a strong tendency to become attached to mast cells through cell surface receptors. When mast cells or basophils, armed with cytophilic IgE antibodies, are re-exposed to the specific allergen, a series of reactions occurs leading to the release of powerful preformed vasoactive mediators (e.g. histamine, eosinophil chemotactic factor of anaphylaxis and neutrophil chemotactic factor), and the release of secondary mediators including leukotrienes (e.g. arachidonic acid metabolites and platelet activating factors).

Type II (cytotoxic) hypersensitivity reactions

This form of hypersensitivity is mediated by antibodies directed towards antigens present on the surfaces of cells or other tissue components. The resultant hypersensitivity reaction results from the binding of antibodies to normal or altered cell surface antigens.

In *complement-mediated cytotoxicity*, antibody (IgG or IgM) reacts with an antigen present on the cell surface, resulting in complement activation with direct cell membrane damage or lysis. The antibody-coated cells also become susceptible to phagocytosis. This type of reaction most commonly involves blood cells, e.g. in blood transfusion reactions, certain drug reactions.

Antibody-dependent cell-mediated cytotoxicity results from target cells being coated with low concentrations of IgG antibody and being killed (but not phagocytosed) by a variety of non-sensitized cells that have Fc receptors. Eosinophils, polymorphonuclear leucocytes, monocytes and K cells are included in these reactions.

Type III (immune complex-mediated) hypersensitivity reactions

This type of hypersensitivity reaction is induced by antigen–antibody complexes that produce tissue damage as a result of their capacity to activate a variety of serum factors, including the complement system, when antigen combines with antibody, either within the circulation or at extravascular sites where antigen may have been deposited. The mere formation of antigen–antibody complexes in the circulation does not lead to disease processes and may in fact represent the normal method of antigen removal. The factors that determine whether the immune complexes formed in the circulation will be pathogenic remain largely obscure. Wherever complexes deposit, there is activation of the complement cascade and the elaboration of biologically active components:

(1) The release of C3b results in opsonization (coating) of particles and micro-organisms facilitating their phagocytosis.
(2) C5 and C5b67 are chemotactic for polymorphonuclear leucocytes and monocytes.
(3) C3a and C5a increase vascular permeability and smooth muscle contraction.
(4) C5–9 cause cell membrane damage and cytolysis.

Phagocytosis of antigen–antibody complexes by polymorphonuclear leucocytes result in the generation and/or release of a variety of substances including:

(1) Prostaglandins.
(2) Vasodilator substances.
(3) Chemotactic substances.
(4) Lysosomal enzymes, including proteases.
(5) Free-oxygen radicals.

Antibody–antigen complexes also cause platelet aggregation and Hageman factor activation.

Type IV (cell-mediated) hypersensitivity reactions

Type IV hypersensitivity reactions are mediated by specifically sensitized T cells and include both delayed-type hypersensitivity and cell-mediated cytotoxic reactions.

Cell-mediated cytotoxicity

In response to certain antigens, e.g. tumour cells, virus-infected cells and incompatible cells, the immune system responds by the generation of cytotoxic T cells. The cytotoxic T cell binds specifically to its target cell (not innocent bystander cells) leading to cell membrane lysis and rupture. The cytotoxic T cell survives and is then recycled to kill other target cells.

Delayed-type hypersensitivity

Delayed hypersensitivity reactions are initiated by specifically sensitized T lymphocytes, generated during initial contact with the antigen. When the individual is re-exposed to the specific antigen, memory T cells are stimulated to divide and release

Table 6.5 Lymphokines

Lymphokine	*Function*
Blastogenic factor	Initiates cell growth
Chemotactic factor	Attracts macrophages
Interferon	Confers host cell protection from viruses
Interleukin 1	Initiates T cell proliferation
Interleukin 2	Promotes continuing T cell proliferation
Lymphotoxin	Destroys target cells
Macrophage-activating factor	Chemotaxis and/or activates macrophages
Macrophage-aggregation factor	Agglutinates macrophages
Migration inhibition factor	Prevents macrophage migration

a variety of biologically active molecules, termed lymphokines. The function of the lymphokines is to amplify the inflammatory response by recruiting inflammatory cells, activating them and maintaining them localized to the site. The lymphokines (*Table 6.5*) include:

(1) Macrophage migration inhibition factor, which maintains macrophages localized to the site.
(2) Interferons, which enhance macrophage cellular activity.
(3) Polymorphonuclear leucocytic, eosinophilic, basophilic, monocytic and lymphocytic chemo-attractive substances, which attract these cells to the particular site.
(4) Interleukin 2, which causes T cell proliferation at the site.

Immune deficiency

Immunodeficiency diseases are characterized by chronic or recurrent infections, or the incomplete response to treatment of the infection. Immunodeficiency diseases are rare, and can generally be divided into:

(1) Primary immunodeficiency disorders, which are almost always genetically generated.
(2) Secondary immunodeficiencies, which arise from complications of infections, malnutrition, ageing, immunosuppression, irradiation, chemotherapy or autoimmune diseases.

In primary immunodeficiency states, either specific immunity (humoral and cell-mediated immunity) or non-specific host defence mechanisms mediated by complement proteins, phagocytes and NK cells are affected. Thus primary immunodeficiencies reflect defects in the differentiation, maturation and function of B, T, K and/or NK lymphocytes, macrophages and polymorphonuclear leucocytes, in addition to defects in the synthesis and function of complement and complement control proteins. Most primary immunodeficiencies manifest themselves in infancy and are characterized by increased susceptibility to infections.

Secondary immunodeficiencies include acquired immune deficiency syndrome (AIDS), and are again characterized by increased susceptibility to infections. These deficiencies accompany a variety of conditions that eventually involve the immune system, including malignancy, overwhelming infection, infection with immunosuppressive viruses, chemotherapy, malnutrition, ageing, autoimmune diseases and AIDS.

The oral cavity

The health of the oral cavity primarily depends on the integrity of the oral mucosa. Provided this mucosa remains intact, few micro-organisms can penetrate the underlying tissues. This partly reflects the function of the keratin barrier.[23] In addition, the basement membrane between the epithelium and connective tissue provides another barrier. In the lamina propria adjacent to the basement membrane there are a few lymphoid cells which may combat micro-organisms that penetrate to this depth. These intra-oral lymphoid aggregations function, together with the extra-oral lymph nodes, for the protection of the oral cavity as a whole.[24]

There are, in fact, several intra-oral lymphoid aggregations.

(1) The *palatine tonsils* comprise paired lymphoid masses, between the glossopalatine and pharyngopalatine arches, covered by squamous epithelium. The component lymphoid tissue contains both B and T cells. In fact, these tonsils resemble lymph nodes, having T and B dependent areas, with IgG-producing cells being the most prominent. There may also be IgA-containing cells in the sub-epithelial location.
(2) The *lingual tonsils* are much less prominent, lying on each side of the tongue just distal to the circumvallate papillae. They comprise lymphoid nodules, some of which have germinal centres, in addition to perifollicular diffuse lymphoid cells.
(3) The *pharyngeal tonsils* comprise a simple mass of lymphoid tissue under the nasopharyngeal mucosa.

There are also scattered collections of lymphoid tissue in other regions of the oral cavity. Lymphocytes and plasma cells are found in small clusters in both major and minor salivary glands. Most of the plasma cells secrete IgA, although a few secrete IgM or IgG. Most of the salivary IgA is probably derived from these plasma cells, with the IgA being dimeric, rather than the serum IgA, which is monomeric.

A few lymphocytes may be found in the normal gingiva although with increasing plaque accumulation the number of B-cell derived plasma cells increases significantly. Clusters of plasma cells are found initially adjacent to the junctional epithelium and near the blood vessels, although the gingival connective tissues subsequently become diffusely infiltrated by these cells. IgG-producing cells predominate, albeit with a few IgA-producing cells and occasional IgM-producing cells. Conceivably, the plasma cell infiltration of the gingiva may be the end-result of a number of complex immune responses, with the immunoglobulins formed by these cells being to a large extent non-specific. It may be that the spread of micro-organisms from the gingival surface may be prevented by coating them with antibodies, immune-complex formation, phagocytosis and bacteriolysis by antibodies and complement. These immune responses, in turn, may elicit host inflammatory reactions through complement activation, phagocytic lysosomal enzyme release and endotoxin release from lysed micro-organisms. In other words, local gingival inflammatory reactions comprise side-reactions to the immune prevention of systemic microbial infections.

Gingival crevicular fluid

With continued plaque accumulation at the cervical surface of the tooth, there is a corresponding increase in crevicular fluid formation. This fluid contains immunoglobulins IgG, IgA and IgM in addition to complement components C3, C4, C5 and C3 pro-activator. Thus the crevicular fluid contains most of the humoral and cellular immune components found in the blood, although salivary sIgA is the predominant component. There are also a number of other components of crevicular fluid, including:

albumin	lysosomal enzymes (derived from phagocytic cells)
transferrin	proteases (formed by bacteria)
haptoglobulins	lysozyme
glycoproteins	hyaluronidase and collagenase.
lipoproteins	

These enzymes not only affect specific tissues, e.g. collagen, but also selective IgA inactivation results from specific protease activity. In addition to the predominant polymorphonuclear cell content, crevicular fluid also contains macrophages and T and B cells which migrate from the underlying blood vessels.

Saliva

In addition to mechanical lavage, the saliva functions as a component of the oral immune system. Saliva combines both non-specific and specific immune components.

Non-specific components

Lysozyme (muramidase)

This is a bactericidal enzyme that splits the bond between *N*-acetyl glucosamine and *N*-acetyl muramic acid in the mucopeptide components of microbial cell walls. Apart from *Streptococcus mutans*, the oral flora is generally resistant to lysozyme.

Peroxidase

In the presence of thiocyanate ions and hydrogen peroxide, peroxidase kills *Lactobacillus acidophilus* by inhibiting lysine uptake and may inhibit some streptococci by limiting the action of their glycolytic enzymes.

Lactoferrin

This has a bacteriostatic effect on a wide microbial spectrum, possibly by depleting local environmental iron required for microbial growth.

Specific components

Secretory IgA

IgA is quantitatively the most important immunoglobulin present in saliva, mainly derived locally from plasma cells. These plasma cells produce not only heavy and light chains of the IgA, but also the J chains which are polypeptides combining the Fc part of the IgA to produce dimeric IgA. The dimeric IgA complexes with SC, the latter being synthesized by the secretory epithelial cells of salivary acini, where complexing of dimeric IgA with SC occurs. The assembled secretory IgA (sIgA) is then transported to the duct lumen and excreted into the oral cavity. sIgA is more resistant to microbial and proteolytic breakdown than other immunoglobulins, so it is particularly suited to saliva, which then functions as an antiseptic paint for the various oral surfaces. sIgA also appears to limit microbial adherence to the mucosal surfaces.

Periodontal disease

The effects of dental plaque on the immune response are both complex and varied.[25,26] This is not surprising in view of the complexity of the plaque itself. The components of dental plaque result in the activation of both complement pathways, lymphocytic stimulation, lymphokine release and macrophage activation.[27] These potent reactions are probably modulated by the immunosuppressive and immunopotentiating effects of the dental plaque components resulting primarily in a localized chronic inflammatory response in the gingiva. This localized gingival inflammatory response may be further exacerbated by the direct toxic effects of the various dental plaque components.[28,29]

Unless meticulous oral hygiene is maintained, dental plaque accumulation ultimately leads to chronic periodontal disease. For ease of description, this disease has been subdivided into four stages. Each stage may be associated with certain immune reactions:

(1) In the initial lesion, there is a localized inflammatory reaction at the base of the gingival sulcus. This correlates with a localized inflammatory response of polymorphonuclear leucocytes, reflecting chemotactic action of plaque antigens, and complement activation.
(2) The subsequent early lesion involves the local gingival tissue infiltration of predominantly T cells with a few B cells. In the circulation, lymphocytes are sensitized, as shown by their ability to release lymphokines.
(3) In the established lesion, there is a characteristic localized plasma cell infiltration of the gingival tissues. Up to this stage, the re-establishment of good oral hygiene measures is still compatible with the restoration of normal gingival health, i.e. the lesions are reversible.
(4) The advanced lesion marks the transition to an advanced irreversible destructive process leading to tooth loss due to periodontal ligament destruction and alveolar bone loss. This phase is characterized by Types I, II, III and IV hypersensitivity reactions, associated with the protective–destructive mechanisms of lymphocytic and macrophagic function, coupled with complement activation. These reactions are associated with immunosuppressive and immunopotentiating forces that serve to prevent the immune reactions from getting out of control.[29]

Periodontal lesions are infections of the supporting tissues of the teeth. It is well established that supragingival plaque causes gingival inflammation.[35] The role of specific Gram-negative micro-organisms in the aetiology and pathogenesis of destructive forms of periodontal diseases is well established.[36] For example:

(1) *Bacteroides gingivalis* has been implicated as a major pathogen in severe adult periodontitis.[37]
(2) *Actinobacillus actinomyecetemcomitans* is a major pathogen in localized juvenile periodontitis.[38]
(3) *Bacteroides intermedius* and intermediate-sized spirochaetes have been implicated in acute necrotizing ulcerative gingivitis.[39]
(4) *Bacteroides intermedius* has been implicated in pregnancy gingivitis.[40]

Many pathogenic micro-organisms e.g. *Bacteroides gingivalis* and *Bacteroides intermedius*, are capable of causing serious and sometimes fatal infections, either systemic or localized to certain organs. Fortunately, such serious extra-oral infections due to periodontopathic organisms occur infrequently, in spite of the fact that infection of the periodontal tissues by these micro-organisms is a common event. It is therefore clear that there are protective mechanisms operating to prevent the spread of pathogenic micro-organisms to extra-oral sites in most individuals. These protective mechanisms effectively localize the infection to the periodontal tissues. In addition, they contribute to the loss of the integrity of periodontal tissues, a loss that characterized periodontal disease.

Either secretory or serum-derived antibodies may impede microbial adherence and so colonization in the initial stages of dental plaque accumulation. Also, in the initial stages of microbial tissue invasion, phagocytes, especially polymorphonuclear leucocytes, acting in concert with opsonic antibody and complement, may play a role in limiting their pathological effects. Invasion of the periodontal tissues by microbial products may also be controlled by complexing with antibody, resulting in the formation of antibody–antigen complexes, which are subsequently ingested by phagocytic cells. In the destructive phases of periodontal disease, it is likely that lymphocytes can lead to tissue destruction, either through direct cytotoxicity or through the elaboration of chemical mediators. Macrophages, collagenase and reactive oxygen species can also effect local tissue destruction. Microbial toxins or enzymes can also lead to direct tissue destruction, although these may be controlled by the production of antitoxic or enzyme-neutralizing antibodies. Finally, it is likely that lymphocytes and macrophages affect the healing and fibrosis phases of periodontal disease, since both lymphocytes and macrophages can stimulate fibroblastic activity. Thus the immune system is directly involved in all phases of the aetiology and pathogenesis of periodontal disease.[41]

Dental caries

Dental caries results from acidic enamel demineralization, primarily caused by microbial (especially *Streptococcus mutans*) utilization of dietary sugars.[30,31] Certainly serum IgA, IgG and IgM antibodies, in addition to sIgA antibodies, as well as cell-mediated immunity, appear to be highly correlated with a patient dental caries experience.[32] But although there is the potential to develop both humoral and cell-mediated immune responses to most cariogenic micro-organisms, they are largely ineffective.[33,34]

Conclusions

The subject of immunology is vast, with the majority of research being focused on the systemic rather than the oral immune system. The reader is urged to visit the nearest library in order to keep abreast of the latest, updated information which is changing our current concepts at an alarming rate.

Review questions

1. Contrast the functions of the various component cells of the immune system.
2. Describe the cellular events of the humoral immune system.
3. Differentiate between Type I and Type IV hypersensitivity reactions.
4. What are the immunological properties of saliva?
5. How does the body reject foreign bodies?

References

1. STANTON, G.J., JOHNSON, H.M. and BARON, S. (1978) Role of interferon in virus infections and antibody formation. In *Pathobiology Annual*, edited by H.L. Ioachin. New York: Raven Press
2. AUSTEN, F. (1978) Homeostasia of effector systems which can also be recruited for immune reactions. *J. Immunol.*, **121**, 793
3. STOSSAL, P.T (1974) Phagocytosis. *New Engl. J. Med.*, **290**, 717, 774, 833
4. VAN FURTH, R. (1975) *Immunity, Infection and Pathology*. Oxford: Blackwell
5. PETERS, H.H. and HEIDENREICH, W. (1980) Spontaneous cell mediated cytotoxicity. *Cancer Immunol. Immunother.*, **8**, 7982
6. VOGLER, L.B., GROSSI, C.E. and COOPER, M.D. (1979) Human lymphocyte subpopulation. In *Progress in Hematology*, edited by E.B. Brown. New York: Grune & Stratton
7. MULLER-EBERHARD, H.J. (1980) Complement reaction pathways. In *Immunology 80*, edited by M. Fougerlave and J. Dausset. London: Academic Press
8. KIRKPATRICK, C.H. (1980) Therapeutic potential of transfer factor. *New Engl. J. Med.*, **303**, 7
9. GELL, P.G.C.H., COOMBS, R.A. and LACHMANN, P. (1974) *Clinical Aspects of Immunology*. Oxford: Blackwell
10. ROITT, I.M. (1977) *Essential Immunology*. Oxford: Blackwell
11. HUDSON, L. and HAY, F.C. (1980) *Practical Immunology*, 2nd edn. Oxford: Blackwell
12. LACHMAN, P.J. and PETERS, K. (1982) *Clinical Aspects of Immunology*. Oxford: Blackwell
13. DICK, G. (1978) *Immunization*. London: Update Books
14. ROITT, I.M. and LEHNER, T. (1983) *Immunology of Oral Diseases*, 2nd edn. Oxford: Blackwell
15. FERGUSON, A. (1985) Immunological responses to food. *Proc. Nutr. Soc.*, **44**, 73–80
16. DE MAEYER, E. (1984) Interferons and the immune system. *Interferon*, **1**, 167–185
17. NESTWENKO, V.G. (1984) Network interactions and the regulation of the immune response. *Folia Biol. (Praha)*, **30**, 231–250
18. MICHEAL, J.G. (1983) Molecular and cellular events in normal and abnormal immune responsiveness. *Clin. Physiol. Biochem.*, **1**, 179–193
19. CORMAN, L.C. (1985) The relationship between nutrition, infection and immunity. *Med. Clin. North Am.*, **69**, 519–531
20. MCCONNELL, I., MUNROE, A. and WALDMANN, H. (1980) *The Immune System: a Course on the Molecular and Cellular Basis of Immunity*, 2nd edn. Oxford: Blackwell
21. GLYNN, L.E. and STEWARD, M.W. (1977) *Immunochemistry: An Advanced Textbook*. Chicester: John Wiley & Son
22. OUTNAM, F.W. (1983) From the first to the last of the immunoglobulins. *Clin. Physiol. Biochem.*, **1**, 63–91
23. JENKINS, G.N. (1978) *Physiology of the Mouth*. Oxford: Blackwell
24. LEHNER, T. (1977) *The Borderland between Caries and Periodontal Disease*. London: Academic Press
25. PAGE, R.C. and SCHROEDER, H.E. (1976) Pathogenesis of inflammatory periodontal disease. *Lab. Invest.*, **33**, 235
26. GENCO, R.J. and MERGENHAGEN, S.E. (1982) *Host-parasite Interactions in Periodontal Diseases*. Washington: American Society for Microbiology
27. NEWMAN, M.G. (1985) Current concepts of the pathogenesis of periodontal disease. *J. Periodontol.*, **56**, 1734–1739
28. LAIRD, W.R. (1983) Dental bacterial plaque. *Int. J. Biochem.*, **15**, 1095–1102
29. VAN HOUTE, J. (1983) Bacterial adherence in the mouth. *Rev. Infect. Dis. (Suppl.)*, **4**, s659–s669
30. SCULLY, C. (1981) Dental caries, progress in microbiology and immunology. *J. Infect. Dis.*, **31**, 107–133
31. ARENDS, J. (1986) The nature of early caries lesions in enamel. *J. Dent. Res.*, **65**, 2–11
32. SMITH, G.E. (1986) The action of fluoride in teeth and bone. *Med. Hypotheses*, **19**, 139–154
33. RIPA, L.W. (1985) The current status of pit and fissure sealants. *Can. Dent. Assoc. J.*, **51**, 367–375, 377–380
34. CIANCO, S.C. (1986) Chemotherapeutic agents and periodontal therapy. *J. Periodontol.*, **57**, 108–111
35. LOE, H., THEILADE, E. and JENSEN, S.R. (1965) Experimental gingivitis in man. *J. Periodontol.*, **36**, 177–187

36. ZAMBON, J.J. (1985) *Actinobacillus actinomycetemcomitans* in human periodontal disease. *J. Clin. Periodontol.*, **12**, 1–20
37. SLOTS, J. (1982) The importance of black-pigmented Bacteroides in human periodontal disease. In *Host-Parasite Interactions in Periodontal Diseases*, edited by R.J. Genco and S.E. Mergenhagen. Washington: ASM Publications
38. ZAMBON, J.J., CHRISTERSSON, L.A. and GENCO, R.J. (1986) Diagnosis and treatment of localized juvenile periodontitis. *J. Am. Dent. Assoc.*, **113**, 295–299
39. LOESCHE, W.J., SYED, S.A., LAUGHON, B.G. and STOLL, J. (1982) The bacteriology of acute necrotizing ulcerative gingivitis. *J. Periodontol.*, **53**, 223–230
40. KORMAN, K.S. and LOESCHE, W.J. (1980) The subgingival microflora during pregnancy. *J. Periodont. Res.*, **15**, 111–122
41. GENCO, R.J., VAN DYKE, T.E., LEVINE, M.J., NELSON, R.D. and WILSON, M.E. (1986) Molecular factors influencing neutrophil defects in periodontal disease. *J. Dent. Res.*, **65**, 1379

7

The blood supply of the oral tissues

Introduction

The blood and lymph vessels that permeate most oral tissues provide essential component homeostatic mechanisms. Most of the gaseous, nutrient and metabolic waste product exchange occurs at the microcirculatory level, in addition to host defence mechanisms. Knowledge of the structure and function of the microcirculatory system is therefore important for the subsequent understanding of the physiology and pathology of the oral tissues. Unfortunately, much of the information concerning the circulation in the oral tissues has to be inferred from data concerning other body tissues, i.e. the circulation of the oral tissues has been subjected to scant investigation.

Microcirculatory system

The microcirculatory system comprises the terminal portions of the vessels between arterioles and venules.[1] This is the key area of the circulatory system. It includes not only the true capillaries, but also the smallest divisions of the arterioles and venules, all components being less than 100 μm in diameter. The blood flow through this microcirculatory system undergoes continuous variation in rate, volume and direction, i.e. the blood flow to the oral tissues is characterized by marked variability.

Based on light[2] and electron[3] microscopic studies, the component microcirculatory unit can be subdivided into a number of endothelial-lined units.

Arteriole

(1) 50–100 μm in diameter.
(2) Subendothelial walls comprising both smooth muscle and elastic tissue.

The basic arteriolar structure comprises a single flattened endothelial cell layer adjacent to an elastic membrane, with an intervening basement membrane. The medial layer comprises up to three smooth muscle coats, arranged in a helical manner, with a few intervening elastic fibres. This layer is then surrounded by an external elastic membrane adjacent to the adventitial connective tissue layer.

Terminal arteriole

(1) Short vessels.
(2) Internal diameter less than 50 μm.
(3) An extensive smooth muscle subendothelial layer indicative of the potential for these vessels to influence blood flow to the peripheral circulation.

The structure of these vessels is similar to that of the arterioles described above, apart from only a single smooth muscle layer in the media and the absence of the internal elastic membrane.

Metarteriole

(1) Small side branch of terminal arteriole.
(2) Discontinuous (incomplete) segmental subendothelial smooth muscle coat.
(3) 5–10 μm lumen, whose diameter may be varied to accommodate functional tissue requirements.
(4) Contributes to vascular resistance by influencing perivascular flow.

True capillary

(1) Endothelial tubes connecting smallest arteriolar and venular segments.
(2) Comprise flattened endothelial cells with a delicate connective tissue framework.
(3) Component endothelial cells are capable of contracting when irritated.
(4) No smooth muscle in these vessel walls, indicative of their being generally passive.
(5) Individual capillaries are small: collectively they form vast networks for transcapillary exchange.
(6) Some are specialized as arteriovenous anastomoses which function to conduct blood from the arterial directly to the venous side of the circulation.

A typical capillary comprises a single layer of flattened endothelial cells, although this layer may be continuous, fenestrated (pores) or discontinuous.[5] This endothelial lining is not a static structure and may be altered by complex local, humoral, extracellular and intracellular factors, depending on the varied functional tissue requirements. These endothelial cells rest on a basement membrane that also exhibits marked variability depending on the tissue's functional requirements. It appears that this basement membrane (basal lamina) may have filtration and storage functions.

Venous capillary

(1) Larger than a true capillary (7–10 μm).
(2) Formed by the union of several true capillaries.

Postcapillary venule

(1) 8–30 μm diameter.
(2) There are a significant number of pericytes on the walls of these vessels (*see* below).

Collecting venule

(1) Formed by the union of venous capillaries.
(2) 30–50 μm diameter.
(3) Complete layer of pericytes on walls in addition to few smooth muscle cells.

Muscular venule

(1) 50–100 μm diameter.
(2) Distinct subendothelial smooth muscle layer.
(3) Unite to form small collecting veins.

The postcapillary venules, muscular venules and small collecting veins are sequentially associated with an increase in luminal diameter, an increase in component pericytes that are gradually replaced by smooth muscle cells, and a number of other detailed changes whose significance has yet to be discerned.

Precapillary sphincter

(1) Short vessels which are analogous in size and structure to arterioles.
(2) Located proximal to a true capillary.
(3) Influence blood flow into capillary networks by their extensive smooth muscle components.

Preferential channel

The terminal portion of a metarteriole that passes directly to the venous side of the microcirculation.

These various components of the microcirculatory unit cannot be detected in all tissues, although many of the components may in fact be potential to accommodate sudden increased functional demands.[4] The flow of blood through a microcirculatory unit appears to be controlled primarily through the arteriole and the arteriovenous anastomoses, with the precapillary sphincters controlling the flow of blood in a particular microcirculatory capillary bed. By contrast, the venules and small veins are concerned primarily with the regulation of vascular capacitance, i.e. the amount of blood stored in the venous system. Precapillary sphincters appear to be most sensitive to changes in the local environment, whereas arterioles are primarily under neural control. In time of acute or overwhelming functional demand, however, the component systems of the microcirculatory unit appear to function in unison.

Vascular microstructure

The endothelial monolayer of all vessels serves three important functions (*Table 7.1*):

(1) It is a selective permeability barrier.
(2) It is a non-thrombogenic surface that insulates circulating blood from highly thrombogenic subendothelial connective tissues.
(3) It is an active synthetic–metabolic–secretory tissue that in the normal state inhibits haemostasis and thrombosis but promotes these two processes when injured.[22]

Table 7.1 Endothelial cell functions

Opposing blood clotting	*Predisposing to blood clotting*
Intact monolayer is barrier between blood and subendothelial thrombogenic elements	With injury, subendothelial elements exposed; initiates clotting and activates platelets
Glycocalyx contains: Anticoagulant heparan sulphate α_2 macroglobulin (an antiprotease)	With injury, tissue factor released; initiates extrinsic pathway clotting
Synthesizes: Plasminogen activators Anti-aggregating and vasodilating prostacyclin (PGI_2), antithrombin III	Synthesizes: Factor VIII (von Willebrand protein) involved in platelet aggregation
Converts pro-aggregating ADP into anti-aggregating adenine nucleotides	

The normal fluid balance between the circulation and the adjacent tissues is maintained by two opposing forces. Those that cause fluid to move out of the circulation are the osmotic pressure of the interstitial fluid and the intravascular hydrostatic pressure; those that cause fluid to move in are the hydrostatic pressure of plasma proteins and the tissue hydrostatic pressure. The balance of these forces is such that there is a net small movement of fluid outward but this fluid normally drains into the lymphatics and no oedema occurs.

Normal fluid exchange is critically dependent on an intact endothelium. Normal endothelium is a thin simple squamous epithelium (endothelium), adapted to permit free rapid exchange of water and small molecules between plasma and interstitium but limit the passage of plasma proteins with increased restriction as the size of the protein increases. The endothelial lining of all arterioles and venules and most capillaries is of the continuous type, having an unbroken cytoplasmic layer with closely apposed intercellular junctions. Fenestrated endothelium is characterized by small pores or slits 6–8 nm wide and large pores up to 25 nm radius, whereas discontinuous endothelial linings characterize the vessels of the spleen, liver and bone marrow.[23] Whereas micropinocytotic vesicles appear to represent the large pores, the morphological form of small pores remains uncertain. One view holds that the small-pore system is represented by continuous transendothelial channels formed by fusing pinocytotic vesicles,[24] whereas a second view contends that the intercellular junctions form the transfer site of molecules up to 40 000 daltons.[25] Whichever the route in capillaries, it is clear that intercellular junctions are less structurally complex and more permeable in small venules.[26] Furthermore, the endothelial junctions are labile rather than static structures and are susceptible to being widened by a variety of physical and chemical factors, e.g. the chemical mediators of inflammation cause increased vascular permeability by opening gaps in intercellular junctions.

There is also evidence that various polyanionic molecules, e.g. sialoglycoproteins and heparan sulphate, are localized in specific domains on the luminal surface of the endothelium (e.g. vesicles, fenestrae and intercellular junctions).[27] These anionic sites may play a role in normal and increased vascular permeability by repelling anionic molecules and facilitating the transport of cationic proteins.

The thromboresistance is pivotal to the initiation and prevention of clotting and thrombosis. The luminal surface of the endothelium is covered by an endocapillary layer representing the glycocalyx. Biochemically, the glycocalyx is a composite of intrinsic membrane glycoproteins and glycolipids, as well as membrane-associated polysaccharides and glycosaminoglycans, among which are sialic acid residues and heparan sulphate. This endothelial layer has a strong net negative charge, which at one time was thought to contribute to thromboresistance by repelling negatively charged elements, although the reduction of the negative charge by sialic acid residues does not alter endothelial blood compatibility. Heparan sulphate in the glycocalyx in concert with antithrombin III synthesized by endothelial cells may in fact inhibit blood clotting.[28] In addition, an α_2 macroglobulin constituting a potent antiprotease is associated with the vascular lining and serves to inhibit the activation of clotting factors in the coagulation sequence. Endothelial cells also inhibit platelet aggregation by several mechanisms. They have the capacity to convert the strongly pro-aggregating adenosine diphosphate (ADP) released from platelets to the potent adenine nucleotide platelet inhibitors.[28] They also have the ability to elaborate anti-aggregating prostacyclin (PGI_2), a prostaglandin that is also a strong vasodilator. If the endothelial cell is injured, the coagulation sequence is activated, resulting in the formation of thrombin at the site of injury. This in turn results in more active synthesis of PGI_2 in the adjacent endothelial cells. Thus, the endothelial cells serve in insulating the blood from highly thrombogenic subendothelial elements. In addition, endothelial cells react against blood clots and thrombi by synthesizing plasminogen activators and inhibitors, which, on balance, promote fibrinolytic activity in the blood, clear fibrin deposits from the endothelial surface and participate in the resolution of intravascular thrombi.

The endothelial cells can also promote haemostasis and thrombosis by their synthetic–metabolic–secretory activities. Their pro-haemostatic functions are mediated by the synthesis and release of substances that act both on the coagulation sequence and on platelets. The extrinsic clotting pathway can be activated by tissue factor (thromboplastin) present in latent form in the endothelium and released by certain pharmacological stimuli, endotoxin and by injury (even if sublethal). Endothelial cells also synthesize and secrete von Willebrand's factor, which is a component of factor VIII coagulant factor.[29] This product is a necessary cofactor for the adherence of platelets to subendothelial components.

The subendothelial connective tissues not only support the endothelial monolayer but are also thrombogenic. Subendothelial cells produce basement membrane collagen, fibrillar collagen, elastin, glycosaminoglycans and fibronectin. Although other components, e.g. basement membrane and elastin, promote platelet adherence, the most potent stimulus is the fibrillar collagen which provides a substrate for attachment and activation of platelets and activation of clotting factors. Fibronectin serves to stabilize cell-to-cell and cell-to-substrate attachments in the normal endothelial lining. It also becomes cross-linked to fibrin and facilitates anchorage of homeostatic plugs.[30] Thus, damage to the endothelial cell barrier exposes the highly thrombogenic subendothelium, initiating thrombosis and haemostasis. Thus, rather than comprising simple cells, the vascular endothelial cells are functionally and metabolically complex, being able to synthesize hormones (prostaglandins), procoagulant (factor VIII), anticoagulant (plasminogen activator) factors, and connective tissue proteins (e.g. fibronectin).[31–33]

Microcirculatory control

The flow of blood to a tissue varies depending primarily upon its functional requirements: lack of blood flow to a tissue, depending upon its duration, may result in ischaemia leading to necrosis. In fact, the flow of blood through a microcirculatory unit depends upon a number of factors.

Vascular geometry

The lumen of any vessel is affected by a number of factors, including circulating hormones and vasoactive substances. The diameter of a vessel is correlated with blood viscosity, i.e. the viscosity of the blood decreases with reduction in vascular lumen. The direction of vascular branching and tortuosity of vascular morphology also affects the flow of blood,[6] so that blood flow through microvascular units exhibits non-Newtonian flow characteristics.

Tissue functional requirements

The precapillary vessels and sphincters, in addition to the capillaries themselves, appear to be sensitive to the metabolic requirements of a particular tissue or organ. Thus the accumulation of many tissue metabolites and ions, especially carbon dioxide, potassium and lactic acid, is reflected by venular dilatation in an attempt to rectify the problem.

Neural control

Neural input to the arterioles, precapillary vessels and precapillary sphincters regulates the flow of blood into the microcirculatory unit (and so the pressure of blood in the unit), whereas neural control to the venular aspect influences the rate of blood flow away from the unit. Under normal resting conditions, there is a basal control of the microcirculatory unit. Such vasomotor control is primarily dependent on the activity of the vasomotor centre in the medulla, although this in turn may be influenced by other higher centres. L-norepinephrine (noradrenaline) appears to be the catecholamine neurotransmitter released from the sympathetic nerve terminals in the microcirculation. This then reacts with specific receptor sites (α receptors) on the vascular smooth muscles, leading to vasoconstriction. There is also experimental evidence that α and β receptors may be stimulated in some instances, leading to a balance between vasoconstriction and vasodilatation following sympathetic stimulation. In addition, there may also be histamine-mediated vasodilatation and purine-mediated vasodilatation. Thus, sympathetic control of the vascular system is far more complex than traditionally envisaged.

Chemical vasoactive substances

The catecholamines, epinephrine and norepinephrine, released from the adrenal medulla, bind to specific α receptors in the microcirculatory unit, leading to vasoconstriction. Certain vascular beds also contain β-adrenergic receptors, so that when bound to epinephrine, vasodilatation is the net result.

Another extremely active vasoconstrictive substance is angiotensin II. This octapeptide is released from angiotensin I in the bloodstream, the latter being derived from circulating angiotensinogen following renin cleavage (renin is an enzyme produced by the kidneys). Angiotensin II is part of the homeostatic mechanism for the maintenance of extracellular fluid volume and local regulation of blood flow; its production is increased in response to a drop in blood pressure or a reduction in the extracellular fluid volume.

Other vasoactive substances include histamine, prostaglandins, serotonin and the kinins, all of which primarily function on the vascular smooth muscle.

Autoregulation

The smooth muscle of a blood vessel can react to distension caused by increased intravascular pressure by contraction. When there is a reduction in blood flow there will be accumulation of the local metabolic products, leading to vasodilatation, and vice versa. It appears that this process of autoregulation occurs independently of neural or chemical influences and is considered not insignificant in the maintenance of homeostasis of an organ or tissue.

Vascular components of host defence mechanisms

Endothelial changes (*see Table 7.1*)

The initial vascular response to tissue injury comprises a rapid transient arteriolar vasoconstriction. This is an inconstant finding: with mild injury it disappears in 3–5 s whereas with severe injury it may last for a few minutes. The method of vasoconstriction is unknown: it may be neurogenic, although chemical vasoconstrictors may also be implicated.

This is then followed by vasodilatation, which first involves the arterioles and then results in opening of new vascular beds in the area. At this stage, the resultant increased blood volume in the vasodilated vessels may result in sufficient increases in local hydrostatic pressure to cause fleeting transudation of protein-poor fluid into the extravascular space.

Slowing of the circulation follows, brought about by increased permeability of the microvasculature, with outpouring of protein-rich fluid into the extravascular tissues. This results in concentration of the red blood corpuscles in small vessels and increased blood viscosity, termed stasis.

As stasis develops, the leucocytes (mainly polymorphonuclear leucocytes) move from the central to the peripheral aspect of the blood flow. This process is termed leucocytic margination. The polymorphs then begin to stick to the endothelium, transiently at first and then more avidly. Soon after, they migrate through the vascular wall into the interstitial tissues.

This process is characterized by changes in vascular permeability. There appear to be a number of processes involved. The first is an immediate-transient response which appears to be primarily dependent on the release of histamine and bradykinin. The venous aspect of the microcirculatory unit appears to be primarily involved in this process, presumably reflecting a higher concentration of high-affinity binding receptors for histamine than the remainder of the circulation.[34,35] The increased vascular permeability in this instance appears to reflect endothelial cell contraction.

Immediate-sustained increased vascular permeability occurs with more severe injury, and appears to be associated with endothelial cell necrosis. Leakage starts immediately after injury and continues for a variable time period, affecting all levels of the microcirculatory unit. In this instance, the mechanism of increased permeability appears to be direct damage by the injurious stimulus.

Delayed-prolonged leakage begins after a delay and lasts for several hours or days.[36] In this instance, there again appears to be direct cellular damage, except that the intercellular junctions of venules and capillaries appear primarily involved.[37]

Cellular changes (*Tables 7.2, 7.3*)

As a result of loss of fluid, increased viscosity and slowing of blood flow, there is a change in the pattern of blood flowing through the affected tissues. Thus, the white blood cells tend to migrate

Table 7.2 Mediators of inflammation

Vasodilatation
Prostaglandins
Increased vascular permeability
Vasoactive amines
C3a and C5a (complement components)
Bradykinin
Leukotriene C,D,E
Chemotaxis
C5a
Leukotriene B_4
Other chemotactic lipids
Neutrophil cationic proteins
Fever
Endogenous pyrogen
Prostaglandins
Pain
Prostaglandins
Bradykinin
Tissue damage
Neutrophil and macrophage lysosomal enzymes
Oxygen metabolites

Table 7.3 Actions of inflammatory mediators

		Action			
		Vascular leakage	*Chemotaxis*		*Other*
Mediator	*Source*		*Neutrophils*	*Monocytes*	
Histamine and Serotonin	Mast cells, basophils, and platelets	+	−	−	
Kinins					
Bradykinin	Plasma substrate	+	−	−	Pain
Kallikrein		−	+	+	
Complement					
C3a	Plasma protein via	+	−	−	Opsonic fragment
C5a	liver macrophages	+	+	+	(C3b)
Prostaglandins	Most cells, from membrane phospholipids	Potentiate other mediators	±	−	Vasodilatation, pain, fever
Leukotrienes					
B_4	Leucocytes	−	+	+	
$C_4D_4E_4$	Leucocytes, mast cells	+	−	−	Bronchoconstriction, vasoconstriction
Lysosomal components					
Cationic proteins	Leucocytes	+	−	−	Immobilization of neutrophils
Neutral proteases	Leucocytes	+			Tissue damage
Oxygen metabolites	Leucocytes	+			Endothelial damage, tissue damage
AGEPC	Mast cells	+	+	?	Bronchoconstriction

from a central location in the vascular stream to a more peripheral location. At the same time, the endothelial cells appear to become sticky. Several mechanisms have been postulated for the increased endothelial adhesiveness.[38]

(1) Both the endothelium and white blood cells are covered with negatively charged cell coats and are thus believed to repel one another. It is possible that injury neutralizes these negative charges causing adhesion.
(2) Divalent ions, e.g. calcium, magnesium and manganese, may serve as bridges between the negative charges on endothelium and white blood cells or as cofactors in some other enzyme reactions or protein interactions necessary for adhesion.[39]
(3) Chemical mediators may not only result in emigration of white blood cells to the site of tissue injury but may also cause increased endothelial adhesiveness.[38]
(4) Arachidonic acid metabolites may also be involved.[40]

The net result is that the polymorphonuclear leucocytes actively migrate through the endothelial lining and basement membrane to the site of tissue injury. This movement of blood cells to the site of tissue injury is the result of chemical inflammatory mediators released from damaged host cells including damaged polymorphonuclear leucocytes. Polymorphonuclear leucocytes have only a short half-life. Thus although they are capable of phagocytosis, their function is subsequently overtaken by the phagocytic activity of macrophages that subsequently migrate through the vascular endothelium and also as a result of mitosis of macrophages native to the host tissues themselves.

If the initial tissue injury resulted from antigenic substances, then the immune system also becomes involved. For instance, if an antigen binds to a B lymphocyte, the B cell will be stimulated to mitosis and the resulting plasma cells release large quantities of humoral antibody, primarily resulting in:

(1) Antigen binding and neutralization.
(2) Promotion of phagocytosis (opsonization).
(3) Complement activation resulting in cellular lysis, leucocyte attraction, bacterial opsonization, histamine release. (Complement is a series of plasma proteins that are activated in sequence when antigen combines with circulating antibody.)

If T lymphocytes are activated by antigens, lymphokines are released resulting in:

(1) Chemotaxis of white cells.
(2) Osteoclastic bone resorption.
(3) Macrophage activation.
(4) Facilitation of B cell activity.

Haemostasis

When a vessel is damaged or cut, there is immediate transient arteriolar vasoconstriction that serves to reduce blood loss. Injury to endothelial cells exposes highly thrombogenic subendothelial connective tissue, to which the platelets adhere and undergo contact activation involving shape change, a release reaction and further aggregation of more platelets. Simultaneously, tissue factors released at the site of injury in combination with platelet factors activate the plasma coagulation sequence. Prostaglandins and derivatives arte synthesized at the site of injury by endothelial cells and platelets modulating the haemostatic response. Ultimately, a permanent haemostatic plug is produced by the combined activities of endothelial cells, platelets and the coagulation sequence, primarily the result of platelet serotonin release.

The initial platelet plug is therefore subsequently replaced by a blood clot and fibrin plug formation. The blood clotting sequence, together with the vessel wall and platelets, is an important homeostatic mechanism. The coagulation sequence essentially involves a cascade in which inactive blood zymogens, the blood clotting factors, are activated into proteolytic enzymes that selectively attack the next zymogen in sequence, converting it into an active enzyme. At each step, there is amplification, so that a small initial stimulus ultimately evokes a significant amount of solid fibrin polymer. The cascade begins as two separate pathways that ultimately converge. One is intrinsic to the blood and probably plays a major role in haemostasis following an injury. The other is extrinsic and triggered by the introduction into the blood of tissue factors containing thromboplastin.

A pivotal reaction is the conversion of prothrombin (factor II) to thrombin (factor IIa), which then activates platelets and contributes to the generation of the definitive secondary aggregation of platelets. Simultaneously, it converts fibrinogen to fibrin. Both pathways lead to the generation of thrombin. In the intrinsic pathway, there is first activation of factor XII (Hageman factor), converting it into a proteolytic enzyme (factor XIIa). Activation of factor XII occurs when fluid blood contacts an abnormal surface (e.g. injured endothelium, collagen). There is also an interaction with high molecular weight kininogen and conversion of prekallikrein into kallikrein. Kallikrein, once formed, activates more factor XII in a positive feedback loop. Factor XIIa can also activate the complement system. The kallikrein likewise converts kininogen precursor into the vasoactive inflammatory mediator bradykinin. Thus, three separate but interrelated systems are triggered into action with the conversion of factor XII to its activated form.

The extrinsic pathway is triggered by a lipoprotein tissue factor (also termed thromboplastin). This substance is present on the surface of virtually all cells, including endothelial cells. Tissue factor complexes with factor VII to activate it, either by a change in shape or proteolytic cleavage, and the complex then interacts with factor X to form Xa. Thereafter, with facilitation of calcium ions and phospholipid, prothrombin is converted to thrombin as the two separate pathways of blood clotting converge.[31] Thus the formation of an insoluble fibrin plug from its soluble plasma protein fibrinogen predecessor involves 12 factors. The principal features of this process include:

(1) Intrinsic and extrinsic thromboplastin formation.
(2) Generation of thrombin from inactive prothrombin, via thromboplastin.
(3) Thrombin catalysed conversion of fibrinogen to fibrin.

The initial loose fibrin network subsequently matures into a dense feltwork with covalent cross-linkage formation.

Lymphatic system

The lymphatic system primarily comprises blind-ended, endothelial-lined tubes which lie in the tissue spaces and fuse into capillaries and ultimately to lymph vessels. These eventually drain into the major veins in the thorax. Unlike blood capillaries, the smaller lymphatic capillaries comprise an endothelial lining with no underlying basement membrane. This endothelial lining is capable of intrinsic contraction and relaxation, thereby signifying an intrinsic luminal control mechanism. The endothelial lining is also virtually continuous, with no fenestrations or pores, although the gap between adjacent endothelial cells increases or decreases with the rhythmic contractions and relaxation of the vascular walls. Finally, the lymphatic capillaries usually have a larger lumen than the corresponding blood capillaries. In addition to smooth muscle in medial lymphatic vessel walls, there are also a series of endothelial valves that ensure a one-way directional flow of lymph fluid. The flow of lymph fluid through the lymph system to the veins in the thorax is primarily the result of rhythmic contraction and relaxation of the vessel walls, with the rate of this contraction increasing with the volume of lymph fluid to be returned to the blood circulation.

In the pulp, the lymphatics appear to originate as blind-ended tubules near the pulpo-odontoblastic border and the odontoblastic zone.[7] These vessels drain into irregular large diameter vessels containing valves that run parallel to the nerves and veins in the centre of the pulp tissue to pass as multiple vessels through the apical foramen.

In the gingival tissues, the lymphatics originate from the connective tissue papillae and connective tissue adjacent to the junctional epithelium.[8] These thin irregular valved vessels then pass through the periodontal membrane towards the tooth apex, communicating freely with those of the periosteum and alveolar bone.[9]

Microcirculation in dental tissues

Dental pulp[10–16]

The dental pulp is a very vascular tissue, with approximately 5% of pulp volume being occupied by vessels, with the drainage vessels outstripping the supplying vessels by about 3:1. The majority (90%) of the capillaries are located close to the odontoblasts in two distinct populations located approximately 50 μm and 200 μm from the predentine, whereas the central pulp tissue contains few capillaries.[47]

Branches of the maxillary artery supply the tooth pulps:

(1) The inferior dental (alveolar) branch enters the mandibular foramen and runs along the inferior dental canal to send branches to the mandibular teeth.
(2) The posterior superior dental artery supplies the maxillary molar and bicuspid (premolar) teeth.
(3) The infraorbital branch runs from the pterygopalatine fossa to the orbital floor via the inferior orbital fissure, subsequently sending an anterior superior dental branch to supply the maxillary incisors and cuspids (canines).

There may be varying degrees of anastomosis between the arteries supplying the maxillary teeth.

The pulp tissue is predominantly supplied by one or two small arteries passing through the apical foramina of the teeth, although in a few instances, tributaries may also pass through accessory foramina, lateral root canals and even in the furcation area of multirooted teeth.

Having passed into the pulp tissue, the arteries pass towards the coronal aspect following a more peripheral path than the venules and lymphatic vessels. The vessels divide into a series of arterioles that subsequently branch to supply the subodontoblastic capillary plexus just beneath the odontoblastic cell layer. These small arteries (less than 150 μm diameter) and arterioles (less than 100 μm diameter) have a thin coat of smooth muscle, with an intervening basement membrane from the endothelial layer. These vessels appear to be surrounded by a dense matrix of collagen fibres interspersed with mucopolysaccharide ground substances. The subodontoblastic capillary plexus subsequently drains to a network of venules and veins passing down the centre of the tooth pulp. These venules and veins tend to have thinner walls and a wider lumen than analogous vessels elsewhere in the body. Arteriovenous anastomoses have also been described in the pulp. Venous blood leaves the apical foramen to drain into the pterygoid venous plexus surrounding the lateral pterygoid muscle, and subsequently passes to the maxillary vein, posterior facial vein and ultimately both internal and external jugular veins.

The subodontoblastic capillary plexus remains predominantly empty at rest, and appears to be arranged in two distinct bands, located 50 μm and 200 μm respectively from the predentine. The central region of the pulp, by contrast, appears to contain scant capillary vessels. These capillaries range from 7 μm to 10 μm in diameter and predominantly comprise an intact endothelial lining resting on a basement membrane. Varying types of fenestrations or pore have been described in the endothelial lining of these capillaries.[17]

Sympathetic nerves innervate the vascular smooth muscle of the pulp,[44] with the receptors being predominantly α- rather than β-adrenergic.[41] By contrast, there is no evidence for parasympathetic pulp vessel innervation. Conceivably, therefore, vasodilatation primarily results from humoral agents, e.g. acetylcholine, bradykinin and histamine, although recent evidence has implicated an important role for the powerful vasodilator polypeptide present at primary afferent neurones, substance P. Axon reflexes may also be involved in vasodilatation.

Pulpal vasodilatation commonly occurs as a result of thermal tooth injury, e.g. during cavity preparation without adequate coolant, or following the placement of a metallic restoration with insufficient lining. The resultant pulpal vasodilatation may not only be associated with increased endothelial permeability, but also the accumulation of interstitial fluid in the pulp, leading to increased intrapulpal pressure, venular and lymphatic collapse and pulpal necrosis. The vasodynamics in the pulp are influenced by the fact that this tissue is surrounded by a rigid layer of dentine with both venous and lymphatic drainage passing through restricted exits.[42] In addition, the non-vascular matrix of the pulp is of a viscous gel-like consistency due to high molecular weight polymers associated with collagen fibres. This relatively immobile matrix serves to localize the accumulation of interstitial fluid associated with increased vascular permeability, i.e. it is possible that only a region of the pulp may be affected by thermal injury or inflammation, the remainder of the pulp remaining normal, viable and healthy. Unfortunately, unless there is prompt remedial treatment, such localized necrosis and inflammation causes tissue breakdown and increased vascularity in the adjacent regions of the pulp,[45] so unless the causative agent is removed, the whole of the pulp often undergoes necrotic changes.

Gingiva and periodontal ligament[18]

The periodontal membrane and gingiva are predominantly supplied by branches of the posterior superior and inferior dental (alveolar) arteries, which are in turn branches of the maxillary artery. Thus, inter-radicular and interseptal branches then enter the radicular and septal bony plates near the tooth apices. As they pass coronally, the branches then pass through the cortical plates to supply the periodontal membrane and both attached and marginal gingivae. Other sources of blood supply include:

(1) Periodontal ligament branches that ascend through the periodontal ligament to supply the marginal gingiva.
(2) Buccinator, lingual, mental and palatine branches that supply the maxillary and mandibular periosteum and adjacent gingival tissues.
(3) The greater palatine artery supplies the palatal gingiva and mucosa.

In fact, there is a marked degree of anastomosis between these arterial branches, although for the most part the gingival arterial blood supply is functionally distinct from that of the periodontal ligament, except in times of functional need.[45,46] The vasculature of the gingival tissues is especially complex, comprising networks of anastomosing capillaries with both fenestrated and continuous endothelial lining being apparent, and a basement membrane.[19,20] The blood supply of the gingival tissues is primarily derived from the supraperiosteal vessels, whereas vessels penetrating the alveolar bone itself form the principal blood supply to the periodontal ligament. The veins and venules of the gingival and periodontal tissues run approximately parallel to the arterial supply.

There is little evidence that the parasympathetic nerves control the diameter of the gingival and periodontal ligament blood vessels, the predominant control being dependent on the sympathetic innervations.[12]

With the accumulation of dental plaque and the onset of gingival inflammation (gingivitis), a number of changes to the gingival vasculature occur.[21]

(1) The gingival vessels become increasingly permeable.
(2) The vessels of the gingiva become increasingly engorged and dilated.
(3) The formed vascular elements migrate through the vessel walls to the adjacent host tissue.
(4) There is a marked increase in the adjacent interstitial fluid, resulting in both gingival swelling (oedema) and increased gingival crevicular fluid flow.

As a result, the gingival tissues become distended, and bleed easily on gentle probing. In addition, the gingival tissues change from the normal pink to a purple colour. This area of inflammatory change increases with the continued accumulation of dental plaque, although this initial inflammation may undergo complete resolution with the removal of plaque and the restoration of correct dental hygiene procedures.

Conclusions

The circulatory system is of paramount importance to the dental tissues and their vitality. Ischaemia is the name given to an inadequate blood supply to the tissues, and results in hypoxia (lack of tissue oxygenation) and/or the accumulation of metabolites. The effects depend on the severity of the reduction in blood supply, the sensitivity of the tissue concerned, the activity of the tissue and its oxygen needs, and the rapidity with which ischaemia develops. Knowledge of such pathological changes hinges on the detailed understanding of the microcirulatory system and its control.

Review questions

1. What factors influence the blood supply to the periodontal ligament?
2. What is the physiological role of the endothelial lining of blood vessels?
3. Contrast the microcirculation of the dental pulp and periodontal tissues.
4. What changes in the microcirculatory system of the dental pulp might be expected with increasing age?
5. What effects do chemical mediators have on the microcirculatory unit?

References

1. SPARKS, H.V. and BELLONI, F.L. (1978) The peripheral circulation: local regulation. *Ann. Rev. Physiol.*, **40**, 67–92
2. CHAMBERS, R. and ZWEIFACH, B.W. (1944) The topography and function of the mesenteric capillary microcirculation. *Am. J. Anat.*, **75**, 173–205

3. RHODIN, J.A.G. (1967) The ultrastructure of mammalian arterioles and pre-capillary sphincters. *J. Ultrastruct. Res.*, **18**, 181–223
4. INTAGLIETTA, M. and ZWEIFACH, B.W. (1974) Microcirculatory basis of fluid exchange. *Adv. Biol. Med. Phys.*, **15**, 111–159
5. WOLFF, J. (1977) Ultrastructure of the terminal vascular bed as related to function. In *Microcirculation*, edited by G. Kaley and B.M. Altura. Baltimore: University Park Press
6. CHIEN, S. (1972) Present state of blood rheology. In *Hemodilution: Theoretical Basis and Clinical Application*, edited by K. Messmer and H. Schmid-Schonbein. Basel: S. Karger
7. BERNICK, S. (1977) Lymphatic vessels of the human dental pulp. *J. Dent. Res.*, **56**, 70–77
8. BERNICK, S. and GRANT, D.A. (1978) Lymphatic vessels of healthy and inflamed gingiva. *J. Dent. Res.*, **57**, 810–817
9. RUBEN, M.P., PRIETO-HERNANDEZ, J.R. and GOTT, F.K. (1971) Visualization of lymphatic microcirculation of oral tissues. II. Vital retrograde lymphography. *J. Periodontol.*, **42**, 774–784
10. MYERS, M.W. (1980) Methodologies for studying pulpal hemodynamics. *J. Endodont.*, **6**, 466–472
11. EDWALL, L. (1972) Nervous control of blood circulation in the dental pulp and the periodontal tissues. In *Oral Physiology*, edited by N. Emmelin and Y. Zotterman. New York: Pergamon
12. EDWALL, L. (1980) Regulation of pulpal blood flow. *J. Endodont.*, **6**, 434–437
13. PASHLEY, D.H. (1979) The influence of dentin permeability and pulpal blood flow on pulpal solute concentrations. *J. Endodont.*, **5**, 355–361
14. KIM, S., FAN, F.C. and CHEN, R.Y.Z. (1980) Effects of changes in systemic hemodynamic parameters of pulpal hemodynamics. *J. Endodont.*, **6**, 392–399
15. TONDER, K.J.H. and NAESS, G. (1979) Microvascular pressure in the dental pulp and gingiva in cats. *Acta Odontol. Scand.*, **37**, 161–168
16. PASHLEY, D.H. (1976) A mechanistic analysis of gingival fluid production. *J. Periodont. Res.*, **11**, 121–134
17. HARRIS, R. and GRIFFEN, C.J. (1971) The ultrastructure of small blood vessels of the normal human dental pulp. *Aust. Dent. J.*, **16**, 220–226
18. LEAK, L.V. (1976) The structure of lymphatic capillaries in lymph formation. *Fed. Proc.*, **35**, 1863–1871
19. EGELBERG, J. (1966) The blood vessels of the dentogingival junction. *J. Periodont. Res.*, **1**, 163–179
20. NUKI, K. and HOCK, J. (1974) The organization of the gingival vasculature. *J. Periodont. Res.*, **9**, 305–313
21. HOCK, J. and NUKI, K. (1971) A vital microscopy study of the morphology of normal and inflamed gingiva. *J. Periodont. Res.*, **6**, 81–88
22. RYAN, G. and MAJNO, G. (1977) *Inflammation*. Kalamazoo, Mich.: Upjohn
23. LANDIS, E.M. and PAPPENHEIMER, J.R. (1963) Exchange of substances through the capillary wall. In *Handbook of Physiology*, edited by W.F. Hamilton and P. Dow, Section 2, Vol II, pp. 961–1043. Washington: American Physiological Society
24. SIMIONESCU, N. (1975) Permeability of muscle capillaries to small hemepeptides. Evidence for the existence of patent transendothelial channels. *J. Cell. Biol.*, **64**, 586
25. KARNOVSKY, M.H. (1970) The ultrastructural basis of transcapillary exchange. *J. Gen. Phys.*, **52**, 645
26. SIMIONESCU, N. (1978) Structural basis of permeability in sequential segments of the microvasculature of the diaphragm. II. Pathways followed by microperoxidase across the endothelium. *Microvasc. Res.*, **15**, 17
27. SIMIONESCU, N. (1981) Differential microdomains on the luminal surface of capillary endothelium. II. Partial characterization of their anionic sites. *J. Cell Biol.*, **90**, 614
28. PEARSON, J.D. and GORDON, J.L. (1979) Vascular endothelial and smooth muscle cells in culture selectively release adenine nucleotides. *Nature*, **281**, 384
29. COLUCCI, M. (1983) Cultured human endothelial cells generate tissue factor in response to endotoxin. *J. Clin. Invest.*, **71**, 1893
30. GAJDUSEK, C. (1980) An endothelial cell-derived growth factor. *J. Cell Biol.*, **85**, 467
31. BAUGH, R.F. and HOUGHIE, C. (1979) The chemistry of blood coagulation. *Clin. Haematol.*, **8**, 3
32. HIRSCH, J. (1977) Hypercoagulability. *Semin. Haematol.*, **14**, 409
33. OGSTON, D. and BENNETT, B. (1977) *Haemostasis: Biochemistry, Physiology and Pathology*. London: John Wiley and Sons
34. HELTIANU, C. (1982) Histamine receptors of the microvascular endothelium revealed *in situ* with a histamine-ferritin conjugate: characteristic high-affinity binding sites in venules. *J. Cell Biol.*, **93**, 357
35. JORIS, I. (1972) Endothelial contraction *in vivo*: a study of the rat mesentery. *Virchows Arch. (Zellpathol.)*, **12**, 73
36. SEVITT, S. (1958) Early and delayed edema and increase in capillary permeability after a burn of the skin. *J. Pathol. Bacteriol.*, **75**, 27
37. HURLEY, J.V. (1967) The mechanism of delayed-prolonged phase of increased vascular permeability in turpentine-induced pleurisy. *J. Pathol. Bacteriol.*, **94**, 1
38. HOOVER, R.L. and KARNOVSKY, M.J. (1982) Leukocyte-endothelial interactions. In *Pathobiology of the Endothelial Cell*, edited by H. Nossel and H. Vogel, New York: Academic Press
39. ATHERTON, A. (1972) Quantitative investigations of adhesiveness of circulating polymorphonuclear leukocytes to blood vessels. *J. Physiol.*, **222**, 447
40. GIMBRONE, M.A. and BUCHANAN, M.R. (1982) Interactions of leukocytes with vascular endothelium. *Ann. N.Y. Acad. Sci.*, **77**, 171
41. TROWBRIDGE, H.O. (1985) Intradental sensory units: physiological and clinical aspects. *J. Endod.*, **11**, 489–498

42. HEYERAAS, K.J. (1985) Pulpal, microvascular and tissue pressure. *J. Dent. Res.*, **64**, 585–589
43. KIM, S. (1985) Microcirculation of the dental pulp in health and disease. *J. Endod.*, **11**, 465–471
44. KIM, S. (1985) Regulation of pulpal blood flow. *J. Dent. Res.*, **64**, 590–596
45. BAAB, D.A. (1986) Gingival blood flow measured with a laser Doppler flowmeter. *J. Periodont. Res.*, **21**, 73–85
46. RUGH, P. (1986) Activation of the vascular system: a main mediator of periodontal fibre remodeling in orthodontic tooth movement. *Am. J. Orthod.*, **89**, 453–468
47. KARLSSON, U. (1980) Quantitative vascularity in normal and denervated feline teeth. *J. Dent. Res.*, **59A**, 396

8

Wound healing

Introduction

Any break in the continuity of the oral mucosa must be followed by healing to prevent the egress of irritants into the underlying tissues. Such irritants may result in continued tissue disruption and/or infection. Wound healing therefore comprises a fundamental biological activity that involves both regenerative and replacement activities.

The ideal function of the reparative process is to restore disrupted or dead tissue to its normal state. The ideal can be achieved in tissues undergoing constant renewal but is least effective in nerve and muscle tissue. Even in severed nerves, however, attempts will be made to restore their continuity if their cell bodies are intact; whereas muscle, including cardiac muscle, is generally repaired by fibrous connective scar tissue, with permanent loss of function.

Wound healing

There are two types of wound healing: primary union (healing by first intention) and secondary union (healing by secondary intention). In effect, the same mechanisms are used for each form of wound healing; they are just subdivided for ease of description.

Primary union

The narrow space between the two cut surfaces of a wound initially undergoes haemorrhage prior to clotting. The margins of the wound subsequently undergo mild acute inflammatory reactions releasing plasma and polymorphonuclear leucocytes into the incised space. After approximately 24 h, capillary blood vessels from the wound margins begin to bud into the wound space and these are followed by both macrophages and fibroblasts. The macrophages are primarily associated with the phagocytosis of the wound debris and haemosiderin from haemoglobin breakdown, whereas the fibroblasts begin to form ground substance. At the same time, or a little earlier, the epithelial cells from the wound margins undergo mitosis and migrate toward the centre of the wound, thereby forming a complete, but thin, epithelial covering. Subsequently, the epithelium undergoes progressive maturation to regain its full thickness, whereas the underlying connective scar tissue becomes increasingly fibrous and relatively avascular. Healing is usually complete by 2–3 weeks, although a longer period may be required before there is complete restoration of the tissue architecture.

Secondary union

In secondary union, the two cut surfaces cannot be approximated so that there are large gaps in the tissue to be repaired. There is initially a degree of haemorrhage, followed by blood clot formation. At this time, mild short-lived acute inflammatory reactions occur in the wound margins. Granulation tissue subsequently begins to move into the wound base and sides, this tissue comprising capillary buds, fibroblasts, macrophages, plasma cells and lymphocytes. The component cells ensure the removal of tissue debris; these cells include macrophages, fibroblasts and polymorphonuclear leucocytes. As fibrous tissue is laid down in the deeper layers of the wound, this granulation tissue tends to heal the wound from the base up.

As successive layers of collagen are formed in the granulation tissue, the wound undergoes contraction, primarily reflecting fibroblastic activity. Thus the space between the two edges of the wound is closed by granulation tissue and wound contraction, thereby facilitating the closure of the wound by epithelial migration and mitosis. Initially, however, excessive granulation tissue is formed, so that the recently healed wound may appear proud of the adjacent tissue; usually this is resolved in a few weeks. It appears that during such wound healing complex interactions occur between the epithelial and connective tissues, since initially connective tissue formation is essential for the restoration of normal epithelial continuity, although, subsequently, epithelial factors may be responsible for the termination of connective tissue scar growth.

Dynamic events of wound healing

In general, a wound of the oral mucosa involves the epithelium, basement membrane and underlying connective tissue. Depending on the agent causing the wound, and the manner in which it is inflicted, the wound may take the form of an incisional space or a cavity, both of which are lined by damaged tissue undergoing necrosis. Immediately following wound formation, an initial and unstable wound cover is obtained by filling the lesion with blood, which eventually clots. The fibrin clot, including entrapped blood cells, forms a scab and provides a preliminary seal. Within the first 24 h after wounding, invading phagocytic cells herald the start of an acute inflammatory response in the margins of the lesion. These phagocytes serve to resorb necrotic tissue and most of the clot. At the same time, migration and mitotic activity by the basal epithelial cells occur, leading to the re-establishment of epithelial continuity. After approximately 48 h, the fundamental processes of wound repair and regeneration begin with the formation of granulation

Table 8.1 Role of platelets in wound repair

Haemostasis
Aggregation
Coagulation
Substance secretion
Vasoactive mediators
Chemotactic factors
Growth factors
Proteases

Table 8.2 Role of endothelial cells in wound repair

Participation in blood flow regulation
Modulation of solute and cell transfer between blood and tissue
Maintenance of non-thrombogenic vascular surface
Angiogenesis
Secretion
Prostacyclin
Growth factors
Proteases and other enzymes
Structural macromolecules

Table 8.3 Role of macrophages in wound repair

Scavenging
Pathogenic micro-organisms
Tissue debris
Secretion of biologically active substances
Vasoactive mediators
Chemotactic factors
Growth factors
Proteases

Table 8.4 Role of epithelial cells in wound repair

Formation of new epithelium
Phenotypic alteration
Retraction of tonofilaments
Dissolution of desmosomes
Formation of peripheral actin bundles
Migration over viable wound surface
Dissection under non-viable wound material
Removal of debris
Reformation of normal phenotype
Restoration of permeability barrier
Restoration of tensile strength
Restoration of basement membrane
Secretion
Vasoactive mediators
Growth factors
Proteases and other enzymes
Structural macromolecules

Table 8.5 Role of fibroblasts in wound repair

Wound contraction
Phenotypic alteration
Migration to wound defect
Deposition of fibronectin and Types I and III collagen
Formation of fibronexus
Contraction
Matrix formation and remodelling
Fibronectin
Hyaluronic acid
Types I and III collagen
Proteoglycans
Proteases and other enzymes

tissue that includes the budding proliferation of capillary blood vessels. This is followed by fibroblastic proliferation and the formation of collagen leading to the restoration of the tensile strength of the wound area. Subsequently, this scar tissue is replaced by normal differentiated epithelial and connective tissues leading to the restoration of normal tissue continuity (*Tables 8.1–8.5*)

Inflammatory stage

During the early inflammatory stage that follows a wound, blood vessel disruption leads to the extravasation of blood constituents (bleeding) and concomitant platelet aggregation, blood coagulation (blood clotting), and generation of bradykinin and complement-derived anaphylatoxins. Activated platelets not only aggregate and trigger blood coagulation to effect haemostasis in disrupted blood vessels, but also release an array of biologically active molecules that promote cell migration and growth into the site of injury. The blood vessel endothelium also exhibits several intrinsic activities that limit the extent of platelet aggregation and blood coagulation to the wounded area.

Although polymorphonuclear leucocytes (PMNs) are considered to be the first leucocytes to infiltrate an area of inflammation and injury, monocytes begin to emigrate at the same time. Both cell types are attracted to the area of tissue injury by a variety of chemotactic factors. The main function of PMNs during this early inflammatory phase of tissue injury is to rid the site of contaminating bacteria, whereas the influx of monocytes and their conversion to macrophages appear critical to the initiation of tissue repair. Macrophages, like PMNs, phagocytose and digest pathogenic organisms, in addition to scavenging tissue debris. Macrophages also release a variety of active substances, whose functions include recruitment of additional inflammatory cells and facilitation of tissue decontamination and débridement, and growth factors for the initiation of wound repair and regeneration. Subsequently, the wound is invaded by granulation tissue, comprising a dense population of macrophages, fibroblasts and neovasculature embedded in a loose collagen, fibronectin and hyaluronic acid matrix. As fibroblasts proliferate and migrate into the wound space, they are aligned along the radial area of the wound and form cell–cell and cell–matrix links (fibronexus) leading to wound contraction. At the same time, blood vessel growth (angiogenesis) into the wound occurs.

Healing stage

When the oral epithelial barrier is disrupted following tissue injury, re-epithelialization must occur as rapidly as possible to re-establish its continuity. This process begins within hours of the injury, resulting in the migration of the free epithelial edges of the wound. If the basement membrane is destroyed, the cells move over a provisional fibronectin and fibrin matrix, gradually reforming the basement membrane. If the basement membrane has not been destroyed, then the hemidesmosomes are disrupted during re-epithelialization. In both cases, the absence of tenacious binding at the epithelial–connective tissue boundary is a prerequisite for epithelial mobility. If large objects or non-viable tissue lie within the wound space, the epithelium will dissect under these structures. Once re-epithelialization is complete, the cells revert to their normal phenotype and firmly attach to the basement membrane through hemidesmosomes.

The final stage of wound healing comprises matrix formation and remodelling. In fact, this stage starts at the same time as the initial reparative phase, although it is a very slow process that involves the accumulation of large fibrous bundles of Type I collagen which provide the residual scar with increasing tensile strength.

Inflammation

The functions of the inflammatory component of wound healing may be considered to include:

(1) The clinical and morphological manifestation of haemostasis and tissue débridement.
(2) The initiation of initial reparative mechanisms.
(3) The delay of wound healing in the case of persistent irritation, especially in the presence of bacteria.

Tissue injury and blood vessel disruption lead to extravasation of blood constituents and concomitant platelet aggregation, blood coagulation, and generation of bradykinin and complement-derived anaphylatoxins. Bradykinin and the anaphylatoxins (C5a and C3a) increase the permeability of undamaged vessels adjacent to the injured area[1] resulting in leakage of plasma proteins[2] and interstitial clot formation in the surrounding tissue. This extravascular gel is an important early component of wound repair. Activated platelets not only aggregate and trigger blood coagulation to effect haemostasis in disrupted blood vessels but also release an array of substances that promote cell migration and ingrowth to the site of injury. Several intrinsic activities of the blood vessel endothelium limit the extent of platelet aggregation and blood coagulation to the wounded area, including:

(1) Prostacyclin production which inhibits platelet aggregation.[3]
(2) Inactivation of thrombin.[4]
(3) Plasminogen activator release, which initiates clot lysis.[5]

Blood clotting factors

The leakage of plasma and formed blood elements from damaged blood vessels results in blood clotting by three major routes:

(1) Hageman factor, activated by adsorption on to fibrillar collagen or other suitable surfaces, together with its co-activators prekallikrein and kininogen induces the intrinsic coagulation system.[6]
(2) Factor VII, activated by tissue procoagulant factor found in the interstitium[7] and released from damaged cells,[8] induces the extrinsic coagulation system.[9]
(3) Platelets, activated by contact with fibrillar collagen or low levels of thrombin, express coagulation factors[10] and phospholipids that include clotting at the levels of factors V and X.[11]

The inciting event in each of these three roles of blood clot formation is the expression of a surface that promotes adsorption and activation of specific coagulation pro-enzymes. Surface adsorption is a prerequisite for pro-enzyme activation, since these proteins are otherwise afloat in a sea of enzyme inhibitors. Although small amounts of pro-enzymes are activated under normal circumstances, the enzymes, once activated, are almost immediately quenched by plasma protease inhibitors. When the pro-enzymes have been adsorbed on to a surface in a micro-environment relatively free of protease inhibitors, however, minute amounts of spontaneous activation are quickly amplified into the physiological response of blood clotting.

Blood clotting can be considered part of the inflammatory response, since Hageman factor activation leads to bradykinin generation,[12] to the initiation of the classic complement cascade,[13] and possibly to the generation of the anaphylatoxins C3a and C5a.[14] The anaphylatoxins, in turn, not only increase blood vessel permeability directly[1] and attract PMNs and monocytes to the sites of tissue injury,[15] but also stimulate the release of vasoactive mediators, histamine[16] and leukotriene C_4 and D_4,[17] from mast cells, as well as the release of granule constituents and biologically active oxygen products from neutrophils[16] and macrophages.[18]

Cellular factors

Both PMNs and macrophages are attracted to sites of tissue injury by a variety of chemotactic factors, including:

(1) Kallikrein from the activated Hageman factor pathway.[19]
(2) Fibrinopeptides generated from fibrin clot formation.[20]
(3) Fibrin lysis products.[21]
(4) C5a from complement activation.[22]
(5) Leukotriene B_4 released by activated PMNs.[23]
(6) Microbial generated formyl methionyl peptides.[24]
(7) Substances released from platelets.[25]

The monocyte influx is also stimulated by fragments of collagen,[26] elastin,[27] fibronectin[28] and thrombin.[29] During this early stage of inflammation, the major function of PMNs centres on the elimination of bacterial contamination, whereas monocytes and their conversion to macrophages mainly serve in the initiation of tissue repair.[30]

If no wound contamination has occurred, the PMN infiltration will resolve after the first few days of tissue injury. By contrast, if wound contamination has occurred, then this acute inflammatory phase will persist and interfere with the next phase of wound healing. In fact, further inflammation and tissue destruction are side-effects of the attempt to rid the injured area of bacteria and other foreign material. As the PMN infiltrate resolves and macrophage accumulation continues, the late phase of wound healing, which primarily centres on macrophage activity, occurs. These cells not only phagocytose and digest pathogenic microorganisms[31] but also scavenge tissue debris, including effete PMNs.[32] Macrophages also release a number of metabolically active substances, e.g. vasoactive mediators,[33] chemotactic and growth factors,[34] and enzymes,[35] including proteases.[36] Thus macrophages are pivotal to the repair phase of wound healing.

Granulation tissue

Granulation tissue comprises a dense population of macrophages, fibroblasts and newly forming blood vessels in a loose matrix of collagen, fibronectin and hyaluronic acid. Re-epithelialization of an oral epithelial wound begins within the first 24 h after injury, i.e. several days prior to granulation tissue formation, although in fact both are intimately associated with one another.

Re-epithelialization of a mucosal wound begins within hours of injury by epithelial cell movement from the free edge of the tissue across the defect.[37] Such epithelial cell movement occurs following the metamorphosis associated with loss of apical–basal polarity and extension of pseudopodia from the free basolateral side into the wound. Such epithelial cell migration does not depend on mitosis[38] but is probably associated with chemotactic factors and active contact guidance, although other factors may also be involved. Within a short period of time the epithelial cells remaining at the edge of the wound begin to proliferate in order to generate an additional population of migrating cells,[39] although whether this is associated with chalones or other local growth factors remains obscure. During re-epithelialization of a wound in which the basement membrane has been disrupted, the basement membrane does not reform until after epithelial migration ceases.[40] As the epithelial cells cease to migrate, type IV collagen and then laminin[41] are produced, beginning at the wound margin, progressing inwards, simulating a zipper mechanism that interlocks the new epithelial and new connective tissue structures. Subsequently, the epithelial cells become firmly attached to the basement membrane by hemidesmosomal formation.

Although the chemical mediators remain obscure, the local proliferation and invasion of fibroblasts into the wound is crucial for healing. Such invasion is predicated on the prior metamorphosis of the fibroblasts to myofibroblasts, where the cells gain motile and contractile properties in addition to their secretory and synthetic capacities. As these myofibroblasts migrate into the wound defect, they concomitantly deposit a loose extracellular matrix comprising predominantly fibronectin.[42] This fibronectin matrix not only appears to be associated with fibroblastic adhesion and growth but is also associated with initial wound contraction and orientation of subsequently produced collagen fibrils.

The invasion of newly formed blood vessels into the site of a wound occurs simultaneously with fibroblastic proliferation, conceivably under the direction of chemical mediators derived from the oral epithelium and underlying connective tissue, in addition to low oxygen tension,[43] lactic acid[44] and biogenic enzymes.[45] Furthermore, whether this vascular invasion centres on mitogenic or migratory cellular activity remains obscure.

The third and final stage of wound healing centres on matrix formation and remodelling. In fact, matrix formation begins at the time of granulation tissue formation, although the matrix is then constantly altered to accommodate functional demands. Such changes involve fibronectin replacement with large fibrous bundles of type I collagen that provide the residual scar with increasing tensile strength.

The initial deposits of extracellular matrix contain predominantly fibronectin, which may serve as a template for collagen deposition.[46] In fact, the fibronectin matrix is replaced by type III and then type I collagen.[47] Although collagen provides a less adherent surface for fibroblasts compared with fibronectin,[48] these types of collagen ultimately form fibrous bundles that greatly enhance the tensile strength.

Hyaluronic acid is another component of granulation tissue that is critical in early fibroblastic proliferation. As granulation tissue matures, however, hyaluronic acid is decreased by tissue hyaluronidase[49] and replaced by proteoglycans.[50] This latter is not so conducive to cell migration but serves to increase tensile strength and resilience. The enormous molecular versatility permits proteoglycans to have many diverse structural and functional tissue activities. These substances promote fibrogenesis by fibroblasts[51] and mediate cellular adhesion and influence the budding of new blood vessels.

At least three classes of collagens occur in connective tissue: fibrillar collagens (types I, II and III); basement membrane collagen (type IV) and pericellular collagens (type V). In addition to providing tensile wound strength, these collagens influence cell activity.

Factors affecting wound healing

Wound healing is a complex process which may be disturbed by malfunctioning of a variety of component events.

Infection

Infection is a major obstacle to wound healing since it not only promotes further inflammation but also tissue destruction (*Table 8.6*).

Table 8.6 Sequence of microbial decontamination of wounds

1. Opsonization of micro-organisms by complement
2. Generation of chemotactic factors
3. Adhesion of polymorphonuclear leucocytes (PMNs) to endothelial cells
4. Emigration of PMNs through blood vessels
5. Attachment of opsonized micro-organisms to PMNs
6. Phagocytosis of micro-organisms
7. Killing and digestion of micro-organisms

Foreign bodies

Foreign bodies within wounds frequently stimulate inflammation, thereby impeding the process of healing. The presence of foreign bodies causes persistent tissue invasion by macrophages and polymorphonuclear leucocytes; this invasion continuing as long as the foreign body remains. The presence of foreign bodies and infection often occur together to delay wound healing (*Table 8.7*).

Table 8.7 Causes of modified host response to micro-organisms

Deficiency	*Causes*
Complement	Hereditary Systemic lupus erythematosus Rheumatoid arthritis Malnutrition
Chemotaxis	Complement deficiency Chediak–Higashi syndrome Diabetes mellitus Cushing's syndrome
Opsonization	Complement deficiency Immunoglobulin deficiency Sickle cell anaemia Diabetes mellitus Severe, prolonged microbial infection Severe viral infection
Phagocytosis-killing	Chronic granulomatous disease Myeloperoxidase deficiency G6PD deficiency Chediak–Higashi syndrome Leukaemia Diabetes mellitus Severe, prolonged microbial infection

Old age

Although, clinically, the healing of wounds is more rapid in the young than the elderly, there have been scant investigations of this problem. It may, in fact, reflect concurrent nutritional and vascular deficiencies, although there is evidence for the efficacy of the immune system deteriorating with age (*Table 8.8*).

Nutritional status

Vitamin C deficiency in addition to many other nutritional deficiencies have been associated with impaired healing, although again there is scant scientific evidence in this regard.

Concurrent disease

Vascular disease

Any disturbance to the blood supply of a tissue will result in delayed or impaired wound healing.

Diabetes mellitus

In poorly controlled diabetic patients the disturbances in wound healing reflect a variety of factors, including impaired blood supply, impaired polymorphonuclear leucocyte function and increased susceptibility to microbial infections.

Uraemia

In patients with persistent high levels of blood urea, wound healing is delayed primarily because of disturbances in the inflammatory response, i.e. diminished polymorphonuclear leucocytic chemotaxis to the site of injury, decreased number of circulating lymphocytes and suppression of delayed hypersensitivity.

Blood diseases

Haemorrhagic diseases are associated with excessive haemorrhage at the site of tissue damage, resulting in large haematomas that predispose to secondary microbial infection. In aplastic anaemia or agranulocytosis, the associated reduction of the number of circulating polymorphonuclear leucocytes and lymphocytes, in addition to the deficiency in red blood corpuscles, contribute to disturbed wound healing. Similarly, while patients with leukaemias may have sufficient numbers of white blood cells, a number of these may in fact be neoplastic and therefore not function effectively in wound healing.

Immunosuppressive drugs

In general, hydrocortisone and prednisone suppress inflammation as a result of:

(1) Inhibited increased vascular permeability and polymorphonuclear leucocyte emigration associated with inflammation.
(2) Stabilized membranes restricting enzymic release from lysosomes.

Table 8.8 Systemic factors associated with delayed wound healing

Endogenous	*Exogenous*

Deficiency states
  Protein
  Vitamin A, C, K
  Zinc
	Corticosteroids
	Anticoagulants
	Antimetabolites

Impaired oxygenation
  Low levels of inspired oxygen
  Pulmonary insufficiency
  Decreased red cell capacity
  Hypovolaemia
  Heart failure
  Fever
  Malignancy
  Thyrotoxicosis	

(3) Inhibited collagen formation due to suppression of protein synthesis.
(4) Impaired polymorphonuclear leucocyte function.

There is increasing awareness of the importance of polymorphonuclear leucocyte function in wound healing, not only for the phagocytosis of microbial and other debris, but also as a component of the immune host defense systems. There are, in fact, a number of defects that may occur with these cells including:

(1) Decreased numbers, e.g. leukaemia, neutropenia.
(2) Disordered microbial killing mechanisms, e.g. impaired hydrogen peroxide production, myeloperoxidase deficiency.
(3) Disorders of phagocytosis, e.g. opsonin or complement deficiencies, impaired degranulation and liberation of lysosomal contents into phagosomes.
(4) Disordered chemotaxis and migration, e.g. deficiencies in chemotactic factors or complement, intrinsic cellular dysfunctions.

Conclusions

Wound healing is a complex process, especially when compromised by local and systemic factors (*Tables 8.6–8.8*). Wound healing is associated with different forms of collagen (*Table 8.9*) and different components of complement (*Table 8.10*). The immune system is also involved (*Table 8.11*).

Table 8.9 Genetically distinct vertebrate collagens

Type	*Native polymer*	*Tissue distribution*	*Distinctive features*
I	Fibril	Skin, tendon, bone, dentine, fascia, widespread	Low content of hydroxylysine, broad fibrils
II	Fibril	Cartilage, nucleus pulposus, notochord, vitreous body	High content of hydroxylysine, heavily glycosylated
III	Fibril	Skin, uterus, blood vessels, reticulin fibres generally	High content of hydroxyproline, low content of hydroxylysine, few sites of hydroxylysine glycosylation
IV	Basement lamina	Kidney glomeruli, lens capsule, basement laminae of all epithelial and endothelial cells	Very high content of hydroxylysine, almost fully glycosylated, retains procollagen extension pieces
V	Unknown	Widespread in small amounts. Basement laminae of smooth and striated muscle cells? Exoskeleton of fibroblasts and other mesenchymal cells?	High content of hydroxylysine, heavily glycosylated, fails to form native fibrils *in vitro*

Table 8.10 Biological effects of complement components

Component	*Effect(s)*
C1	Initiation of classic pathway Increase in affinity of some antibodies Promotion antigen-antibody complexes aggregation
C4b	Amplification of complement system Virus neutralization Immune adherence (opsonin)
C2b	Kinin activity
C3a	Anaphylatoxin Chemotactic activity Leucocyte mobilization Amplification of complement system
C3b	Immune adherence (opsonin) Activation of alternate pathway
C5a	Same effects as C3a
C5b67	Chemotactic activity Initiation of reactive lysis
C8	Slow membrane damage
C9	Rapid membrane damage

Table 8.11 Possible relationships between immune system component areas

Type of immune system	*Components*
Humoral immunity:	
Anaphylactic Type I hypersensitivity	Plasma cells IgE Mast cells Histamine and other vasoactive amines
Immune complex-mediated Type III hypersensitivity	Plasma cells Antigen-antibody complexes Complement Polymorphonuclear leucocytes Macrophages Extracellular lysosomes
Cell-mediated immunity:	
Delayed Type IV hypersensitivity	Plaque antigens Lymphocytes Lymphokines Macrophages Immunological memory

Review questions

1. What might be the consequences of inadequate haemorrhage following a wound?
2. What is the role of granulation tissue in wound healing?
3. Why are blood platelets so important in wound healing?
4. Why would you expect a foreign body to delay wound healing?

References

1. WILLIAMS, T.J. and JOSE, P.J. (1981) Mediation of increased vascular permeability after complement activation: histamine independent action of C5a. *J. Exp. Med.*, **153**, 136–153
2. WILLIAMS, T.J. (1973) Simultaneous measurement of local plasma exudation and blood flow changes induced by intradermal injection of vasoactive substances using ^{131}I-albumin and ^{133}Xe. *J. Physiol. (Lond.)*, **246**, 215–217
3. MONCADA, S., GRYGLEWSKI, R., BUNTING, S. and VANCE. J.R. ((1976) An enzyme isolated from arteries transforms prostaglandin endoperoxidases to an unstable substance that inhibits platelet aggregation. *Nature*, **263**, 663–665
4. BAKER, J.B., LOW, D.A., SIMMER, R.L. and CUNNINGHAM, D.D. (1980) Protease-nexin: a cellular component that links thrombin and plasminogen activator and mediates their binding to cells. *Cell*, **21**, 37–45
5. BINDER, B.R., SPRAGG, J. and AUSTEN, K.F. (1979) Purification and characterization of human vascular plasminogen activator derived from blood vessel perfusates. *J. Biol. Chem.*, **254**, 1998–2003
6. KAPLAN, A.P. (1983) Hageman factor-dependent pathways: mechanism of initiation and bradykinin formation. *Fed. Proc.*, **42**, 3123–3127
7. DVORAK, H.F., SENGER, D.R. and DVORAK, A.M. (1985) Regulation of extravascular coagulation by microvascular permeability. *Science*, **227**, 1059–1061
8. MAYNARD, J.R., HECKMAN, C.A., PITLICK, F.A. and NEMERSON, Y. (1975) Association of tissue factor activity with the surface of cultured cells. *J. Clin. Invest.*, **55**, 814–824
9. MARLAR, R., KLEISS, A. and GRIFFIN, J.H. (1982) An alternative extrinsic pathway of human blood coagulation. *Blood*, **60**, 1353–1358
10. SIXMA, J.J. (1978) Platelet coagulant activities. *Thromb. Haemost.*, **40**, 163–167
11. BODE, A.P., DOMBROSE, E.A., LENTZ, B.R. and ROBERTS, H.R. (1981) The platelet membrane as a catalytic surface in thrombin generation. *Ann. N.Y. Acad. Sci.*, **370**, 348–358
12. KAPLAN, A.P. and AUSTEN, K.F. (1971) A prealbumin activator or prekallikrein. *J. Exp. Med.*, **133**, 696–712
13. GHEBREHIWET, B., SILVERBERG, M. and KAPLAN, A.P. (1981) Activation of classic pathway of complement by Hageman factor fragment. *J. Exp. Med.*, **153**, 665–676
14. CRADDOCK, P., FEHR, J. and DALMASSO, A. (1977) Hemodialysis leukopenia. *J. Clin. Invest.*, **59**, 879–888
15. SNYDERMAN, R., ALTMAN, L., HAUSMAN, M.S. and MERGENHAGEN, S.E. (1972) Human mononuclear leukocyte chemotaxis. *J. Immunol.*, **108**, 857–860
16. HUGLI, T.E. and MULLER-EBERHARD, H.J. (1978) Anaphylotoxins, C3A and C5A. *Adv. Immunol.*, **26**, 1–53
17. STIMLER, N.P., BACH, M.K., BLOOR, C.M. and HUGLI, T.E. (1982) Release of leukotrienes from guinea pig lung stimulated by C5a des Arg anaphylatoxin. *J. Immunol.*, 2247–2257
18. MCCARTHY, K. and HENSON, P.M. (1979) Induction of lyosomal enzyme secretion by macrophages in response to the purified complement fragments C5a and C5a des Arg. *J. Immunol.*, **123**, 2511–2517
19. GALLIN, J.I. and KAPLAN, A.P. (1974) Mononuclear cell chemotactic activity of kallikrein and plasminogen activator and its inhibition by C1 inhibitor and macroglobulin. *J. Immunol.*, **113**, 1928–1934
20. KAY, A.B., PAPPER, D.S. and EWART, M.R. (1973) Generation of chemotactic activity for leukocytes by the action of thrombin on human fibrinogen. *Nature*, **243**, 56–57
21. STECHER, V.J. and SORKIN, E. (1972) The chemotactic activity of fibrin lysis products. *Int. Arch. Allergy Appl. Immunol.*, **43**, 879–886
22. FERNADEZ, H.N., HENSON, P.M., OTANI, A. and HUGLI, T.E. (1978) Chemotactic response to human C3a and C5a leukotaxis *in vitro* and under simulated *in vivo* conditions. *J. Immunol.*, **120**, 109–115
23. FORD-HUTCHINSON, A.W., BRAY, M.A. and DOIG, M.V. (1980) Leukotriene B, a potent chemokinetic and aggregating substance released from polymorphonuclear leukocytes. *Nature*, **286**, 264–265
24. FREER, R.J., DAY, A.R. and RADDING, J.A. (1980) Further studies on the structural requirement for synthetic peptide chemoattractants. *Biochemistry*, **19**, 2402–2410
25. DUEL, T.F., SENIOR, R.M., HUANG, J.S. and GRIFFIN, G.I. (1982) Chemotaxis of monocytes and neutrophils to platelet-derived growth factor. *J. Clin. Invest.*, **69**, 1046–1049
26. POSTLETHWAITE, A.E. and KANG, A.H. (1976) Collagen and collagen-peptide induced chemotaxis of human blood monocytes. *J. Exp. Med.*, **143**, 1299–1307
27. SENOIR, R.M., GRIFFIN, G.L. and MECHAM, R.P. (1980) Chemotactic activity of elastin-derived peptides. *J. Clin. Invest.*, **66**, 859–862
28. NORRIS, D.A., CLARK, R.A.F. and SWIGART, L.M. (1982) Fibronectin fragments are chemotactic for human peripheral blood monocytes. *J. Immunol.*, **129**, 1612–1618
29. BAR-SHAVIT, R., KAHN, A., FENTON, J.W. and WILMER, G.D. (1983) Chemotactic response of monocytes to thrombin. *J. Cell. Biol.*, **96**, 282–285
30. LEIBOVITCH, S.J. and ROSS, R. (1975) The role of the macrophage in wound repair. *Am. J. Pathol.*, **78**, 71–100

31. LOOSE, L.D. and TURINSKY, J. (1979) Macrophage dysfunction after burn injury. *Infect. Immunol.*, **26**, 157–162
32. NEWMAN, S.L., HENSON, J.E. and HENSON, P.M. (1982) Phagocytosis of senescent neutrophilis by human monocyte derived macrophages and rabbit inflammatory macrophages. *J. Exp. Med.*, **156**, 430–442
33. HUMES, J.L., BONNEY, R.J. and PELUS, L. (1977) Macrophages synthesize and release prostaglandins in response to local inflammatory stimuli. *Nature*, **269**, 149–151
34. LACHMAN, L.B. (1983) Human interleukin. *Fed. Proc.*, **42**, 2639–2645
35. SCHROFF, G., NEWMAN, C. and SONG, C. (1981) Transglutaminase as a marker for subsets of murine macrophages. *Eur. J. Immunol.*, **11**, 637–642
36. MORLAN, B. and KAPLAN, G. (1977) Macrophage activation *in vivo* and *in vitro*. *Exp. Cell Res.*, **108**, 279–288
37. WINTER, G.D. (1962) Formation of the scab and the rate of epithelialization of superficial wounds of the young domestic pig. *Nature*, **193**, 293–294
38. KRAWCZYK, W.S. (1971) A pattern of epidermal cell migration during wound healing. *J. Cell Biol.*, **49**, 247–263
39. WINTER, G.D. (1972) Epidermal regeneration studied in the domestic pig. In *Epidermal Wound Healing*, edited by H.I. Maibach and D.T. Rovee. Chicago: Yearbook Medical
40. CLARK, R.A.F., LANIGAN, J.M. and DELLEPELLA, P. (1982) Fibronectin and fibrin provide a provisional matrix for epidermal cell migration during wound reepithelialization. *J. Invest. Dermatol.*, **70**, 264–269
41. HINTER, H., FRITSCH, P.O. and FOIDART, J.M. (1980) Expression of basement membrane zone antigens at the dermo-epibolic function in organ culture of human skin. *J. Invest. Dermatol.*, **74**, 200–205
42. GRINNELL, F., BILLINGHAM, R.E. and BURGESS, L. (1981) Distribution of fibronectin during wound healing *in vivo*. *J. Invest. Dermatol.*, **76**, 181–189
43. REMENSNYDER, J.P. and MAJNO, G. (1968) Oxygen gradient in healing wounds. *Am. J. Pathol.*, **52**, 301–319
44. IMRE, G. (1964) Studies on the mechanism of retinal neovascularization. *Br. J. Ophthalmol.*, **48**, 75–82
45. ZAUBERMAN, H., MICHAELSON, I.C., BERGMANN, F. and MAURICE, D.M. (1969) Stimulation of neovascularization of the cornea by biogenic amines. *Exp. Eye Res.*, **8**, 77–83
46. CLARK, R.A.F., DELLEPELLA, P. and MANSEAU, E. (1982) Blood vessel fibronectin increases in conjunction with endothelial cell proliferation and capillary ingrowth during wound healing. *J. Invest. Dermatol.*, **79**, 269–276
47. GAY, S., VILJANTO, J., RAEKALLIO, J. and PENTTINEN, R. (1978) Collagen types in early phases of wound healing in children. *Acta Chir. Scand.*, **144**, 205–211
48. PEARLSTEIN, E. (1976) Plasma membrane glycoprotein which mediates adhesion of fibroblasts to collagen. *Nature*, **262**, 497–500
49. BERTOLAMI, C.N. and DONOFF, R.B. (1982) Identification characterization and partial purification of mammalian skin wound hyaluronidase. *J. Invest. Dermatol.*, **79**, 417–421
50. HASCALL, V.C. and HASCALL, G.K. (1981) Proteoglycans. In *Cell Biology of Extracellular Matrix*, edited by E.B. Hay. New York: Plenum Press
51. TOMIDA, M., KOYAMA, H. and ONO, T. (1975) Induction of hyaluronic acid synthetase activity in rat fibroblasts by medium change of confluent cultures. *J. Cell Physiol.*, **86**, 121–130

9

Gingiva and periodontal ligament

Introduction

In 1971, an estimated 23 million North Americans were endentulous. This endentulous condition increases dramatically with age, affecting approximately one-third of the population up to 45 years of age but 50% by 65 years of age. The primary cause of tooth loss, over 35 years of age, is an insidious destruction of the gingiva and periodontal supporting teeth structures termed periodontal disease. The most common destructive periodontal disease is a progressive disorder (chronic periodontitis) that begins with gingivitis (inflammation of the gingival tissues). This inflammation is the body's response to bacterial infection harboured in the dental plaque. This thin film coats the exposed tooth surfaces and predominantly comprises bacteria. If unchecked, these micro-organisms proliferate, with their products eroding healthy tissue, creating periodontal pockets and separating the tooth from its supporting structures. At the same time, the body's immune defence system rallies to combat the infecting bacteria and their products. Unfortunately, the interaction between the bacteria and their products with the white blood cells and antibodies attracted to the area may exacerbate the problem. Indeed, unless the plaque is removed, the defending cells accumulate at the site, creating a state of chronic inflammation. They may even become subverted to attack the body's own periodontal tissues. In time, the destructive process may spread from the gingiva to the periodontal tissues. The result may be tooth mobility, painful abscesses, ulcers and eventual tooth loss.

While all patients with periodontitis have had earlier signs of gingivitis, not all patients with untreated gingivitis develop periodontitis. Gingivitis can exist as a chronic disorder in some people, reversible if treated. Gingivitis can also develop in association with changes in hormones, diet or in reactions to drugs. Presumably such changes alter the host's immune system, or affect local conditions in the mouth in other ways.

In North America, gingivitis and periodontitis are endemic, affecting 75% of adults, 68% of youths and 39% of children. Typically, the younger age groups have milder reversible disease affecting one or several teeth, whereas both the incidence and severity of periodontal disease increase with age, paralleling the rise in edentulousness. In addition to pain, bleeding, loss of function and diminished appearance that accompany advanced disease and tooth loss, periodontal disease is responsible for bad breath (halitosis). Thus, knowledge of the periodontal supporting tissues is crucial to understanding and preventing this endemic problem.

Gingiva

The gingiva is the part of the oral mucosa that covers the alveolar processes and surrounds the cervical (neck) region of the teeth. The gingiva may be anatomically divided into three regions: the marginal, attached and interdental regions.

Marginal (unattached) gingiva

The marginal (unattached) gingiva is the border (or terminal edge) of the gingiva surrounding the teeth in a collar fashion. In about 50% of cases, it is demarcated from the adjacent attached gingiva by a shallow linear depression, the free gingival groove.[1] It forms the soft tissue wall of the gingival sulcus that may be separated from the tooth surface by a periodontal probe.

Gingival sulcus

The gingival sulcus is the shallow crevice around the tooth, bounded by the surface of the tooth on one side and the epithelium lining the free margin of the gingiva on the other. The clinical determination of the depth of this groove provides an important index of periodontal health. Under normal healthy conditions, the depth of this sulcus is up to 2 mm,[2] although depths of 1.5–1.8 mm are clinically regarded as healthy.[3,4]

Attached gingiva

The attached gingiva is continuous with the marginal gingiva. It is firm, resilient and tightly bound to the underlying alveolar periosteum, i.e. it is a mucoperiosteum. The facial aspect of this gingiva extends to the relatively loose and movable alveolar mucosa, from which it is demarcated by the mucogingival junction.

The width of the attached gingiva provides an important clinical parameter. It is defined as the distance between the mucogingival junction and the projection of the bottom of the gingival sulcus (or the periodontal pocket) on the external tooth surface. The width of the attached gingiva on the facial aspect differs between different regions of the mouth,[5] being 3.5–4.5 mm in the maxilla and 3.3–3.9 mm in the mandible. It is less in the posterior (molar) than anterior (incisor) regions of the mouth and least in the premolar region (1.9 mm in the maxilla and 1.8 mm in the mandible).[1]

The mucogingival junction remains in a standard location throughout adult life.[6] Thus any changes in the width of the attached gingiva are due to modifications in the position of its coronal end. The width of the attached gingiva increases with age[7] and in supererupted teeth.[8] On the lingual aspect of the mandible the attached gingiva terminates at the junction with the lingual alveolar mucosa, which is continuous with the mucosa of the mouth floor. The palatal surface of the attached gingiva in the maxilla blends imperceptibly with the equally firm and resilient palatal mucoperiosteum.

Interdental gingiva

The interproximal space between the areas of adjacent tooth contact, the gingival embrasure, is occupied by the interdental gingiva. In the healthy mouth it comprises two papillae separated by a central col. The latter comprises a valley-like depression that conforms to the shape of the interproximal tooth contact. When teeth are not in contact the col is often absent, although it may also be absent even when teeth are in contact in some individuals. Each interdental papilla is pyramidal in shape, with the facial and lingual surfaces tapered towards the interproximal col area. The lateral borders and tip of the interdental papillae are formed by continuation of the marginal gingiva from the adjacent teeth. In the absence of proximal tooth contact the gingiva is firmly bound over the interdental bone and forms a smooth, rounded surface without interdental papillae or col.

Microscopic anatomy of the gingiva

The gingiva comprises a central connective tissue core covered by stratified squamous epithelium, the latter being subdivided into a number of different regions.

Oral epithelium

The oral (outer) epithelium covers the crest and outer surface of the marginal gingiva and the surface of the attached gingiva. It comprises a keratinized or parakeratinized stratified squamous epithelium, which may be subdivided into a number of different layers.

(1) A cuboidal or columnar basal layer.
(2) A spinous polygonal cell layer
(3) A granular cell layer comprising flattened cells with basophilic keratohyaline granules and a shrunken hyperchromic nucleus; this cell layer is not always present.
(4) A superficial keratinized or parakeratinized cell layer.

The cells of the oral epithelium are connected by desmosomes,[9] comprising two dense attachment plaques into which tonofilaments insert, radiating from the cellular cytoplasm and an intermediate electron-dense line in the extracellular space. The outline of each cell membrane is highly irregular, forming projections that either extend into the intercellular space or interdigitate with those of the adjacent cells.

The epithelium is joined to the underlying connective tissue by a basal lamina comprising a lamina lucida adjacent to the basal epithelial cells and a largely glycoprotein lamina densa.[10,11] The basal lamina may be synthesized in part by the basal epithelial cells and may be permeable to fluids but not particulate matter.

Sulcular epithelium

The sulcular epithelium lines the gingival sulcus. This is a thin layer of non-keratinized squamous epithelium that extends from the coronal limit of the junctional epithelium to the crest of the gingival margin. Although non-keratinized under normal conditions, it may become keratinized following intensive antibacterial therapy.[12] It is through this semipermeable layer that bacterial irritants pass to the underlying tissues.[13]

Junctional epithelium

The junctional epithelium comprises a collar-like band of non-keratinized squamous epithelium 3–20 cells thick and 0.25–1.35 long. The attachment of this epithelial layer to the underlying connective tissue comprises a lamina densa adjacent to the enamel or cementum and a lamina lucida into which hemidesmosomes are attached. This junctional epithelium has been divided into three zones:

(1) The apical zone, comprising basal germinal cells.
(2) The middle zone, which has predominantly adhesive properties.
(3) The coronal zone, which is quite permeable.[14]

The attachment of the junctional epithelium to the tooth is reinforced by the gingival fibres that brace the marginal gingiva against the tooth surface. The junctional epithelium and gingival fibres of the periodontal ligament are therefore referred to as the dentogingival unit.

Gingival sulcular development

After the completion of amelogenesis the enamel is covered by the reduced enamel epithelium, which is attached to the tooth by a basal lamina.[15] When the tooth erupts through the oral mucosa, the reduced epithelium unites with the oral epithelium to form the epithelial attachment.[16] During this process, the cells of the reduced enamel epithelium are gradually replaced by squamous epithelial cells. The junctional epithelium is, however, undergoing continuing renewal, with mitoses occurring in all cell layers.[17] The regenerating epithelial cells move towards the tooth surface in a coronal direction to the gingival sulcus, where they are shed.[18] The gingival sulcus is then formed when the tooth erupts into the oral cavity.

The gingival epithelium also differentiates to form two epithelial types:

(1) The epithelium which covers the outer surface of the marginal gingiva and the attached gingiva and comprises keratinized and/or parakeratinized layers.[19]
(2) The gingival sulcular epithelium which is usually non-keratinized, although keratinization may occur when it is experimentally reflected and exposed to the oral cavity.[8]

The oral epithelium undergoes continuous renewal, with the cells lost due to attrition and abrasion being balanced by mitosis at the basal layer. The mitotic rate varies not only with a diurnal cycle (being greater in the morning and evening) but also with the region of the mouth (being greater in the palatal mucoperiosteal region than in the sulcular, junctional epithelium or attached gingiva).[20,21] The mitotic rate also appears to be greater in the non-keratinized than keratinized mucosa and increases with gingivitis.

Gingival fluid

The gingival sulcus contains a fluid which seeps through the thin sulcular epithelium.[22] There is still debate as to whether this is a continuous transudate or an inflammatory exudate. Certainly not only does the amount of gingival (crevicular) fluid increase with inflammation[23] but also with the eating of coarse foods, tooth brushing, ovulation and the consumption of hormonal oral contraceptives.[24,25] In addition to desquammated epithelial cells, polymorphonuclear leucocytes, lymphocytes and monocytes may be found in this fluid, together with potassium, sodium and chloride ions. The total protein content of this fluid is much lower than that of serum.[26] IgG, IgA, IgM, complement components C3 and C4, in addition to plasma proteins albumin and fibrinogen, have been detected. A number of other substances have been found in this gingival fluid; these include:

(1) Lactic acid.
(2) Urea.

(3) Hydroxyproline.
(4) Hydrogen sulphide.
(5) Acid phosphatase.
(6) Lysozyme.
(7) Alkaline phosphatase.
(8) Lactic dehydrogenase.
(9) Proteases.

A number of functions have been assigned to this crevicular fluid, including:

(1) Lavage of material from the gingival sulcus.
(2) Antibacterial, based on the presence of antibodies against plaque bacteria, in addition to viable leucocytes.
(3) Adhesive, based on the presence of sticky plasma proteins that may augment adhesion between junctional epithelium and tooth surface.

Gingival connective tissue

The connective tissue of the gingiva is termed the lamina propria. It is densely collagenous, comprising two layers:

(1) A papillary layer subjacent to the epithelium consisting of papillary projections between the epithelial rete pegs.
(2) A reticular layer contiguous with the periosteum of the alveolar bone.

The connective tissue of the marginal gingiva contains prominent collagenous bundles, the gingival fibres, which serve the following functions:

(1) To brace the marginal gingiva firmly against the tooth.
(2) To provide rigidity necessary to withstand displacement of the gingiva from the tooth surface during mastication.
(3) To unite the free marginal gingiva with the cemental tooth surface and the adjacent attached gingiva.

These gingival fibres are arranged in three groups:

(1) *The gingivodental group* is embedded into the cementum just beneath the epithelium at the base of the gingival sulcus. The fibres then spread in fan-like fashion into the periosteum of the facial and lingual alveolar periosteum, crest of the interdental gingiva and attached gingiva.
(2) *The circular group* courses through the marginal and interdental gingival connective tissue to encircle the tooth in a ring-like fashion.
(3) *The trans-septal group* of fibres forms horizontal bundles between the cementum of approximating teeth into which they are embedded. They lie in the area between the epithelium at the base of the gingival sulcus and the crest of the interdental bone. They are sometimes classified as one of the principal groups of fibres of the periodontal ligament.

In addition to fibroblasts and occasional macrophages, the gingival connective tissue often contains polymorphonuclear leucocytes, lymphocytes and plasma cells. These latter, however, cannot be detected if gingival normalcy is judged by very strict clinical criteria.[27] These cells are then embedded in a non-collagenous ground substance comprising predominantly glycoproteins and glycosaminoglycans.

Gingival vascular supply

There are three sources of blood supply to the gingiva:

(1) The supraperiosteal arterioles along the facial and lingual alveolar bone surfaces, from which capillaries extend along the sulcular epithelium and between the epithelial rete pegs.
(2) The vessels of the periodontal ligament, which extend into the gingiva to anastomose with capillaries in the sulcus area.
(3) Arterioles emerging from the crest of the interdental septa[28] to anastomose with capillaries of the periodontal ligament, gingival crevicular areas and vessels that run over the alveolar crest.

Beneath the epithelium, on the outer gingival surface, the capillaries extend into the papillary connective tissue between the epithelial rete pegs in the form of terminal anastomosing hairpin loops,[29] some of which lie dormant unless irritated. Along the sulcular epithelium, the capillaries are arranged in a flat anastomosing plexus extending from the base of the sulcus to the gingival margin,[30] parallel to the enamel.

The lymphatic drainage of the gingiva progresses into the collecting network external to the alveolar periosteum and then to the regional (especially sublingual) lymph nodes.[31] The lymphatic vessels just beneath the junctional epithelium extend into the periodontal ligament along with the blood vessels.

Gingival innervation

The gingival tissues are innervated by fibres arising from the periodontal ligament, as well as those from the labial, buccal and lingual nerves. In addition to unspecialized nerve endings, Meissner-type and Krause-type specialized nerve endings have been reported (*see* Chapters 1 and 2).

Gingival morphology

Colour

The coral pink colour of the marginal and attached gingivae is generally a reflection of a rich blood supply, a degree of epithelial pigmentation and keratinization. The attached gingiva is demarcated from the adjacent alveolar mucosa by a clearly defined mucogingival line, with the alveolar mucosa being red, smooth and shiny as opposed to the pink and stippled gingiva.

Pigmentation

The melanin pigmentation of the gingiva is derived from the activity of the neural-crest derived melanocytes in the basal and spinous layers of the epithelium. This pigment is synthesized by the intracellular premelanosomes or melanosomes[32] containing tyrosinase, which hydrolyses tyrosine to hydroxyphenylalanine (dopa), that is then progressively converted to melanin. Melanin granules are phagocytosed by adjacent epithelial and connective tissue cells (termed melanophages or melanophores). Gingival pigmentation occurs as a diffuse deep purple discoloration, or irregular brown pigmented areas.

Contour

The contour of the gingiva depends on the shape of the teeth, the alignment of the teeth within the arch, the location and size of the proximal contact between adjacent teeth and the dimensions of the facial and lingual gingival embrasures. The marginal gingiva follows a scalloped line on the facial and lingual surfaces of the teeth, although where there is a pronounced mesiodistal concavity (e.g. the maxillary canines), this contour is greatly exaggerated. By contrast, the marginal gingiva follows a relatively straight line where the tooth surface is flat.

Consistency

The gingiva is generally firm and resilient and attached to the underlying periosteum, except in the region of the free gingival margin. In cases of gingivitis, the gingiva may be swollen, oedematous and soft, reflecting the underlying inflammatory process.

Surface texture

The surface of the gingiva is said to be stippled, a feature that applies to the attached rather than marginal gingiva. The pattern and extent of the stippling depends on the region of the mouth,[33] being less prominent on the lingual than facial surfaces, although there may be no stippling in some mouths. Microscopic examination reveals that stippling is reflected by alternate rounded protuberances and depressions in the gingival surface in concert with undulations in the underlying connective tissue. One of the earliest signs of gingivitis is that this stippling is lost and replaced by a smooth shiny surface.

Location

When the tooth erupts into the oral cavity, the margin and sulcus are at the tip of the crown although, with eruption, the level of the free gingival margin migrates cervically along the tooth surface. Thus, the free gingival margin in the healthy mouth is said to be at the level of the amelocemental junction, although with chronic periodontitis the free gingival margin may descend down the cementum, resulting in the affected teeth being sensitive to thermal (especially cold) changes.

Cementum

Cementum is the calcified mesenchymal tissue that covers the dentine surface of the tooth root. Acellular (or primary) cementum and cellular (or secondary) cementum are the two component types found around human tooth roots, although the distinction between the two is frequently not readily apparent. The coronal part of the root is usually covered by acellular cementum whereas the apical portion is usually covered by cellular cementum. With advancing age, the amount of cellular cementum tends to increase, especially when there is exposure of root furcations following chronic periodontitis. Cellular cementum, however, contains cementocytes which communicate with one another by anastomosing canaliculi. Both acellular and cellular cementum are arranged in lamellae separated by incremental lines parallel to the long axis of the tooth. These lamellae represent periods of cemental formation and are more highly calcified than the adjacent cementum.[34] Cementoblasts not only form a glycoprotein ground substance but also part of the collagenous framework of the cementum itself.[35] In addition, cementum, especially the acellular layer, contains the embedded portions of the principal fibres of the periodontal ligament, Sharpey's fibres.[36] Sharpey's fibres are the predominant inclusion of acellular cementum, with most being at right angles to the tooth surface, although others appear to enter at diverse angles. The size, number and distribution of these fibres varies with tooth function.[37] By contrast, Sharpey's fibres occupy a smaller portion of cellular cementum. In acellular cementum, the Sharpey's fibres are completely calcified, except in a 10–50 μm wide zone near the cementodentinary junction, where they are only partly calcified.[38] By contrast, some of the Sharpey's fibres are completely calcified in cellular cementum, others are partly calcified and in some there is a central uncalcified core surrounded by a calcified border.[38] The cellular remnants of Hertwig's epithelial root sheath may sometimes be seen on microscopic examination of the cementodentinary junction of some teeth.

The inorganic portion of cementum in the form of hydroxyapatite (45–50%) is less than that of bone (65%), dentine (70%) and enamel (97%).[39] There are also many detailed differences in the composition of cementum matrix compared with that of bone.[40]

At the coronal portion of the tooth root, the cementum is 16–60 μm thick, whereas this may be 150–200 μm thick at the apical portion.[41] Moreover, the cementum increases in thickness with advancing age,[42] although there have been scant investigations to determine the forensic significance of this fact.

Amelocemental junction

Three types of relationships between enamel and cementum have been described at the cervical margin of a tooth:

(1) Cementum overlaps the enamel in 60–65% of cases.
(2) There is a butt joint between cementum and enamel in 30% of cases.
(3) Cementum and enamel do not meet in 5–10% of cases, leaving exposed root dentine, a feature that may cause unpleasant symptoms with the apical migration of the free gingiva in chronic periodontal disease.

Cementogenesis

Cementoblasts are of mesenchymal origin in the tooth germ. As with bone, cementogenesis starts with the deposition of an irregular collagenous matrix with an interfibrillar matrix, termed cementoid. Progressive mineralization of the matrix begins at the cementodentinary junction, and is associated with the inclusion of the principal periodontal fibres as Sharpey's fibres. Also, with progressive cementum formation, some of the cementoblasts become incorporated in a manner analogous to osteocytes.

Cementogenesis does not cease with tooth eruption but may continue throughout life, although often at miniscule rates. Interestingly, certain people, especially female Negroes, have a genetic predisposition to hypercementosis.[43] Although all the teeth may be affected, usually the mandibular incisors are predominantly involved, leading to ankylosis between tooth roots and adjacent alveolar bone. There may also be attempted hypercementosis in areas of root fracture, although there is little documentation in this regard.

Cementum may also undergo resorption, e.g. in occlusal trauma,[44] orthodontic therapy,[45] pressure from adjacent teeth, cysts or tumours,[46] teeth without functional antagonists, transplanted or replanted teeth, periodontal disease and low-grade periapical inflammation. A number of systemic factors have also been associated with cemental resorption, including deficiencies of calcium, vitamin D and vitamin A,[47,48] in addition to hypothyroidism[49] and Paget's disease.[50]

Periodontal ligament

The periodontal ligament is the connective tissue that connects the tooth root to the adjacent alveolar bone. The most important elements are the principal periodontal fibres, which comprise collagen bundles arranged in specific groups. The terminal portions are inserted into cementum and alveolar bone as Sharpey's fibres.

Principal periodontal fibre groups

Transeptal fibres

These fibres are embedded into the cementum of adjacent teeth and extend interproximally over the alveolar crest.

Alveolar crest fibres

These fibres extend obliquely from the cementum beneath the junctional epithelium to the alveolar crest.

Horizontal fibres

These fibres extend at right angles to the long axis of the tooth between cementum and alveolar bone.

Oblique fibres

This is the largest group of principal periodontal fibres, extending from the cementum obliquely to the alveolar bone.

Apical fibres

The apical group of fibres radiates from the apical cementum to the alveolar bone at the base of the socket.

In addition, there are numerous smaller groups of collagen fibres that contain blood vessels, nerves and lymphatics, as well as elastin[51] and oxytalan[52] fibres.

Cells of the periodontal ligament

In addition to fibroblasts, numerous other cell types may occur in the periodontal tissues, including cementoblasts, osteoblasts, osteoclasts, macrophages and strands of epithelial cells termed 'epithelial rests of Malassez'. These latter form a lattice or network and are considered to be derived from Hertwig's epithelial root sheath which disintegrates during development. These cells remain viable and capable of undergoing mitosis if irritated.[53] In addition to procollagen synthesis,[54] the periodontal ligament fibroblasts have been shown to undertake a phagocytic function,[55] so that these cells may be responsible for the formation and replacement of periodontal fibres.

Periodontal organogenesis

The periodontal ligament develops from the circular connective tissue surrounding the tooth bud.[56] This dental follicle is continuous with the ectomesenchyme of the dental papilla and comprises:

(1) Undifferentiated fibroblastic cells that give rise to fibroblasts, cementoblasts and osteoblasts.
(2) Undifferentiated perivascular mesenchymal cells that also give rise to fibroblasts.

During tooth eruption and function, the principal fibres of the periodontal ligament become more regularly arranged and thicker.

Periodontal vascular supply

The blood supply of the periodontal ligament is derived from:

(1) Apical vessels entering the periodontal ligament at the apical region and extending to the gingiva, giving branches to the cementum and bone; within the periodontal ligament, this vascular network runs closer to the bone than cementum.
(2) Penetrating vessels from the alveolar bone, an important contribution to this tissue.
(3) Anastomosing vessels from the gingiva, derived from branches of deep vessels in the lamina propria.

Venous drainage follows a similar course.

The lymphatic drainage supplements the venous drainage system. The lymphatic drainage just beneath the junctional epithelium passes into the periodontal ligament, to accompany the blood vessels to the root apex. From there it passes through the alveolar bone, mainly to the submandibular lymph nodes.

Periodontal innervation

The periodontal ligament has an abundant sensory innervation, particularly touch, pressure, proprioception and pain, via the trigeminal nerve[57] as both specialized and unspecialized nerve endings. The nerves pass into the periodontal ligament from the periapical region and through channels in the alveolar bone. The nerves generally follow the course of the blood vessels.

Periodontal functions

Formative

The periodontal ligament serves as the periosteum for cementum and alveolar bone in that the component cells participate in the formation and resorption of these tissues with orthodontic tooth movement, repair following injury and the accommodation of occlusal forces. Collagen turnover in the periodontal ligament is greatest at the apical and crestal regions of the periodontal ligament, whereas fibroblastic activity is greatest adjacent to the alveolar bone and least at the cemental aspect.[58]

Physical

The physical functions of the periodontal ligament include:

(1) Transmission of occlusal forces to the alveolar bone.
(2) Attachment of teeth to the jaws.
(3) Maintenance of gingival tissue location to the teeth.
(4) Shock absorption for occlusal forces.
(5) Protection of vessels and nerves from mechanical injury during function.

The tensional theory of tooth support contends that the principal periodontal ligament fibres primarily function for tooth support and transmission of forces to the alveolar bone. Certainly, the principal periodontal ligament fibres change from a wavy to a straight form when forces are applied to the tooth crown, and revert to a wavy form when the tooth is at rest. An alternative view contends that the displacement of a tooth in the alveolar socket is controlled by movement of the extracellular fluid, with the principal periodontal fibres having but a secondary role.[59] A third theory contends that the periodontal ligament exhibits the rheological behaviour of a thixotropic gel.[60]

When a horizontal or tipping force is applied to a tooth, the tooth will tend to rotate within the confines of the periodontal ligament, with the apical region of the root tending to move in an opposite direction to the coronal portion.[61] In single rooted teeth, the axis of rotation is slightly apical to the middle one third of the root, which corresponds to the morphology of the periodontal ligament, with its narrowest portion in the region of the axis of rotation.[62] In multirooted teeth, the axis of rotation is located in the bone between the roots. Conceivably, therefore, there are two characteristic phases of tooth movement, the first embracing the confines of the periodontal ligament and the second resulting in displacement of the alveolar bone with increasing rotation.[63]

Just as the tooth depends on the periodontal ligament for support during function, the periodontal ligament depends on stimulation from occlusal forces to maintain its structure. Within physiological limits, increased function is accommodated by increased principal fibre size, Sharpey's fibre thickness and number, in addition to increased width of the periodontal ligament as a whole. Necrosis of the periodontal ligament occurs when these forces are exceeded, whereas when function is diminished or absent, the periodontal ligament is thinned and the component principal fibres become disorganized.[64]

Sensory and nutritional

The innervation of the periodontal ligament, in the form of proprioception and tactile sensitivity, is crucial to the neuromuscular control of masticatory function.[65,66] In addition, the periodontal ligament provides nutrients for the cementum, alveolar bone and gingiva by its component blood vessels as well as lymphatic drainage.

Alveolar bone

The alveolar bone forms and supports the tooth sockets. It comprises a thin inner socket wall of compact bone, termed the cribriform plate or lamina dura, surrounded by cancellous bone and the facial and lingual plates of compact bone. The cancellous portion of the alveolar bone comprises trabeculae, whose form and direction are determined by occlusal forces.[67] The cribriform plate, however, contains numerous Sharpey's fibres, again their number, size and location being dependent upon functional forces. Thus the alveolar bone is a dynamic structure, whose detailed morphology is largely governed by function. Thus the height and thickness of the facial and lingual cortical plates are affected by tooth alignment, root angulation and occlusal forces. Alveolar bone undergoes constant remodelling activity, with bone removed where it is no longer needed and added to regions with increased demand. Within physiological limits, increased tooth function results in forces being transmitted via the periodontal ligament to the alveolar bone, leading to its increased bone mass. By contrast, decreased function, in the form of tooth extraction, is associated with progressive alveolar bone resorption.

Periodontal assessment

The evaluation of clinical signs and dental radiographs are the principal clues for the assessment of the periodontal health of an individual.

Gingival inflammation

A reddening of the gingivae and bleeding upon gentle probing both provide an index of gingival inflammation. The assessment of colour is, however, rather subjective, whereas the degree of bleeding on probing is partly dependent upon probing force.

Soft tissue destruction

The periodontal probe is the primary tool for measuring the depth of the gingival sulcus, although variation in the probing force and angulation may compromise such assessments.

Bone destruction

Dental radiographs are frequently used to assess the degree of periodontal support for a tooth, in addition to the status of the alveolar bone. Variation in angulation, ray direction and film processing may compromise their evaluation.

Crevicular fluid assessment

Gingival crevicular fluid correlates well with the clinical and microscopic assessment of gingivitis, although the problems of such fluid collection have so far hampered its evaluative potential.

Plaque analysis

While micro-organisms in dental plaque are the acknowledged culprits in gingivitis and periodontal disease, the organisms responsible for the initiation or promotion of the disease have yet to be discerned. Thus the diagnosis of gingivitis and chronic periodontal disease is hampered by a dearth of objective assessment criteria.

Plaque control is not only essential for the patient who has had periodontal disease; it is the cornerstone of all programmes aimed at preventing gum disease in the first instance. Mechanical means of plaque control are the most common approach, aimed at the non-selective removal of plaque from all tooth surfaces. Such measures include the use of the tooth brush, tooth pick, dental floss and irrigational devices, although chemical agents in the form of antibiotics and antimicrobials (e.g. chlorhexidine, cetylpyridinium chloride (CPC), domiphen bromide (DB) and cetyltrimethylammonium chloride (CTAB)) have proved effective in some instances. Dietary substitutes and additives (e.g. xylitol and sorbitol in place of sucrose) can reduce plaque activity. However, effective prevention and treatment of periodontal and gingival disease is presently curtailed, not only by the lack of understanding of the basic physiology of the supporting tissues as a whole, but also of the causative factors of these diseases and the resulting host responses.

Conclusions

As will be evident from Chapter 10, the periodontal ligament is a complex entity, which is intimately associated with the health of the gingival and alveolar bone supporting tissues. Further information on the structure and function of the normal supporting tissues is, however, required before we can fully understand the disease processes.

Review questions

1. How do the vascular systems of the gingiva, periodontal ligament and alveolar bone communicate with one another?
2. Describe the clinical methods for the assessment of the periodontal health of a tooth.
3. Why do gingivitis and periodontal disease start in the gingival sulcus?
4. What is the role of the various component periodontal ligament fibres in the support of the tooth in the alveolar socket?
5. What is the origin of gingival fluid?

References

1. AINAMO, A. and LOE, H. (1966) Anatomical characteristics of gingiva. A clinical and microscopic study of the free and attached gingiva. *J. Periodontol.*, **37**, 5
2. GOTTLIEB, B. (1926) What is a normal pocket? *J. Am. Dent. Assoc.*, **13**, 214
3. ORBAN, B. and KOHLER, J. (1924) The physiologic gingival sulcus. *Z. Stomatol.*, **22**, 353
4. GARGIULO, A.W. and WENTZ. F.M. (1961) Dimensions and relations of the dentogingival junction in humans. *J. Periodontol.*, **32**, 261
5. BOWERS, G.M. (1963) A study of the width of the attached gingiva. *J. Periodontol.*, **34**, 210
6. AINAMO, A. (1978) Influence of age on the location of the maxillary mucogingival junction. *J. Periodontol. Res.*, **13**, 189
7. EICHEL, B., SHAHRIK, H.A. and LISANTI, V.F. (1964) Cytochemical demonstration and metabolic significance of reduced diphospho-pyridine-nucleotide and triphospho-pyridine-nucleotide reductases in human gingiva. *J. Dent. Res.*, **43**, 92
8. BRAL, M.M. and STAHL, S.S. (1977) Keratinizing potential of human crevicular epithelium. *J. Periodontol.*, **48**, 381
9. LISTGARTEN, M.A. (1964) The ultrastructure of human gingival epithelium. *Am. J. Anat.*, **114**, 49
10. KURAHASHI, Y. and TAKUMA, S. (1962) Electron microscopy of human gingival epithelium. *Bull. Tokyo. Dent. Col.*, **3**, 29
11. STERN, I.B. (1965) Electron microscopic observations of oral epithelium. I. Basal cells and the basement membrane. *Periodontics.*, **3**, 224
12. CAFFESSE, R.G., KORMAN, T. and NASJLETI, C.E. (1980) The effect of intense antibacterial therapy on the sulcular environment in monkeys. *J. Periodontol.*, **51**, 155
13. THILANDER, H. (1964) Permeability of the gingival pocket epithelium. *Int. Dent. J.*, **14**, 416
14. SAGLIE, R., SABAG, N. and MERY, C. (1979) Ultrastructure of the normal epithelial attachment. *J. Periodontol.*, **50**, 544
15. STERN, I.B. (1966) The fine structure of the ameloblast–enamel junction in rat incisors, epithelial attachment and cuticular membrane. *5th Int. Cong. Electron Microscop.*, 6
16. GOTTLIEB, B. (1921) Der Epithelansatz am Zahns. *Dtsch. Monatsschr. Zahnheilk.*, **39**, 142
17. MCHUGH, W.D. and ZANDER, H.A. (1965) Cell division in the periodontium of developing and erupted teeth. *Dent. Pract.*, **15**, 451
18. BEAGRIE, G.S. and SKOUGAARD, M.R. (1962) Observations on the life cycle of the gingival crevicular epithelial cells of mice as revealed by autoradiography. *Acta Odontol. Scand.*, **20**, 15
19. WEINMANN, J.P. and MEYER, J. (1959) Types of keratinization in the human gingiva. *J. Invest. Dermatol.*, **32**, 409
20. ANDERSON, G.S. and STERN, I. (1966) The proliferation and migration of the attachment epithelium on the cemental surface of the rat incisor. *Periodontics*, **4**, 115
21. TROTT, J.R. (1957) An investigation into the glycogen content of the gingiva. *Dent. Pract.*, **7**, 234
22. BRILL, N. and KRASSE, B. (1958) The passage of tissue fluid into the clinically healthy gingival pocket. *Acta Odontol. Scand.*, **16**, 223
23. GARNICK, J.J., PEARSON, R. and HARRELL, D. (1979) The evaluation of the peritron. *J. Periodontol.*, **50**, 424
24. LINDHE, J. and ATTSTROM, R. (1967) Gingival exudation during the menstrual cycle. *J. Periodont. Res.*, **2**, 194
25. LINDHE, J. and BJORN, A.L. (1967) Influence of hormonal contraceptives on the gingiva of women. *J. Periodont. Res.*, **2**, 1
26. GIBBONS, R.J. and VAN HOUTE, J. (1973) On the formation of dental plaques. *J. Periodontol.*, **44**, 347
27. OLIVER, R.C., HOLM-PEDERSEN, P. and LOE, H. (1969) The correlation between clinical scoring, exudate

measurements and microscopic evaluation of inflammation in the gingiva. *J. Periodontol.*, **40**, 201
28. FOLKE, L.E.A. and STALLARD, R.E. (1967) Periodontal microcirculation as revealed by plastic microspheres. *J. Periodont. Res.*, **2**, 53
29. ITOIZ, M.E., CARRANZA, F.A., GIMENEZ, I. and CABRINI, R.L. (1972) Microspectrophotometric analysis of succinic dehydrogenase and glucose-6-phosphate dehydrogenase in human oral epithelium. *J. Periodont. Res.*, **7**, 14
30. CARRANZA, F.A., ITOIZ, M.E., CABRINI, R.L. and DOTTO, C.A. (1966) A study of periodontal vascularization in different laboratory animals. *J. Periodont. Res.*, **1**, 120
31. STILLMAN, P.R. and MCCALL, J.O. (1922) *Textbook of Clinical Periodontics*. New York: Macmillan
32. COHEN, B. (1959) ATPase and dopa oxidase activity in human gingival epithelium. *Arch. Oral Biol.*, **12**, 1241
33. QUITARELLI, G. and CHERASKIN, E. (1961) Histochemistry of the gingiva. *J. Periodontol.*, **32**, 339
34. YAMAMOTO, H. (1962) Microradiographic and histopathological study of the cementum. *Bull. Tokyo Dent. Univ.*, **9**, 141
35. SELVIG, K. (1965) The fine structure of human cementum. *Acta Odontol. Scand.*, **23**, 423
36. ROMANIUK, K. (1967) Some observations of the fine structure of human cementum. *J. Dent. Res.*, **46**, 152
37. INOUE, M. and AKIYOSHI, M. (1962) Histological investigation on Sharpey's fibres in cementum of teeth in abnormal function. *J. Dent. Res.*, **41**, 503
38. JONES, S.J. and BOYDE, A. (1972) A study of human root cementum surfaces as prepared for and examined in the scanning electron microscope. *Z. Zellforsch.*, **130**, 318
39. ZIPKIN, I. (1970) The inorganic composition of bones and teeth. In *Biological Calcification*, edited by H. Schraer. New York: Appleton-Century-Crofts
40. SELVIG, K.A. (1977) Structure and metabolism of the normal periodontium. *Int. Conf. Res. Biology of Periodontal Diseases*. Chicago: University of Illinois, p.5
41. ORBAN, B. (1944) *Oral Histology and Embryology*. St Louis: C.V. Mosby
42. ZANDER, H.A. and HURZELER, B. (1958) Continuous cementum apposition. *J. Dent. Res.*, **37**, 1035
43. ZEMSKY, J.L. (1931) Hypercementosis and heredity: an introduction and plan of investigation. *Dent. Items Int.*, **53**, 355
44. ORBAN, B. (1928) Tissue changes in traumatic occlusion. *J. Am. Dent. Assoc.*, **15**, 2090
45. KETCHAM, A.H. (1929) A progress report of an investigation of apical root resorption of permanent teeth. *Int. J. Orthod.*, **15**, 310
46. KRONFELD, R. (1938) Biology of cementum. *J. Am. Dent. Assoc.*, **25**, 1451
47. BURN, C.G., ORTEN, A.I., GROETZINGER, G. and DEWITT, T.F. (1940-1941) Changes in the structure of the developing tooth in rats maintained on a diet deficient in vitamin A. *Yale J. Biol. Med.*, **13**, 817
48. JONES, M.R. and SIMONTON, F.V. (1928) Mineral metabolism in relation to alveolar atrophy in dogs. *J. Am. Dent. Assoc.*, **15**, 881
49. BECKS, H. (1936) Root resorptions and their relation to pathologic bone formation. *Int. J. Orthod.*, **22**, 445
50. RUSHTON, M.A. (1938) Dental tissues in osteitis deformans. *Guys Hosp. Rep.*, **88**, 163
51. THOMAS, N.G. (1927) Elastic fibres in periodontal membrane and pulp. *J. Dent. Res.*, **7**, 325
52. GOGGINS, J.F. (1966) The distribution of oxytalan connective tissue fibres in periodontal ligaments of deciduous teeth. *Periodontics*, **4**, 182
53. TROWBRIDGE, H.O. and SHIBATA, F. (1967) Mitotic activity in epithelial rests of Malassez. *Periodontics*, **5**, 109
54. WEINSTOCK, M. (1972) Collagen formation – observations on its intracellular packaging and transport. *Z. Zellforsch.*, **129**, 455
55. TEN CATE, R., DEPORTER, D.A. (1975) The degradative role of the fibroblast in the remodelling and turnover of collagen in soft connective tissue. *Anat. Rec.*, **182**, 1
56. TEN CATE, R. (1969) The development of the periodontium. In *Biology of the Periodontium*, edited by A.H. Melcher and W.H. Bowen. New York: Academic Press
57. AVERY, J.K. and RAPP, R. (1959) Pain conduction in human dental tissues. *Dent. Clin. North Am.*, **March**, 489
58. STALLARD, R.E. (1963) The utilization of H3-proline by the connective tissues of the periodontium. *Periodontics*, **1**, 185
59. BOYLE, P.E. (1938) Tooth suspension. *J. Dent. Res.*, **17**, 37
60. KARDOS, T.B. and SIMPSON, L.D. (1979) A theoretical consideration of the periodontal membrane as a collagenous thixotropic system and its relationship to tooth eruption. *J. Periodont. Res.*, **14**, 444
61. PICTON, D.C.S. and DAVIES, W.I.R. (1967) Dimensional changes in the periodontal membrane of monkeys. (*Macaca irus*) due to horizontal thrusts applied to the tooth. *Arch. Oral Biol.*, **12**, 1635
62. COOLIDGE, E.D. (1937) The thickness of the human periodontal membrane. *J. Am. Dent. Assoc.*, **24**, 1260
63. DAVIES, R. and PICTON, D.C.S. (1967) Dimensional changes in the periodontal membrane of monkey's teeth with horizontal thrusts. *J. Dent. Res.*, **46**, 114
64. ANNEROTH, G. and ERICSSON, S.G. (1967) An experimental histological study of monkey teeth without antagonist. *Odontol. Revy*, **18**, 345
65. KIZIOR, J.E., CUOZZO, J.W. and BOWMAN, D.C. (1968) Functional and histologic assessment of the sensory innervation of the periodontal ligament of the cat. *J. Dent. Res.*, **47**, 59
66. TRYDE, G., FRYDENBERG, O. and BRILL, N. (1962) An assessment of the tactile sensibility in human teeth. *Acta Odontol. Scand.*, **20**, 233
67. PARFITT, G.J. (1962) An investigation of the normal variations in alveolar bone trabeculation. *Oral Surg.*, **15**, 1453

10

Dental plaque

Introduction

The oral cavity harbours a large diverse microbial population. This population originates from micro-organisms in the air, water, food and other environmental segments that regularly come into contact with the oral cavity. The majority of these micro-organisms are rapidly eliminated by the host defence mechanisms. Alternatively, they may not survive the hostile oral environment. Some species colonize one or more regions of the oral cavity (econiches), however, to become established as the oral flora. Most of the micro-organisms that successfully colonize the mouth are acquired directly from other individuals, rather than the environment as a whole.

The oral environment is unique, comprising both mineralized and epithelial tissues. These tissues, together with a constant salivary flow, provide a variety of econiches for microbial colonization. This diverse and dynamic oral flora comprises species (opportunistic pathogens) that are also capable of causing disease if the host defence mechanisms become impaired. For instance, dental caries and periodontal disease are infectious diseases that result from excessive normal oral microbial accumulation exceeding the capacity of the host defence mechanisms to cope with the insult. Alternatively, endogenous infections may arise when component members of the normal oral flora are introduced into tissues to which they normally have no access, e.g. subacute bacterial endocarditis may result from an oral flora bacteraemia leading to permanent heart valve impairment and sometimes death.

Oral microflora

The cheeks, lips, palate and tongue comprise relatively aerobic epithelial surfaces, bathed in saliva and exposed intermittently to dietary nutrients. Similarly, the buccal and lingual tooth surfaces are also relatively smooth aerobic surfaces bathed in saliva. The interproximal tooth surfaces, along with the occlusal pits and fissures, exhibit similar environments, apart from the absence of the natural salivary cleansing activities, i.e. micro-organisms tend to accumulate at these sites. The gingival sulcus presents a rather unique environment:

(1) The tissues are bathed by gingival (crevicular) fluid whose composition differs from that of saliva.
(2) The micro-organisms of the gingival sulcus are not subjected to salivary lavage.

Interestingly, the saliva itself may comprise an intraoral econiche, although its constituent microbial population generally originates from other oral surfaces (econiches).

Oral bacterial colonization begins at, or shortly after, birth, and proceeds discontinuously until 5–6 years of age. The composition then generally remains relatively stable until adulthood, except for a few nutritionally fastidious anaerobes, e.g. spirochaetes, *Bacteroides melaninogenicus*. The variation in number and species of micro-organisms that can be isolated from analogous sites at different time periods,[1] however, attests to the dynamic nature of the oral environment. Such environmental variations, in part, reflect:

(1) Changes in the host (e.g. tooth eruption or exfoliation, dietary or nutritional changes, dental treatment or xerostomia).
(2) Metabolic activity of the established oral flora. For example:
    (a) toxic microbial metabolic end-product production and removal;
    (b) depletion of nutrients essential for microbial retention;
    (c) biosynthesis of substances required for the growth of other species.

The oral econiches therefore undergo constant flux which is reflected in their variable microbial composition.[2] There are, however, some general overall trends. For instance, *Streptococcus salivarius* tends to predominate on the dorsal surface of the tongue, whereas *S. sanguis*, and *S. mutans* accumulate on the occlusal tooth surfaces.[3] Gram-positive filamentous bacteria tend to be distributed throughout the mouth, but are especially numerous on the tooth surfaces. *Bacteroides melaninogenicus*, vibrios and spirochaetes are most frequently isolated from the gingival sulcus. The gingival sulcus comprises a unique environment that is not only protected from the normal oral cleansing mechanisms but also contains gingival fluid with a high protein concentration.[4,5] The relatively low gingival fluid oxygen concentration[6] and oxidation–reduction potential[7] facilitates anaerobic microbial growth.[7,8]

Effect of oral flora on the host

The presence, growth and reproduction of the normal oral microflora have both beneficial and detrimental effects. These interactions reflect, in part, functional host defence activity and the oral microbial burden.

The normal oral microflora comprise opportunists exhibiting three types of host parasite interaction.

Mutualism

Mutualism occurs when the host provides a suitable environment for microbial growth and reproduction, and the host receives some beneficial product(s) in exchange. For example, vitamin K is synthesized by the coliform gastrointestinal bacteria, so in return the host receives a vitamin for prothrombin formation which would otherwise have been entirely dietary in origin.

Commensualism

Commensualism is a relationship in which neither host nor parasite is harmed, although either the parasite or host generally receives most benefit.

Parasitism

Parasitism is a host–parasite relationship detrimental to the host in the form of a disease.

The normal oral microbial flora has both detrimental and beneficial effects on the host, and these may vary depending on the microbial burden and functional host defence activity. The detrimental effects of the normal oral microflora on the host may be summarized as follows:

(1) Provide a source of endogenous infection when the host defence mechanisms are impaired, e.g. when poor oral hygiene results in excessive microbial overload.
(2) Predispose the host to an infection by an exogenous pathogen that could not itself otherwise have become established in the normal oral flora, e.g. by changing the local physical environment to facilitate exogenous microbial survival.[9]
(3) Host sensitization to oral microbial antigens, leading to an accentuated response to subsequent specific antigenic encounters.

The beneficial effects of the normal oral flora on the host include:

(1) Disease prevention by bacterial antagonism, nutrient competition, and/or inhibitory substance production, e.g. mucosal candidal overgrowth is often associated with antibiotic therapy-induced reduced oral microbial species.
(2) Host immune response stimulation.
(3) Essential nutrients provision required by the host, e.g. biotin, pathonate, pyridoxine, riboflavin and vitamin K, may be partly microbial in origin.
(4) Enhancement of renewal and maturation rates of host gastrointestinal epithelium.

The variability of the oral microflora is partly a reflection of the plethora of oral econiches. The intraoral temperature and pH are relatively stable at 37°C and 7 respectively, along with the general physical and nutritional environment. There are, however, detailed environmental differences between the component econiches of the oral cavity. These are associated with qualitative and quantitative variations in their respective resident microfloras.

When exogenous micro-organisms enter the oral cavity, they first make contact with saliva and then colonize the various oral surfaces (*Table 10.1*). If one of these surfaces cannot be colonized, then the particular micro-organism will be eliminated by swallowing. Adherence is therefore the first necessary prerequisite for microbial colonization. Adherence depends on a number of factors:

Table 10.1 Colonization criteria

Criterion	*Factors*
Adherence	Adsorption Contact Dose Frequency of exposure
Retention	Accumulation Adaptation Growth Reproduction

(1) *Contact:* contact between host and micro-organism must be sufficiently close for interactions to occur.
(2) *Dose:* a certain number of micro-organisms are required for colonization, e.g. *Streptococcus mutans* requires more cells to become adsorbed onto enamel than *S. sanguis.*[10]
(3) *Frequency of exposure:* this may influence the initial or subsequent colonization of certain microbial species.
(4) *Adsorption:* bacteria adsorb directly on the acquired pellicle, comprising salivary glycoprotein, rather than the actual surface of enamel.[11]

Subsequent microbial survival then depends on their adaptive capacity to both the particular econiche and to changes in such a niche. Changes in such econiches may result from a variety of factors including host defence products, microbial competition and changes resulting from their component microbial growth. Microbial succession is the term used to describe new microbial species superseding others, reflecting adaptive failure of the original flora. Subsequent oral microbial retention then depends on four intimately related factors: adaptation; growth; reproduction and accumulation.

The different intra-oral distributions of the various microbial genera suggest that microbial adsorption to the various oral surfaces (econiches) involve one of two specific mechanisms:[12]

(1) Oral micro-organisms may possess specific receptor sites on their cell surfaces or on their fibrillar appendages extending from the cell surfaces. These must then match up to complementary receptor sites on the colonized surface.[13] Such microbial receptor sites appear to be sensitive to proteolytic enzymatic degradation, whereas the complementary host receptor sites appear to be sensitive to lipases.[14] Whether these latter occur on both oral mucosal cells and/or acquired pellicle has yet to be confirmed.[15,16]
(2) There may be electrostatic interactions between the oral microflora and host tissues,[17] possibly involving calcium ions or hydrogen bonds bridging between negative charges on the acquired pellicle and microbial lipoteichoic acids.

These two theories may not be mutually exclusive, however, in that electrostatic attraction may be responsible for initial colonization, with specific receptor sites being involved in mature colonization.

The oral micro-organisms do not occur as discrete isolated entities but tend to aggregate together in varying clusters or colonies. Such microbial aggregation is mediated by a number of factors, including:

(1) Salivary components, e.g. oral streptococci agglutinate in the presence of secretory immunoglobulin A (sIgA) and high-molecular weight salivary mucoproteins.[18]
(2) Associations between specific receptor sites on oral microbial surfaces.[19,20]
(3) Microbial polymers, e.g. glucan-induced *S. mutans* agglutination.

There may also be other symbiotic and antagonistic associations between the constituent oral microbial flora, although such relationships have yet to be fully determined. As a result, the dental plaque is very complex and contains a wide variety of micro-organisms, including those with little or no specific affinity for the true host oral surfaces but colonizing on the pre-existing flora.

Following adsorption on to either an oral surface or other micro-organisms, their subsequent retention depends on continued metabolic and biosynthetic activity.[13] Only those species that can adjust their growth requirements to changing environmental conditions in a particular oral econiche are retained. Thus, the vast majority are quickly desorbed and eliminated by salivary lavage or epithelial cell desquammation.[13] Subsequent microbial growth will also depend on a variety of other factors, including:

(1) The diet of the host providing sufficient microbial nutrients.[3]
(2) Host-derived nutrients present in desquammated epithelial cells, gingival fluid and saliva.[4,5]

(3) Microbial interaction whereby the nutritional requirements of one microbial species are partially satisfied by metabolites and end-products of other oral species.

Each micro-organism colonizing a specific oral econiche alters the immediate chemical and physical environment by its own metabolism. The particular econiche may also be altered by the temperature, pH, oxidation–reduction potential and quality and quantity of gases. For example, a low pH caused by high acid concentrations may result in microbial shifts from an acidogenic to an aciduric flora, e.g. from streptococci to lactobacilli.

The environment of a particular econiche may also be affected by host-derived factors. For instance, acquired pellicle salivary glycoproteins[16] and salivary immunoglobulins (especially sIgA) may inhibit initial microbial colonization of specific oral econiches. For example, sIgA may combine with receptor sites on microbial surfaces, although the oral flora may circumvent such host defence mechanisms by altering their antigenic composition. Colonization may also be impeded by continual epithelial desquammation, in addition to the salivary lysozyme and lactoperoxidase–thiocyanate–hydrogen peroxide system.[3] Also, hydrogen peroxide, volatile fatty acids and protein toxins (bacteriocins) from other micro-organisms may inhibit microbial growth. The role of auto-inhibition wherein the oral floras liberate substances that control their own growth and survival has yet to be fully investigated.

The plaque microbial composition therefore undergoes constant flux, although there are some more retentive areas than others, e.g. occlusal fissures and pits, interproximal areas and the gingival sulcus. A more stable oral flora is established in such retentive areas.

Dental plaque

Dental plaque comprises a soft non-mineralized deposit of micro-organisms embedded in an adhesive glycoprotein and extracellular microbial polymer matrix. It is deposited on both the surface of the teeth and intra-oral prostheses. Dental caries and periodontal disease follow dental plaque accumulation, although both diseases are preventable by thorough and meticulous oral hygiene.

On initial eruption, the teeth are plaque free. Subsequently a salivary-derived glycoprotein film is deposited on their exposed surfaces. This is subsequently colonized by the oral flora. As more micro-organisms are adsorbed and retained on the tooth surface, the microbial colonies fuse together to form mature plaque. Muture dental plaque comprises approximately 80% water and 20% solids.[21] The major organic components comprise proteins (40–50%), carbohydrates (13–18%) and lipids (10–14%).[22]

The protein is both microbial and host in origin, the former comprising hyaluronidase and proteases, whereas host-derived salivary and gingival fluid proteins include sIgA, IgG, albumin, amylase and lysozyme. Plaque carbohydrates are mostly of microbial origin, including glucans produced by *Streptococcus mutans*. With patients consuming diets containing large quantities of sucrose, this facilitates microbial aggregation and surface colonization. In addition to such adhesive polymers, some oral micro-organisms synthesize extracellular levans. These may furnish sources of fermentable carbohydrates for micro-organisms embedded deep within the plaque.[23] Plaque microbial nutrition may also be augmented by salivary glycoprotein degradation.

The pathogenicity of dental plaque is dependent upon both the quality and quantity of its component microbial flora.[24] Early plaque comprises mainly Gram-positive cocci but this gradually gives way to a more filamentous Gram-positive flora. Subsequently plaque matures to contain a very complex microflora comprising a high proportion of Gram-negative micro-organisms. Once this climax community is established, it remains relatively stable unless there is a sudden environmental change.

The plaque microflora may elaborate a series of carbohydrate and protein catabolic products that can directly or indirectly cause dental carious or periodontal lesions to develop. For instance, plaque-derived lactic acid may result in enamel dissolution and cavity formation. Alternatively, the host defence mechanisms may be stimulated by plaque-derived products which indirectly result in periodontal disease.

Dental caries

Dental plaque develops on the tooth surface as the result of the succession of microbial populations which leads to a microbial community. The composition of this community will depend on two main factors:

(1) The ability of micro-organisms to colonize either the acquired pellicle covering enamel surfaces or other micro-organisms that have previously colonized the tooth surfaces.
(2) The ability of micro-organisms to grow on the surface in competition with the other members of the community.

Micro-organisms can be successful within the dental plaque community when they have special characteristics which either enable them to suppress their competitors, e.g. bacteriocins, or allow them to take advantage of an environmental feature, e.g. acidogenicity. In some situations one species may have such an advantage that it becomes a major component of the community in an econiche. This is termed dominance of one microbial species over others. The pathogenic potential of a species may be more obviously expressed when it is dominant than when it comprises a minor component of the community. In achieving dominance, the species may cause a reduction of, or even eliminate, other members of the community.

The species (or group of species) *Streptococcus mutans* is undoubtedly the most significant cariogenic micro-organism in the mouth. The genus Lactobacillus also has a significant cariogenic role, together with other micro-organisms to a lesser extent. Microbial dominance by itself may not necessarily be sufficient to cause a carious lesion; environmental factors also play a major role in the carious process, independent of micro-organisms.

Thus dental caries appears to be initiated by acid fermentation products, formed by plaque micro-organisms from dietary carbohydrates. The resultant acid demineralization of the enamel leads to the characteristic 'white spot' formation on the outer enamel surface. Such a spot frequently occurs on the approximal tooth surface. The subsequent fate of such an enamel white spot is that it may subsequently lead to cavity formation on the enamel surface, or it may be remineralized following plaque removal, rather than lead to cavity formation. The carious process is in fact very complex, being also influenced by two groups of host-associated factors: artificial and genetic.

Artificial factors

(1) Oral hygiene practice.
(2) Dietary consistency and composition (diets containing organically-bound or inorganic phosphates may reduce the incidence of caries, along with trace dietary molybdenum and vanadium); increasing the proportion of dietary fat may reduce the cariogenic effect of sugars, possibly by physical effect.
(3) Mouth breathing.
(4) Antibiotic therapy.
(5) Xerostomia.

Genetic factors

(1) Tooth morphology, including enamel composition, solubility and enamel fluoride composition; enamel hypoplasia or hypomineralization; deep occlusal fissures, pits.
(2) Dental overcrowding within the arch predisposing to plaque accumulation or inhibiting effective oral hygiene measures.
(3) Salivary composition including the presence of antimicrobial agents such as urea and lysozymes, buffering capacity, viscosity and flow rate.
(4) Immune host defence mechanisms.

The phenomena of microbial adherence and retention are important to dental caries, with some micro-organisms contributing to the retention of other non-adherent species or strains.[25] A pH lower than 5.5 at the tooth surface will result in enamel demineralization and such a critical pH may occur within 5 minutes following glucose exposure.[26] In the presence of dental plaque, acids formed by microbial carbohydrate metabolism accumulate more rapidly than they can be neutralized, further metabolized or removed by diffusion. In addition to causing enamel demineralization, acids may also facilitate further microbial adhesion to the tooth surface.[27] In fact, the acidogenic capacity of the dental plaque varies, depending on the component microbial flora in addition to dietary composition.

The plaque microflora varies between different sites of the mouth and even between different locations on a tooth. This suggests that a degree of microbial specificity may be involved in the aetiology of different forms of carious lesions. For instance, root surface caries is predominantly associated with Actinomyces,[28] whereas deep dentinal caries shows a predominance of Lactobacillus organisms, along with several other species of Gram-positive rods and filaments and sometimes Gram-positive cocci.[29] The extent of the microbial aetiology of carious lesions is, however, beyond the scope of this chapter, and the reader is referred to Nolte,[30] Newbrun[31] and Menaker.[32] It is sufficient to state that the carious lesions may be classified by site of attack into:

(1) *Pit* or *fissure* caries that primarily affects the occlusal surfaces of molar and bicuspid teeth and the lingual surface of the maxillary incisors.
(2) *Smooth surface* caries that occurs on the proximal surfaces and gingival third of the buccal and lingual surfaces.
(3) *Cemental (root)* caries that occurs following cemental exposure associated with chronic periodontal disease.
(4) *Recurrent* caries that occurs at the margin or base of previously existing restorations.

Alternatively, carious lesions may be classified by the rate of progression into the following:

(1) *Acute (rampant)* caries, whereby there is rapid caries even on those tooth surfaces that are normally immune to such lesions: the rapid coronal destruction leads to early pulp involvement.
(2) *Chronic (slowly progressive)* caries: this slow carious progression allows time for dentinal sclerosis and secondary dentine formation.

(3) *Arrested* caries, whereby enamel or dentinal caries shows little or no tendency for progression.

The concentrated localization of micro-organisms on the tooth surface results in the placement of a large amount of metabolic potential at sites where interactions with ingested substrates can readily occur. In the anaerobic environment of plaque, the fermentative capacity of the micro-organisms is not only localized but very efficient in converting dietary carbohydrates to acidic metabolic end-products. Thus, plaque has the capacity to convert carbohydrates to acids very rapidly. This leads to a sudden drop in pH. As the plaque pH falls, a concentration of acid will eventually be reached that will cause demineralization of enamel adjacent to the plaque. This critical pH is somewhere in the range of pH 6.0–5.0, although this value may vary between different tooth surfaces depending on the complexity of local factors. The production of acid by dental plaque favours the survival of certain oral microflora and the elimination of others. With the passage of time and repeated rounds of acid production, a highly acidogenic and aciduric microbial population is selected. This may dominate the mature plaque microbial community in some patients. Thus *Streptococcus mutans* and Lactobacillus have been implicated as the predominant cariogenic micro-organisms, and assays of these micro-organisms may soon be used to indicate the future caries potential of a particular patient.

The reader is referred to standard textbooks of oral pathology for the pathology of the carious process in enamel, dentine and cementum.

Periodontal disease

Periodontal disease is a collective term. It embraces a number of pathological (mainly inflammatory) states of the cementum, gingiva, periodontal ligament and alveolar bone (*Table 10.2*). Inflammatory destruction of these tissues ultimately leads to tooth loosening and exfoliation. There are therefore many forms of periodontal disease, although there is much confusion caused by their varying forms of classification (*Table 10.3*). These classifications are beyond the scope of this book. From an oral physiological viewpoint, periodontal diseases may be categorized thus:

(1) Acute and chronic gingivitis.
(2) Acute necrotizing ulcerative gingivitis (ANUG).
(3) Adult chronic or rapidly destructive periodontitis.
(4) Adult generalized and localized juvenile periodontitis (periodontosis).

It is firmly established that supragingival plaque causes gingivitis and that the active pathogenic agent in dental plaque is microbial in origin (*Tables 10.4–10.6*). Although plaque formation in man is

Table 10.2 Classification of periodontal inflammatory lesions

Lesion	*Classification*
Gingivitis	Acute Chronic Acute necrotizing ulcerative

Periodontitis	Adult
	  Chronic
	  Rapidly destructive
	Adolescent
	  Generalized
	  Localized juvenile (periodontosis)

Table 10.3 Specific bacteria associated with various forms of periodontal disease

Periodontal disease	*Micro-organism(s)*
Adult periodontitis	*Bacteroides gingivalis*
Localized juvenile periodontitis (periodontosis)	*Actinobacillus actinomycetemcomitans*, Capnocytophaga
Periodontitis in juvenile diabetics	Capnocytophaga, *Actinobacillus actinomycetemcomitans*
Periodontitis in granulocytopenic hosts	Capnocytophaga
Gingivitis in pregnancy	*Bacteroides intermedius*
Acute necrotizing ulcerative gingivitis	*Bacteroides intermedius*, intermediate-sized spirochaetes

Table 10.4 Characteristics of subgingival plaque

Subgingival plaque	*Characteristics*
Attached zone	Gram-positive microflora Not extended to junctional epithelium Not in contact with gingival sulcular epithelium Periodontopathic microbial content Associated with calculus formation areas Root surface caries Continuous with supragingival plaque
Unattached zone	Gram-negative microflora In contact with gingival sulcular and junctional epithelia Periodontopathic microbial content The 'advancing front' of the periodontal lesion

Table 10.5 Effect of subgingival products

Microbial product	*Effect*
Hydrolytic enzymes	
Collagenase, Proteases, Hyaluronidase, Fibrinolysin, Chondroitin sulphatase	Pathological alterations of periodontal tissues
Bacterial envelope components	
Endotoxin	Complement activation, inflammation
Mucopeptides	Complement activation, inflammation hypersensitivity
Lipoteichoic acids	Hypersensitivity, stimulation of bone resorption, inflammation
Capsules	Inhibition of phagocytosis, facilitation of adherence
Metabolic end-products	
Organic acids, Hydrogen sulphide, Indole	Toxic to gingival tissue cells
Ammonia	
Toxins	
Leucotoxin	Cytolytic for neutrophils and monocytes
Antineutrophil factor	Dysfunctions in neutrophil chemotaxis

ubiquitous, there are strong indications that microbial colonization of teeth and gingivae is characterized by a certain degree of selectivity, and the establishment of particular microbial species is associated with different periodontal disease states. Thus, the microflora of subgingival plaque associated with chronic gingivitis differs from the microbial composition of plaque associated with gingiva in health. The supragingival plaques associated with slow-developing loss of periodontal attachment and periodontal pocket formation are significantly different from the supragingival varieties of plaque. All supragingival plaques have been found to elicit inflammatory reactions in the gingiva. There is, however, ample evidence to show that absence of plaque is consistent with gingival health and a reduction of dental plaque may be associated with a reduction of gingivitis. Thus good oral care, combined with professional cleaning and/or the use of antimicrobial compounds, can control dental plaque and therefore prevent periodontal disease.

Generally, the initial gingival lesion is confined to the tissues of the marginal gingiva and does not involve the periodontal ligament or alveolar bone. Gingivitis, therefore, represents the initial (and often reversible) clinical stage in the development of a periodontal lesion. Progressive destruction of connective tissue and alveolar bone only occurs in areas exhibiting overt gingivitis. This does not suggest that all gingivitis proceeds to periodontitis. In fact, in some cases, long-standing inflamed gingiva may be quite compatible with the normal maintenance of periodontal attachment and alveolar bone levels. The questions to be asked therefore include:

(1) Why do some gingival lesions progress to advanced lesions, and others do not?
(2) What are the microbial and/or host mechanisms responsible for the progression of the periodontal lesion during adult life?
(3) What factors determine the progression and remission of gingivitis and periodontal disease?

The multifactorial aetiology of periodontal disease involves an interaction between the periodontal microflora and the defence mechanisms of the host, albeit modified by certain predisposing conditions. The primary aetiological agent for all forms of periodontal disease centres on the subgingival microflora, which is derived from the dental plaque. These micro-organisms produce lytic enzymes, metabolic end-products and antigenic components that are either potentially harmful or initiate damage to the periodontium.[33] Thus micro-organisms in the dental plaque, which accumulate at the gingival margin, cause the early forms of gingivitis and also possibly slow-moving periodontitis, although unusual forms of gingivitis and rapidly advancing forms of periodontal disease are probably associated with specific micro-organisms (or combinations of micro-organisms) found mainly in the subgingival microflora. In fact, a number of diseases of the periodontium have been associated with a specific microbial aetiology.[34,35] Many of the specific micro-organisms associated with periodontal disease are Gram-negative anaerobes, which cause

Table 10.6 Contrasts between subgingival and supragingival plaques

Property	*Subgingival plaque*	*Supragingival plaque*
Cleansing	None	Saliva and abrasion
Retention	Mechanical	Attachment
Metabolism	Carbohydrate and protein	Mostly carbohydrate
Environment	Facultative and anaerobic	Aerobic and facultative
Motile micro-organisms	Many	Few
Host defences	Crevicular fluid	Saliva

periodontal destruction. These micro-organisms are also virulent when they enter the body and affect tissues other than the periodontal tissues, e.g. *Actinobacillus actinomycetemcomitans* has been associated with subacute bacterial endocarditis and brain abscesses; *Bacteroides gingivalis* may cause brain and lung abscesses in addition to dissecting infections of the head and neck. This means that the host defence mechanisms must usually be very effective in localizing and confining these potentially serious pathogens to the periodontal tissues, preventing their spreading to other areas of the body where they may cause fulminating and possibly fatal infections. The result of these host responses is often the localized destruction of the gingiva and alveolar bone support, which together are termed periodontal disease. The net effect of such host responses to the organisms causing periodontal infections is, however, protection from serious systemic infection with these organisms.

Table 10.7 Host responses operative in the pathogenesis of periodontal diseases

Disease stage	*Host factors*
Colonization	Antibody-mediated inhibition of adherence; sIgA, and gingival fluid antibodies prevent adherence and co-adherence
Invasion	Neutrophil chemotaxis, phagocytosis, and bactericidal activity, with opsonic effects of antibody protect against periodontal infections. Macrophage bactericidal activity and extracellular killing may also be protective
Destruction	(1) Toxic effects on tissues of lymphocytes and macrophages exerted via lymphokines and toxic macrophage products such as collagenase and reactive oxygen species (2) Direct toxic effects of bacteria controlled by antibodies which neutralize toxins and enzymes
Healing	(1) Lymphocytes and macrophages produce fibroblast chemotactic factors and fibroblast activating factors which result in repair of connective tissue and epithelium (2) Bacteria and bacterial products removed by phagocytes

Stages of periodontal disease

Recent research data and investigation has led to the categorization of several stages of periodontal disease.[34,35] These stages are, however, not discrete entities but merge one with another. Also the time sequence of each of these stages is complex. Microbial colonization must precede all other stages but microbial tissue invasion and tissue destruction may occur together. Microbial tissue invasion may be transient, immediately preceding the tissue destructive phase. Alternatively, tissue invasion may be continuous, resulting in progressive periodontal destruction. The healing stage is, however, distinct from microbial colonization and tissue invasion, and terminates tissue destruction. Such complex changes may be occurring at different stages, even in the periodontium of a single tooth (*Tables 10.7, 10.8*).

Table 10.8 Components of the immune system affecting periodontal infections

System	*Main function(s) in periodontal diseases*	*Cells*	*Humoral components*	*Mediators*
Secretory immune	Reduce bacterial colonization of mucosal surfaces	Mucosal-associated lymphoid tissues (eg. Peyer's Patch) and local IgA-plasma cells	Secretory antibodies, mainly sIgA	—
Neutrophil–antibody–complement	Bacterial, also secretory, producing extracellular enzymes and reactive oxygen species	Neutrophils	IgG antibodies, complement, especially C3	Bactericidal activity, mediated by reactive oxygen species, and granule components
Lymphocyte–macrophage–lymphokine	Tissue destruction	T and B effector cells, macrophages and monocytes	—	Lymphokines (LT, OAF, I 1, I 2), macrophage enzymes (eg. collagenase), and reactive oxygen species

Colonization

A salivary pellicle is initially deposited on to the enamel or cemental surface, which soon becomes colonized by micro-organisms, e.g. *Streptococcus sanguis* binds both specifically and non-specifically to the pellicle-coated surface by adherence. Also, other micro-organisms bind to these initial plaque forms by co-adherence. Co-adherence may be:

(1) Intergenic, in which cells of different microbial species bind to one another.
(2) Intragenic, in which cells of the same genus or species bind to each other.

Once attached to the tooth surface, organisms proliferate apically, reflecting both microbial growth and apical migration. The gingival fluid contains growth factors, which:

(1) Facilitate microbial development and chemotactic factors.
(2) Direct micro-organisms to migrate into the gingival crevice or periodontal pocket, e.g. spirochaetes.

The micro-organisms' motility also contributes to their migration down the side of the tooth, e.g. gliding action of Capnocytophaga or the flagella of anaerobic vibrios.

Invasion

In this stage, either the whole organism and/or its products invade the gingiva through the sulcus or periodontal pocket epithelium and pass to the adjacent connective tissues, including alveolar bone.[36,37] Such invasion implies that microbial antigens must penetrate or adhere to the tissues, thereby stimulating an immune response. Indeed, the connective tissues underlying the gingival crevice and pocket epithelium exhibit a marked inflammatory cell migration, further disrupting their normal histological appearance. Since these microbial antigens penetrate the tissue, it is likely that other molecules, e.g. collagenase and endotoxins, also penetrate the gingival and pocket epithelium, conceivably as a consequence of epithelial disruption and ulceration.

Destruction

Once the micro-organisms and/or their products have penetrated the gingival crevicular epithelium, further tissue destruction occurs. Such tissue destruction may result from:

(1) Direct microbial toxic effects due to:
 (a) exotoxins;
 (b) endotoxins;
 (c) histolytic enzymes, e.g. collagenase.
(2) Indirect (host-mediated) effects due to:
 (a) endotoxin-triggering of macrophages to produce collagenases;
 (b) endotoxin-triggering of cellular immune responses to release lymphokines, e.g. lymphotoxin kills fibroblasts.

Healing

At the same time that tissue destruction is occurring in the subepithelial gingival crevicular tissues, there is also inflammatory resolution and periodontal tissue healing.

Characteristically, healing and destruction occur simultaneously. This is reflected by periodontal disease being characterized by periods of remission and exacerbation. Periods of remission are characterized by the reduction of inflammation, the restoration of gingival collagenous tissues and fibrosis (scarring) of the subepithelial tissues. These periods of exacerbation and remission reflect the dynamic balance between the microbial burden and the host defence mechanisms.

Host defence mechanisms

One of the major components of the host defence mechanisms in periodontal disease centres on the immune system. In fact, the following components of the immune system are implicated.

Secretory immune system

The secretory immune system comprises mucosal associated lymphoid tissues (e.g. local IgA-containing tissue, Peyer's patches), with the IgA antibodies comprising prominent antibodies in the secretions which bathe the mucosal surfaces.

In the microbial colonization stage, antibody-mediated inhibition of adherence may play a role in influencing the microbial content of both dental plaque and the subgingival microflora. Initially, such defence mechanisms may centre around sIgA antibodies from saliva, although serum-derived and gingival crevicular fluid antibodies may subsequently influence the gingival microflora. Such antibody activity may include disruption of colonization, microbial aggregation or enhancement of microbial phagocytosis.

Neutrophil–antibody–complement system

The neutrophil–antibody–complement system comprises phagocytic blood and tissue polymorphonuclear leucocytes (PMNs) which are not only highly motile but also migrate in large numbers from the gingival blood vessels, through the gingival connective tissues and epithelium into the gingival crevice or periodontal pockets, and so to the oral cavity. In fact, the majority of the cells of crevicular fluid comprise PMNs and these serve as powerful host defence mechanisms to combat the colonization and invasion by the oral microbial flora. The PMNs do not work in isolation, however, but in concert with IgG or IgM antibodies and complement. The IgG antibody coats the micro-organism, and the IgG-coated micro-organism then binds to PMN surface receptors for the Fc portion of the IgG to enhance phagocytosis. IgM, and to some extent IgG, antibodies may also coat the micro-organisms. When this occurs, the coated micro-organisms bind components of the complement system, particularly the third component. The result is enhanced phagocytosis of the complement-coated micro-organism, compared with phagocytosis of the non-coated micro-organism. Once the micro-organism has been phagocytosed by the PMN it can be killed by:

(1) *Oxidative mechanisms:* these involve reactive oxygen species, e.g. hydrogen peroxide, superoxide ion, hydroxyl radicals. (Catalase produced by either the micro-organisms or PMNs inhibit the peroxide effects, whereas myeloperoxidase may enhance hydrogen peroxide microbial lysis in the presence of chloride.)
(2) *Non-oxidative mechanisms:* these important mechanisms result from PMN-derived lysozyme, lactoferrin and cathepsins which kill micro-organisms directly in the absence of oxygen, i.e. under anaerobic conditions which typify the gingival crevice and particularly the periodontal pocket.

The neutrophil–antibody–complement axis appears to function primarily to limit microbial tissue invasion,[38,39] although the virulence of the oral microflora may result in their evasion of such defence mechanisms.

Lymphocyte–macrophage–lymphokine system

The lymphocyte–macrophage–lymphokine axis mainly comprises effector T lymphocytes, whose functions include the following:

(1) T helper and T suppressor lymphocytes regulate T effector cell activity and antibody production by B lymphocytes.
(2) T lymphocyte modulation of macrophage activity.
(3) Specific lymphocyte stimulation by antigens or non-specific lymphocyte stimulation by mitogens. This results in lymphokine production (*Table 10.9*), which includes:
   (a) osteoclast activating factor (OAF); lymphotoxin (LT) which results in fibroblastic necrosis;
   (b) macrophage activating factor (MAF) which not only enhances macrophagic phagocytosis function but also the release of interleukin 1 and macrophagic enzymes and reactive-oxygen species which cause tissue destruction.

Table 10.9 Lymphokines and periodontal disease

Lymphokine	*Action*
Mononuclear phagocyte chemotactic factor (CF)	Macrophage localization
Migration inhibition factor (MIF)	Macrophage localization
Macrophage activation factor (MAF)	Increased macrophage aggression
Lymphotoxin	Cytotoxic for gingival fibroblasts
Lymphocyte inhibitory factor	T cell suppression
Osteoclast activating factor (OAF)	Osteoclastic bone resorption
Interferon	Inhibition of viral replication

The lymphocyte–macrophage–lymphokine axis has a potential to exert marked pathological effects on the host tissues. For instance, antigenic or mitogenic lymphocytic stimulation may result in the release of lymphotoxin to kill fibroblasts, and osteoclast activating factor to result in alveolar bone resorption.[35] Microbial or lymphokine (interleukin 2) macrophagic stimulation may result in the release of collagenase and reactive-oxygen species, both capable of resulting in marked tissue destruction.

The healing stage of periodontal disease may be associated with macrophagic phagocytosis of micro-organisms and tissue debris, whereas there are also lymphokines, e.g. fibroblast activating factor, that stimulate both fibroblastic proliferation and collagen formation.

The reader is referred to standard textbooks of periodontology and oral pathology for the pathology of periodontal disease and gingivitis.

Calculus

Calculus is mineralization of the dental plaque. It is a facet of the complex regulatory systems involved in maintaining oral calcium and phosphorus homeostasis. Such homeostatic mechanisms centre on the encouragement of remineralization rather than demineralization. Usually, this is achieved without provoking an undue deposition of calculus on the tooth crowns. In the main, this mission is carried out effectively, which may also be a reflection of efficient oral hygiene limiting dental plaque formation. In some individuals, particularly where oral hygiene measures are less than adequate, the plaque deposits become calcified. Thus, calculus tends to accumulate on those tooth surfaces opposite the salivary glands, i.e. the lingual aspect of the mandibular incisors and the buccal aspect of the maxillary molars. It has, however, still to be unequivocally determined that the presence of such mineralized calculus deposits results in a greater degree of gingivitis compared with other regions of the same patient's mouth.[40] Calculus may affect the supra- and subgingival plaque. Further, it is generally held that supragingival calculus leads to exacerbation of periodontal disease by the retention of new plaque accumulations. Certainly the generally porous nature of calculus deposits tends to favour microbial toxic product retention. This suggests that calculus has an active, rather than a passive, aetiologic role in periodontal disease.[41] In addition, supra- and subgingival calculus tend to limit natural self-cleansing mechanisms, to make oral hygiene more difficult and to impede crevicular drainage.

Professional calculus removal may be required to remove both the increased microbial burden of supra- and subgingival calculus and the source of mechanical irritation to facilitate the return and/or maintenance of gingival health. Supra- and subgingival calculus deposits may also result in mechanical displacement of the adjacent junctional epithelium. Moreover, since the toxic stimulators of bone resorption produced by microbial plaque have a finite radius of function,[42] mineralization of dental plaque may serve to extend the radius of alveolar bone destruction from the overlying dental plaque.

Conclusions

Dental plaque is detrimental to the health of the host, not only in the initiation of dental caries and periodontal diseases, but also in providing the potential for serious systemic and local infections. Obviously, the principal actions of the immune system function to protect the host tissues, although these defence mechanisms are also responsible for periodontal destruction.

Review questions

1. Why might the accumulation of calculus be associated with severe periodontal tissue destruction in some patients and not in others?
2. What is the evidence for periodontal disease being of infective aetiology?
3. Describe the host defence mechanisms against the oral microflora.
4. What are the differences between the dental plaque in different sites of the same oral cavity?
5. What is calculus?

References

1. RITZ, H.L. (1967) Microbial population shifts in developing human dental plaque. *Arch. Oral Biol.*, **12**, 1561–1568
2. GIBBONS, R.J. and VAN HOUTE, J. (1973) On the formation of dental plaques. *J. Periodontol.*, **44**, 347–360
3. GIBBONS, R.J. and VAN HOUTE, J. (1975) Bacterial adherence in oral microbial ecology. *Annu. Rev. Microbiol.*, **29**, 19–44
4. CIMASONI, G. (1974) The crevicular fluid. In *Monographs in Oral Science*, edited by H.M. Meyer, Vol 3. Basel: S. Karger
5. LOESCHE, W.J. (1968) Importance of nutrition in gingival crevice microbial ecology. *Periodontics*, **6**, 245–249
6. LOESCHE, W.J. (1969) Oxygen sensitivity of various anaerobic bacteria. *Appl. Microbiol.*, **18**, 723–727
7. KENNEY, E.B. and ASH, M.M. (1969) Oxidation reduction potential of developing plaque, periodontal pockets and gingival sulci. *J. Periodontol.*, **40**, 630–633
8. SOCRANSKY, S.S. (1977) Microbiology of periodontal disease – present status and future considerations. *J. Periodontol.*, **48**, 497–504
9. PLAUT, A.G., GENCO, R.J. and TOMASI, T.B. (1974) Production of an Fc fragment from human immunoglobulin A by an IgA-specific bacterial protease. *Adv. Exp. Med. Biol.*, **45**, 245–249
10. VAN HOUTE, J. and GREEN, D.B. (1974) Relationship between concentration of bacteria in saliva and the colonization of teeth in humans. *Infect. Immun.*, **11**, 711–718
11. MAYHALL, C.W. (1970) Concerning the composition and source of the acquired pellicle in human teeth. *Arch. Oral Biol.*, **15**, 1327–1341
12. GIBBONS, R.J., SPINELL, D.M. and SKOBE, Z. (1976) Selective adherence as a determinant of the host tropism of certain indigenous and pathogenic bacteria. *Infect. Immun.*, **13**, 238–246
13. GIBBONS, R.J. and VAN HOUTE, J. (1973) On the formation of dental plaques. *J. Periodontol.*, **44**, 347–360
14. GIBBONS, R.J., VAN HOUTE, J. and LILJEMARK, W.F. (1972) Parameters that affect the adherence of *Streptococcus salivarius* to oral epithelial surfaces. *J. Dent. Res.*, **51**, 424–435
15. STAAT, R.H., LANGLEY, S.D. and DOYLE, R.J. (1980) *Streptococcus mutans* adherence: presumptive evidence for protein-mediated attachment followed by glucan-dependent cellular accumulation. *Infect. Immun.*, **27**, 675–681
16. WILLIAMS, R.C. and GIBBONS, R.J. (1975) Inhibition of streptococcal attachment to receptors on human buccal epithelial cells by antigenically similar salivary glycoproteins. *Infect. Immun.*, **11**, 711–718
17. ROLLA, G. (1977) Formation of dental integuments–some basic chemical considerations. *Swed. Dent. J.*, **1**, 241–251

18. HAMADA, S. and SLADE, H.D. (1980) Biology, immunology and cariogenicity of *Streptococcus mutans*. *Microbiol. Rev.*, **44**, 331–384
19. GIBBONS, R.J. and NYGAARD, M. (1970) Interbacterial aggregation of plaque bacteria. *Arch. Oral Biol.*, **15**, 1397–1400
20. MILLER, C.H. and KLEINMAN, J.L. (1974) Effect of microbiological interactions on *in vivo* plaque formation by *Streptococcus mutans*. *J. Dent. Res.*, **53**, 427–434
21. HOTZ, P., GUGGENHEIM, B. and SCHMID, R. (1972) Carbohydrates in pooled dental plaque. *Caries Res.*, **6**, 103–121
22. SHARMA, M.L. and NEWBURN, E. (1974) Chemical composition of the washed cells of *Streptococcus sanguis* (804) and *Streptococcus mutans* (B-14). *J. Dent. Res.*, **54**, 482–486
23. SCHACHTELE, C.F., LOKEN, A.E. and SCHMITT, M.K. (1972) Use of specifically labelled sucrose for comparison of extracellular glucan and fructan metabolism by oral streptococci. *Infect. Immun.*, **5**, 263–266
24. THEILADE, E. and THEILADE, J. (1976) Role of plaque in the etiology of periodontal disease and caries. *Oral Sci. Rev.*, **9**, 23–63
25. RUSSELL, C. and AHMED, F.I.K. (1978) Interrelationships between lactobacilli and streptococci in plaque formation on a tooth in an artificial mouth. *J. Appl. Bacteriol.*, **45**, 373–382
26. STEPHAN, R.M. (1944) Intra-oral hydrogen-ion concentrations associated with dental caries activity. *J. Dent. Res.*, **23**, 257–266
27. OLSSON, F.J. and GLANTZ, P.O. (1977) Effect of pH and counter ions on the zeta-potential of oral streptococci. *Arch. Oral Biol.*, **22**, 461–466
28. SYED, S.A., LOESCHE, W.J., PAPE, H.L. and GRENIER, E. (1975) Predominant cultivatable flora from human root surface caries plaque. *Infect. Immun.*, **11**, 727–731
29. EDWARDSSON, S. (1974) Bacteriological studies on deep areas of carious dentine. *Odontol. Revy*, **25**, Suppl. 32
30. NOLTE, W.A. (1977) *Oral Microbiology*, 3rd ed. St Louis: C.V. Mosby
31. NEWBURN, E. (1978) *Cariology*. Baltimore: Williams & Wilkins
32. MENAKER, L. (1980) *The Biologic Basis of Dental Caries*. New York: Harper & Row
33. SOCRANSKY, S.S. (1970) Relationship of bacteria to the etiology of periodontal disease. *J. Dent. Res.*, **49**, 497–504
34. SLOTS, J. and GENCO, R.J. (1984) Black-pigmented Bacteroides species, Capnocytophaga species and *Actinobacillus actinomycetemcomitans* in human periodontal disease. *J. Dent. Res.*, **63**, 412
35. GENCO, R.J. and SLOTS, J. (1984) Host responses in periodontal diseases. *J. Dent. Res.*, **63**, 441
36. GILLETT, R. and JOHNSON, N.W. (1982) Bacterial invasion of the periodontium in a case of juvenile periodontitis. *J. Clin. Periodontol.*, **9**, 93–100
37. SLOTS, J. (1979) Subgingival microflora and periodontal disease. *J. Clin. Periodontol.*, **6**, 351–382
38. VAN DYKE, T.E., LEVINE, M.J. and GENCO, R.J. (1984) Neutrophil function and oral disease. *J. Oral Pathol.*, **14**, 95–120
39. CIANCIOLA, L.J., GENCO, R.J., PATTERS, M.R., MCKENNA, J. and VAN OSS C.J. (1977) Defective polymorphonuclear leukocyte function in a human periodontal disease. *Nature*, **265**, 445–447
40. SCHROEDER, H.E. (1969) *Formation and Inhibition of Dental Calculus*. Vienna: Hans Huber
41. SCHWARTZ, H.E. and LINDHE, J. (1975) Conversion of stable established gingivitis in the dog into destructive periodontitis. *Arch. Oral Biol.*, **20**, 775–782
42. WAERHAUG, J. (1979) The infrabony pocket and its relationship to trauma from occlusion and subgingival plaque. *J. Periodontol.*, **50**, 355–365

11

Nutrition

Introduction

In this world, avoidance or reduction of calorie consumption is the focus for vast segments of society, while many less fortunate populations are dying from lack of food.[1] Half of all deaths in these starving populations occur in children under five years of age. For optimal health, 45–48 dietary nutrients are currently considered essential, including:

(1) Vitamins.
(2) Nine amino acids – lysine, threonine, leucine, isoleucine, methionine, tryptophan, valine, phenylalanine, and histidine.
(3) Two polyunsaturated fatty acids – linoleic and arachidonic acid.
(4) A large number of elements, including sodium, potassium, calcium, magnesium, phosphorus, chlorine, sulphur, carbon, hydrogen, oxygen, iron and nitrogen.
(5) A number of trace elements, including zinc, copper, iodine, cobalt, molybdenum, selenium, vanadium, nickel, silicon, fluorine, tin and arsenic.[2]

Nutritional diseases may be primary or secondary in origin (*Table 11.1*). Primary malnutrition is caused by lack of a reasonably balanced diet, and is largely a socio-economic problem that tends to be endemic in the underprivileged and war-torn regions of the world, e.g. Africa, Asia, Central and South America. Even in Western societies, however, primary malnutrition may occur in poverty-stricken families. Secondary, or conditioned, malnutrition is usually a sporadic condition that arises in the midst of dietary plenty. In fact, secondary malnutrition may reflect a number of factors, including:

(1) Aberrant or fad diets (e.g. chronic alcoholism).
(2) Increased metabolic requirements (e.g. during puberty, pregnancy).
(3) Inability to ingest or absorb diet (e.g. inadequate dentition, severe gastrointestinal disease).
(4) Impaired utilization (e.g. uncontrolled diabetes mellitus).
(5) Excessive losses (e.g. profuse sweating, diarrhoea).
(6) Drug therapy (e.g. oral contraceptive medication may result in increased vitamin B_6 requirements and folic acid metabolic impairment).

Protein–energy malnutrition

Marasmus/Kwashiorkor

Protein–energy malnutrition is a global problem of staggering dimensions. Although all ages may be affected, infants and children exhibit the major manifestations. Two forms are manifested.

Table 11.1 Effects of nutritional deficiencies

Deficiency	*Effect*
Calories	Underweight, underheight, weight loss, lethargy, anaemia, oedema, marasmus
Protein	As above; fatty liver, kwashiorkor
Fat	Dermatoses in infants, deficiencies of the fat soluble vitamins, A, D, E, and K
Water	Thirst, dehydration, oliguria, mental changes progressing to coma
Inorganic	
Iron	Anaemia, achlorhydria, glossitis
Iodine	Simple goitre
Fluorine	Dental caries
Calcium	Osteomalacia; a role in the production of senile osteoporosis has been suggested but not proved
Magnesium	Neuromuscular irritability, tetany
Potassium	Alkalosis, muscle weakness and paralysis, cardiac disturbances
Salt (NaCl)	Anorexia, nausea, vomiting, lassitude, asthenia, muscle cramps, circulatory collapse
Vitamins	
Vitamin A	Growth failure, follicular hyperkeratosis, night blindness, xerophthalmia, keratomalacia
Vitamin D	Rickets, tetany, osteomalacia
Vitamin K	Decreased plasma prothrombin activity with prolonged coagulation time and haemorrhages
Thiamine	Anorexia, beriberi, polyneuropathy, toxic amblyopia, heart disease, the ophthalmoplegia of Wernicke's syndrome
Riboflavin	Photophobia, corneal vascularization, angular stomatitis, glossitis, dermatitis
Niacin	Pellagra, dermatitis, glossitis, diarrhoea, mental confusion and deterioration, encephalopathy
Pyridoxine	Anaemia, convulsions, polyneuropathy, seborrhoeic eczema
Pantothenic acid	Nutritional melalgia
Folic acid	Glossitis, achrestic anaemia, megaloblastic anaemia of infancy, megaloblastic anaemia of pregnancy, nutritional macrocytic anaemia, sprue
Vitamin B_{12}	Glossitis, macrocytic anaemia, peripheral neuropathy, combined system disease – mental changes and deterioration
Biotin	Seborrhoeic dermatitis
Choline, inositol and carnitine	Unknown
Ascorbic acid	Scurvy, gingivitis, subperiosteal haemorrhages, petechial haemorrhages, anaemia, impaired wound healing

Marasmus

Marasmus is the consequence of a deficiency in total calories and is encountered in mild-to-severe starvation. Adipose tissue and muscle are lost in a graduated fashion. The marasmic child is obviously wasted, with the face wizened, imparting a prematurely aged appearance. In contrast to kwashiorkor, the children remain alert and hungry, and will eat ravenously if given food.

Kwashiorkor

Kwashiorkor is the consequence of a relative or absolute protein deficiency, despite sometimes adequate total calories. The clinical manifestations vary, but include growth failure, oedema, liver enlargement due to the fat accumulation, anaemia, hair changes and dermatoses. The child is often apathetic and anorexic, withdrawn and irritable. The oedema may be generalized or localized to the upper or lower extremities. There is always hypoalbuminaemia, and a reduction in total serum protein. It has been suggested that along with the loss of serum albumin, there is a concomitant loss of trace elements, of which vanadium may be involved in the regulation of water and sodium metabolism.[3] A change in skin pigmentation, in addition to scaling, may occur, although the associated anaemia (normocytic, normochromic type) may be particularly important.

Controvesy persists as to whether clinical and anatomical changes induced by protein–energy malnutrition are totally reversible with the restoration of a normal diet. There is a general consensus that dietary impairment in infancy or early childhood may result in irreversible impairment in the level of intellectual performance and attainment,[4] i.e. protein–energy malnutrition during the early growth phases may have long-lasting consequences.

Vitamins

Water-soluble vitamins

Thiamine

Thiamine deficiency principally damages the nervous system (dry beriberi) and the cardiovascular system (wet beriberi). The vitamin is a highly water soluble nutrient, comprising a substituted pyrimidine linked to a substituted thiazole by a methylene bridge. It is widely distributed in the cells, where it undergoes phosphorylation into the co-enzyme thiamine pyrophosphate, also known as co-carboxylase. In this form, it participates in the oxidative decarboxylation of α-keto acids. The pyrophosphate is also a cofactor for the enzyme transketolase, which is the key component of the pentose pathway of carbohydrate metabolism. In addition, thiamine, or its derivatives, may participate in neural conduction by mechanisms independent of its enzymatic functions. The vitamin or its esters can be found in axonal membranes of nerves.

Thiamine is widely available in a variety of foods, with absorption mainly occurring through the upper intestinal tract. Absorption is unaffected by most intestinal disorders, except those that produce severe anorexia and vomiting or marked gastrointestinal hypermobility. A primary deficiency state of thiamine is mainly encountered where populations subsist largely on polished rice or milled grains from which the vitamin has been depleted by removal of the outer husks. In addition, thiamine deficiency is encountered in alcoholics, and in renal dialysis patients. In thiamine deficiency, pyruvic acid tends to accumulate, which may itself be toxic and damage neurones and nerve trunks. Alternatively, nervous tissues are heavily dependent on carbohydrate for energy requirements, and so may suffer because of the important role of thiamine pyrophosphate in carbohydrate metabolism. The basis of the associated myocardial injuries are obscure.

Beriberi may occur in a chronic or subacute form, usually dominated by involvement of the nervous system or in an acute, virtually fulminating, form, dominated by cardiovascular manifestations. Neurological manifestations without cardiac decompensation and peripheral oedema constitute dry beriberi. This syndrome is manifested by numbness and tingling of the legs, sensory disturbances in the affected parts, atrophy and weakness of the muscles of the extremities, depression and loss of reflexes. Such neuropathy is most often encountered in malnourished chronic alcoholics. Cardiovascular involvement of thiamine deficiency may lead to peripheral vasodilatation, which, in some cases, is followed by myocardial failure and peripheral oedema (wet beriberi). The peripheral oedema is usually striking, especially in the lower extremities, although the trunk, face and body cavities may also be involved.

Riboflavin

Riboflavin is widely distributed in both plant and animal foods as riboflavin, riboflavin phosphate or as a constituent of the flavoproteins. Ariboflavinosis occurs in economically deprived developing countries and is frequently accompanied by other vitamin and protein deficiencies. In industrialized countries, a deficiency is most likely to occur in alcoholics, and individuals with chronic infections, advanced cancer and other debilitating diseases. Riboflavin is critical to the function of cytochrome c reductase, succinate dehydrogenase, monoamine oxidase and other enzymes, with deficiencies resulting in the following signs:

(1) Angular cheilosis (pallor followed by fissures at the angles of the mouth tending to become secondarily infected and macerated).
(2) Glossitis (resulting from atrophy of the lingual mucosa).
(3) Dermatitis (greasy, scaling of the skin occurring in a generalized fashion or in the nasal fold, cheeks or ears).
(4) Ocular lesions (characterized by corneal opacities and ulceration in addition to conjunctivitis).
(5) Bone marrow suppression.

None of these findings is specific for riboflavin deficiency, since similar lesions are encountered, for instance, with pyridoxine deficiency.[5]

Niacin

Niacin is the generic term for nicotinic acid and its derivatives, having the functional activity of nicotinic acid. Unlike the other B vitamins, niacin can be endogenously synthesized from dietary tryptophan. Niacin is a component of the two important co-enzymes nicotinamide adenine dinucleotide (NAD) and nicotinamide adenine dinucleotide phosphate (NADP), which are involved in a great variety of oxidation–reduction reactions, especially the electron transport of cellular respiratory reactions. It is widely distributed in most foods, although deficiencies are encountered in alcoholics and those suffering from chronic debilitating diseases, e.g. cirrhosis of the liver and advanced cancer. Persistent fatigue and weakness are the dominant complaints of patients who are niacin deficient, although dementia (resulting from central nervous system degeneration), diarrhoea (due to desquammation of the gastric mucosa) and dermatitis (symmetrical scaling, desquammation and inflammation of the skin) may also occur.

Vitamin B_6

Whereas a primary, clinically overt, vitamin B_6 deficiency is rare, subclinical conditioned deficiencies are thought to be common. The components of vitamin B_6 are converted in the tissues to the co-enzyme form, pyridoxal 5-phosphate, which participates as a cofactor in a number of enzymes involved in transaminations, carboxylations, and deaminations involving lipids, amino acids, nucleic acid and glycogen in the brain.[6] Clinical manifestations of pyridoxine deficiency include seborrheic dermatitis, cheilosis, glossitis, angular stomatitis, peripheral neuropathy and sometimes convulsions. The vitamin is, however, abundantly available in the usual diet, although secondary hypovitaminosis B_6 may be precipitated during pregnancy, hyperthyroidism and with high-protein diets.

Folic acid

A deficiency of this nutrient induces a megaloblastic anaemia, although lack of vitamin B_{12} produces an analogous haematological picture. A deficiency of vitamin B_{12}, however, also leads to neurological damage, i.e. anaemia and neurological disease. Folic acid is the common name for pteroylmonoglutamic acid, with the term folic acid and folates being used for all derivatives of folic acid. They essentially serve as co-enzymes in a wide variety of intracellular metabolic processes. Largely in the form of polyglutamate conjugates, folates are abundant in virtually all raw foods, particularly vegetables and fruits. Despite the abundance of folates in raw foods, however, cooking may deplete their content, especially when coupled with a marginal diet such as may be encountered in many chronic alcoholics and the single elderly. Inadequate absorption may also occur, especially in patients with disease of the gastrointestinal tract, e.g. after gut resection for carcinoma.[7] Many drugs, e.g. some anticonvulsants (phenytoin), oestrogens and antineoplastic chemotherapeutic agents, may also serve as folate antagonists. Folate deficiency impairs purine and thus DNA synthesis. As a consequence, rapidly dividing cells, e.g. red cell precursors in the bone marrow, suffer from retarded DNA synthesis relative to the cytoplasm (asynchrony). Thus the cells become large but cannot undergo mitosis. Such cellular asynchrony may also be detected in the rapidly dividing population of the oral mucosal epithelium, resulting in large atypical cells.

Vitamin B_{12}

A lack of vitamin B_{12} results in megaloblastic anaemia. Vitamin B_{12} or cobalamin, is a complex metallo-organic compound synthesized only by a variety of micro-organisms, including some found in the intestinal flora of humans. A deficiency of cobalamin, whether primary or conditioned, leads to megaloblastic anaemia, characterized by haematological anomalies and changes in the rapidly dividing cells of the gastrointestinal tract, and damage to the nervous system. This is frequently termed 'combined systems disease'. A lack of vitamin B_{12} inhibits DNA synthesis and concomitantly deranges lipid metabolism, with the formation of abnormal fatty acids. Incorporation of these fatty acids into myelin may underlie the neurological abnormalities of vitamin B_{12} deficiency.

In industrialized countries, vitamin B_{12} deficiency is generally a conditioned deficiency resulting from cobalamin malabsorption.[8] This may result from lack of intrinsic factor (mainly due to a genetic defect of the gastric mucosa), chronic pancreatitis, small intestine bacterial overgrowth and ileal disorders, such as Crohn's disease or ileal resections. Whatever the basis, the lack of B_{12} is manifested by a megaloblastic anaemia, alteration of the mucosal cells (identical to those produced by folate deficiency) and notably by demyelination followed by axonal degeneration and possibly neuronal death. Peripheral neuropathy and degeneration of the posterior and lateral spinal columns are the typical sites of involvement. Only rarely is the cerebrum involved.[9]

Vitamin C

Vitamin C is richly abundant in many foodstuffs and is quite resistant to most methods of food processing. Vitamin C deficiency is, however, encountered endemically among the grossly malnourished poor of developing countries. The function of vitamin C (ascorbic acid) and ascorbates involves the synthesis of collagen.[10] Specifically, ascorbate is required for:

(1) Activation of prolyl and lysyl hydroxylase from inactive precursors.
(2) Hydroxylation of proline and lysine residues in already synthesized collagen polypeptides.
(3) Aggregation of hydroxylated polypeptide chains into the triple helix of collagen, prior to its secretion from the cell.

With a deficiency of ascorbate and failure of hydroxylation, there is incomplete intra- and intermolecular cross-linkage, yielding collagen fibrils that lack tensile strength, have increased solubility and are more vulnerable to enzymatic degradation.[11] The collagen in blood vessel adventitia, media and basal laminae are primarily affected, due to their high hydroxyproline content. A number of other functions have been ascribed to ascorbic acid, including interaction with folate metabolism[12] along with neutrophil and macrophage mobility and activity.[13] Ascorbic acid also appears to play a role in iron metabolism, including iron storage and absorption.

Scorbutic adults typically manifest hyperkeratotic and perifollicular skin lesions. They also have a haemorrhagic diathesis and often develop a skin purpura or ecchymoses. There is poor wound healing and dehiscence of recently healed wounds. The teeth may become loosened, accompanied by gingivitis and bleeding into the gingiva. The healing of bone fractures may be impaired, with the primary deficiency being in the formation of the osteoid matrix rather than in the mineralization or calcification as in rickets. Thus fibroblasts proliferate into the defect to produce a loose, disorganized connection, but this tissue is weakened by the lack of a mature collagen matrix. Finally, the gingival inflammation and tooth loosening in scorbutic patients is associated with host defence mechanism impairment, i.e. PMN and macrophage activity, in addition to disturbed collagen metabolism.

Fat-soluble vitamins

Avitaminoses of the fat-soluble vitamins, A, D, E and K, may occur as primary deficiency states or as secondary conditioned deficiencies, including biliary and pancreatic dysfunction, malabsorption syndromes and liver diseases. The normal reserves of fat-soluble vitamins are, however, considerable, so deficiency states develop only after protracted negative balances.

Vitamin A

Vitamin A deficiency results in blindness, conjunctival keratinization, corneal conjunctival opacity, follicular (papular) hyperkeratosis of the skin, metaplasia of the mucosal linings of the respiratory, gastrointestinal and genito-urinary tracts and of the ducts of glands. In addition to predisposition to epithelial cancers of the skin, lungs, bladder and colorectum, avitaminosis A may lead to retarded skeletal growth in infancy and childhood anaemia.

Vitamin A is essential for the maturation and differentiation of specialized epithelial surfaces of the body, e.g. the oral and respiratory mucosae, although the reasons are obscure. Thus, specialized keratinized epithelial surfaces become excessively keratinized, whereas non-keratinized surfaces become keratinized in vitamin A deficiency. Also, the ducts of glands may become plugged by keratin debris, which may also contribute to the formation of stones either in the salivary glands or, particularly, in the kidneys. There is some evidence that vitamin A deficiency may contribute to the aetiology of lung cancer,[14] and even more uncertain is the suggestion that vitamin A deficiency may result in retarded skeletal growth and anaemia.[15]

The detailed metabolic interactions of this vitamin remain obscure, although it is known to be involved in intracellular glycosylation reactions that help to maintain the integrity of mucus secreting cells. Other functions include vitamin A in the maintenance of intracellular organelles and the regulation of prostaglandin synthesis and a regulatory role of the immune system.

Vitamin D

A deficiency of vitamin D, if sufficiently protracted, leads to two classic skeletal disorders:

(1) *Rickets* in growing infants and children whose epiphyses have not yet fused.
(2) *Osteomalacia* in adults.

Both conditions are characterized by inadequate or delayed mineralization of newly laid-down osteoid and therefore an excess of osteoid. In rickets there is also defective mineralization of epiphyseal cartilage. Since vitamin D plays a critical role in the maintenance of normal calcium metabolism, vitamin D deficiency will induce hyperfunction of the parathyroid glands, and the excess of parathyroid hormone causes a skeletal disorder, osteitis fibrosa cystica. Thus a deficiency of vitamin D induces not only abnormal serum levels of calcium and phosphate, but also secondary hyperparathyroidism and so skeletal morphological changes that constitute a combination of rickets (or osteomalacia) and osteitis fibrosa cystica. In fact, there are two generic causes of rickets and osteomalacia:

(1) Vitamin D deficiency or abnormal metabolism of the vitamin.
(2) A deficiency or deranged utilization of inorganic phosporus.[16]

Both aetiologies are associated with deranged skeletal calcification.

There are two native forms of the vitamin, vitamin D_3 (cholecalciferol) and vitamin D_2 (ergocalciferol). Both are essentially steroids. Vitamin D_3 may be endogenously derived from 7-dehydrocholesterol, an intermediate in cholesterol biosynthesis. Upon exposure to sunlight (ultraviolet light), 7-dehydrocholesterol (provitamin D_3) in the skin is transformed first into previtamin D_3, which, without further exposure to light, slowly equilibrates into vitamin D_3.[17] Vitamin D_3 may also be derived from a variety of animal products, especially liver, although with sufficient exposure to sunlight, no dietary source of vitamin D is required.

Vitamin D_3 is absorbed in the small intestine, requiring normal biliary function, as with other fats. After absorption or endogenous synthesis, it is transported and stored in the liver before passing to the kidney where it undergoes final evolution to vitamin D hormone or calciferol. As with all steroid hormones, cellular receptors appear to mediate the intracellular function of calciferol.[18] High-affinity receptors have been located in the nuclei of the villus cells of the small intestine, osteoblasts, osteocytes, chondrocytes, parathyroid glands, distal kidney tubules, podocytes of the glomerulus, basal cells of the skin, endocrine cells of the stomach and the TSH-producing cells of the pituitary.[19] In the intestinal mucosal cells, the hormone calciferol stimulates the synthesis of a calcium-binding protein, although whether this protein facilitates calcium transport across the cell membrane or initiates absorption remains obscure. Once within the mucosal cells, the calcium is transferred across the cell to the blood. The hormone participates in the active transport of phosphate by a process that is independent of calcium transport. In this manner, calciferol serves to elevate the plasma calcium and phosphorus concentrations to supersaturated levels required for mineralization of newly formed bone. Whether the hormone is also directly involved in the mineralization of osteoid is surprisingly uncertain. Normal calcium levels in the blood are also necessary for the normal functioning of nerve and muscle (including the myocardium) and normal membrane permeability and blood clotting. Calciferol is also involved in the mobilization of calcium and phosphate from the blood–fluid interface, together with parathormone.

There are many disturbances in vitamin D, calcium or phosporus metabolism that may lead to defective skeletal mineralization:[20]

(1) Vitamin D deficiency resulting from insufficient endogenous synthesis; primary dietary deficiency; secondary deficiency due to malabsorption of the lipid-soluble vitamin. Collectively, such deficiencies occur in economically-deprived populations: the elderly who live on restricted diets and shun sunlight, and patients with defective absorption syndromes, including pancreatic and biliary diseases and following gastrectomy.
(2) Chronic renal failure, with the associated acidosis also contributing to the disturbance in mineral metabolism.
(3) Hypophosphataemia, due to primary dietary deficiency and also secondary to long-term antacid medication for peptic ulcers, in addition to renal tubular diseases, e.g. Fanconi syndrome.
(4) Hereditary diseases, e.g. X-linked hypophosphataemia (also known as vitamin D-resistant rickets) – an autosomal dominant disorder, and vitamin D-dependent rickets – an autosomal recessive disorder.
(5) Drug-induced rickets and osteomalacia, resulting from a variety of drugs including anticonvulsive agents.

The basic derangement is the same in osteomalacia and rickets, i.e. delayed and/or inadequate mineralization and hence excessive osteoid. Basically osteomalacia comprises a subtle loss of skeleton and is one of a group of metabolic bone diseases including osteopenia. In rickets, there is failure of mineral deposition into the mature cartilagenous spicules at the metaphyseal interface; failure of the cartilage cells to mature and disintegrate with the resultant overgrowth of cartilage; persistence of distorted irregular masses of unmineralized cartilage, many of which project into the marrow cavity; deposition of unmineralized osteoid matrix on cartilagenous remnants with the formation of a disorderly, totally disrupted osteochondral junction; abnormal overgrowth of capillaries and fibroblasts into the disorganized zone; bending, compression and microfracture of the weakly supported osteoid and cartilaginous tissue, with the resultant skeletal deformities. The degree of the skeletal deformity depends on the severity of the disorder, but the cranial disturbances may lead to frontal bossing, in addition to cranial base and mid-face deformity.

Vitamin E

Vitamin E plays an important role as an anti-oxidant in that it protects labile vitamin A from oxidation, DNA from denaturation by free radicals and the phospholipids within cellular and organelle membranes against peroxidative attack by free radicals. Vitamin E may thus control the amounts of lipofuschin and ceroid (both peroxidation products of membrane lipids) which accumulate within cells with ageing, injury and atrophy.[21] The requirement for the anti-oxidant activity of vitamin E depends to an extent on the level of easily peroxidized polyunsaturated fatty acids in the diet, i.e. the greater the intake of polyunsaturated fatty acids in the diet, the greater the need for vitamin E. Absorption of vitamin E is essentially dependent on normal biliary, pancreatic and intestinal function, so that a deficiency of this vitamin is frequently a sequel of gastrointestinal disorders.

Vitamin K

The fat-soluble vitamin K is necessary for the synthesis of the functionally active clotting factors II (prothrombin), VII, X and XI. In vitamin K deficiency, therefore, there may be persistent haemorrhage following tooth extraction, nosebleeds, haematuria, melaena, and intracranial haemorrhage. Such haemorrhagic disorders can, however, be quickly rectified by intravenous vitamin K injections.

Three closely related compounds all possess vitamin K activity:

(1) K_1 (phylloquinone) widely distributed in leafy green vegetables;
(2) K_2 (menaquinone) synthesized by microorganisms including the intestinal flora;
(3) K_3 (menadione) a synthetic product.

Prolonged administration of antibiotics, which may destroy the intestinal flora, in association with a marginal dietary intake or malabsorption syndrome, is a frequent cause of vitamin K deficiency.[22]

Minerals

A number of minerals are no less essential for health than the vitamins. Some are required in large amounts, e.g. iron, whereas others are required as trace elements.

Iron

As a global cause of deficiency disease, iron is probably no less important a nutrient than protein. In the USA, iron deficiency anaemia related principally to inadequate intake is said to be present in 25% of infants, 15–20% of menstruating women, and 30–40% of pregnant women. Less severe levels of iron lack, insufficient to produce anaemia, may be present in 50% of all infants, menstruating women and pregnant women. In contrast, only about 3% of adult males are similarly affected.[23]

The possible origins of an iron deficiency state include:

(1) An inadequate diet, especially when associated with chronic alcoholism or food faddism.
(2) Impaired adsorption, e.g. gastrointestinal malabsorption syndromes.
(3) Increased requirement, e.g. during adolescence or pregnancy.
(4) Loss of blood, especially following major surgery.

In practical terms, an iron deficiency in adult males and postmenopausal females in the Western world should be considered to be caused by gastrointestinal blood loss.

Trace elements

Trace elements play critical roles in many vital homeostatic functions. For instance, copper, manganese, selenium and zinc are crucial components of a variety of enzymes ranging from oxidase and dehydrogenases to DNA and RNA polymerases. Other trace elements, e.g. iodine, are essential for the synthesis of thyroid hormone.

A deficiency of a trace element may have the same origins as a lack of a vitamin. Alternatively, dietary, parenteral, nutritional and gastrointestinal malabsorptional deficiencies are the principal aetiological factors.

Zinc is an essential component of one or more of the 20 metallo-enzymes, including DNA and RNA polymerases, carbonic anhydrase, alcohol dehydrogenase and alkaline phosphatase. With children and adults, chronic zinc deficiency may be associated with anaemia, retarded growth and sexual maturation. In adults, retarded growth, poor wound healing, testicular atrophy with hypogonadism, anaemia and skin lesions have been attributed to zinc deficiency, together with diarrhoea, mental lethargy and depression.

Copper in appropriate amounts is critical to health, although excess copper may lead to a genetic disease, Wilson's disease. Copper deficiency has been associated with anaemia, neutropenia and osteoporosis, in addition to mental disturbances resulting from malfunctioning of intraneuronal enzymes.

Selenium deficiency has been incriminated as a cause of cardiomyopathy. Certainly selenium is a component of glutathione peroxidase, an enzyme that plays a role in scavenging free oxygen radicals, although the reason for targeting cardiac muscle remains obscure.

Obesity

Obesity is the result of the intake of calories in excess of utilization; in essence, the storage of unneeded energy in fat cells. Obesity is defined as a body weight 20% or more above the norm, and by these standards, 20% of middle-aged males and 40% of middle-aged females in the USA are obese. Although mild obesity may not be harmful to health, marked obesity predisposes to hypertension,[24] adult onset (non-insulin-dependent) diabetes, hyperlipoproteinaemia, cholelithiasis (gallstones), hypoventilation, strokes, osteoarthritis and other forms of skeletal degeneration. In addition, in many instances of marked obesity, dental treatment may be compromised by the lack of space in the oral cavity.

Conclusions

The mouth mirrors general ill-health in many nutritional deficiencies. For instance, the tongue becomes pale in iron deficiency, the corners of the lips develop painful ulcers in riboflavin deficiency and taste may be affected by lack of zinc. The mouth also mirrors good health, so that determination of the quality and quantity of nutrients appropriate for good health can be aided by observing the effects of particular nutrients on the oral tissues. In effect, the mouth is a sensitive barometer, reacting to nutritional imbalances as well as reflecting a diet conducive to the health and well-being of the individual. If imposed early in life, protein-calorie malnutrition may not only lead to changes in the size and composition of the brain but can also affect any developing tissue, e.g. the tooth germ. Inadequate vitamin A has been associated with craniofacial abnormalities, including cleft lip and palate in addition to increased dental caries susceptibility. Vitamin D deficiency may lead to enamel hypoplasia due to disturbances in enamel mineralization and maturation, whereas zinc deficiency has been associated with micrognathia and hydrocephalus. Nutrients may also affect the course of disease by exacerbating or antagonizing pathological processes. For instance, gingival enlargement and inflammation frequently accompany oral contraceptive usage, although significant improvement is obtained with folic acid supplementation. Excessive use of alcohol has been associated with oral, oesophageal, heart, liver and neurological diseases. Nutritionally related ill-effects of chronic excessive alcohol intake may occur because of the effect of ethanol on appetite or because it displaces or interferes with food in the diet. Ethanol may also strip protective barrier proteins from the oral mucosal surface. Epidemiological and experimental studies support the hypothesis that infectious diseases and nutritional deficiencies during tooth development increase susceptibility to dental caries. Pre-eruptive protein-calorie malnutrition and vitamin A deficiency have each been shown to increase the susceptibility to caries. Post-eruptive provision of foods high in refined sugar can enhance the establishment, colonization and metabolic activity of cariogenic micro-organisms in dental plaque, despite the beneficial effects that may have been contributed pre-eruptively by a healthy diet. Proteins can also affect plaque by providing basic amino acids that can neutralize the products of bacterial metabolism of sugars and also stimulate the rate of salivary flow. Saliva, in turn, can buffer acids produced by plaque bacteria or reduce the residence time of foods in the mouth and thus limit the availability of fermentable substrate to the plaque. Overall, nutritional deficiencies affect the severity and extent of periodontal diseases by modulating the response and repair properties of the tissues. Inadequate nutrient intake could also affect the metabolism of plaque flora in the gingival crevice as well as systemic responses to microbial antigens. The periodontal tissues may also be subject to local end-organ nutritional influences, e.g. the ability of foods to stimulate salivary flow and the effects of masticatory action as a stimulant to periodontal tissue and alveolar bone. Antigens in food may also elicit local immunological responses in periodontal tissues. Nutritional deficiency also affects cell-mediated immunity, metabolic and bactericidal functions of polymorphonuclear leucocytes and macrophages, and the function of the complement and secretory antibody system. Oral mucosal diseases, e.g. herpes infections and aphthous ulceration, poor-fitting dentures and oral surgical problems may also interfere with eating and compromise the general health and nutritional status of a patient. Salivary gland disease can affect the nutritional status of a patient by altering salivary composition and flow, which may affect taste, digestion and influence food preference. Thus, nutrition is intimately associated with oral health and disease.

Review questions

1. What minerals are essential, and why?
2. What are the manifestations of obesity?
3. What is the evidence for Vitamin D being considered a hormone?
4. What deficiencies are likely to be prevalent in a refugee camp?
5. Is Vitamin C essential for life?

References

1. BROWN, C.B. (1971) The incidence of protein-energy (calorie) malnutrition of early childhood. *Guys Hosp. Rep.*, **120**, 129
2. CASEY, C.E. and HAMBIDGE, K.M. (1980) Trace element deficiencies in man. *Adv. Nutr. Res.*, **3**, 23
3. EDITORIAL (1981) Nutritional oedema, albumin and vanadate. *Lancet*, **i**, 646
4. EVANS, D. (1980) Intellectual development and nutrition. *J. Pediatr.*, **97**, 358
5. PERRY, G.M. (1980) The effect of riboflavin on red-cell vitamin B_6 metabolism and globin synthesis. *Biomedicine*, **33**, 36
6. MINNS, R. (1980) Vitamin B_6 deficiency and dependency. *Dev. Med. Child. Neurol.*, **22**, 795
7. CHANARIN, I. and BENNETT, M.C. (1962) Absorption of folic acid and D-xylose as tests for small intestinal function. *Br. Med. J.*, **5283**, 985
8. HERBERT, V. (1980) The nutritional anemias. *Hosp. Pract.*, **15**, 65
9. SHORVON, F.D. (1980) The neuropsychiatry of megaloblastic anemia. *Br. Med. J.*, **281**, 1036
10. EDITORIAL (1978) The function of ascorbic acid in collagen formation. *Nutr. Rev.*, **36**, 118
11. LEVENE, C.I. (1977) Scurvy: a comparison between ultrastructural and biochemical changes observed in cultured fibroblasts and the collagen they synthesize. *Virchows Arch. (Zell. pathol.)*, **23**, 825
12. CHATTERJEE, I.B. (1975) Effect of ascorbic acid on histamine metabolism in scorbutic guinea pigs. *J. Physiol. (Lond.)*, **251**, 271
13. THOMAS, W.R. and HOLT, P.G. (1978) Vitamin C and immunity: an assessment of the evidence. *Clin. Exp. Immunol.*, **32**, 370
14. HARISIADIS, L. (1978) A vitamin A analogue inhibits radiation-induced oncogenic transformation. *Nature*, **274**, 486
15. EDITORIAL (1979) Vitamin A deficiency and anemia. *Clin. Nutr.*, **37**, 38
16. TEITELBAUM, S.L. (1980) Pathological manifestations of osteomalacia and rickets. *Clin. Endocrinol. Metab.*, **9**, 43

17. HOLICK, M.G. and CLARK, M.G. (1978) The photobiogenesis and metabolism of vitamin D. *Fed. Proc.*, **37**, 2567
18. ROTH, S.P. and HENRY, H.L. (1980) Recent advances in the understanding of the metabolism and functions of vitamin D. *Clin. Orthop.*, **149**, 249
19. STUMPF, W.E. (1979) Target cells for 1,25-dihydroxyvitamin D_3 in the intestinal tract, stomach, kidney, skin, pituitary and parathyroid. *Science*, **206**, 1188
20. MARIE, P.J. (1982) Histological osteomalacia due to dietary calcium deficiency in children. *N. Engl. J. Med.*, **307**, 584
21. OSKI, F.A. (1980) Vitamin E: a radical defense. *N. Engl. J. Med.*, **303**, 454
22. ANSELL, J.E. (1979) The spectrum of vitamin K deficiency. *JAMA*, **238**, 40
23. DAVIDSON, L.S.P. and PASSMORE, R. (1969) *Human Nutrition and Dietetics*, 4th edn. Edinburgh: Livingstone
24. DUSTAN, H.P. (1980) Obesity and hypertension. *Compr. Ther.*, **6**, 29

12

Age (gerontology)

Introduction

It is a well known fact that the percentage of edentulous patients increases with age, with caries being the principal cause of tooth loss in the earlier age groups, whereas periodontal disease accounts for the majority of tooth loss over 35 years of age. In the Western world, the percentage of old people in the population as a whole is beginning to show progressive increases, reflecting a reduction in family size and an increase in life-expectancy; both, in part, consequences of the advances in modern medicine. The question is, to what extent are the deleterious changes in the oral cavity related to true age changes, rather than the ravages reflecting years of chronic irritation, including dental plaque accumulation? The problem is that, although the number of elderly in the population is increasing, knowledge of the cause(s) of age changes remains obscure. Currently, age changes are generally considered to reflect one or more of the following:

(1) Decline in efficacy of the immune host defence system.
(2) Malfunctioning of the neuro-endocrine system.
(3) Genetic determination of life span of both cells and tissues.
(4) Metabolic error accumulation.
(5) Effects of free radicals, cross-linking or molecular instability.
(6) Changes in entropy.
(7) Lipofuscin accumulation.
(8) Cell loss exceeding cellular renewal.

In fact, there may not be a single cause, since, as with so many other biological phenomena, the ageing process is almost certainly multifactorial in nature. Moreover, any therapy current today is likely to be overtaken by more plausible theories developed in the light of future research data. Only when the causes of ageing are well delineated will it be possible to prevent or minimize some of the associated signs and symptoms.

In this chapter the current theories of ageing are briefly considered, followed by a short summary of the current data related to the age changes seen in the oral cavity.

Theories of ageing

The ageing of a person may be regarded as the composite effect of ageing of cells. As a result, most of the theories as to the cause of ageing centre on cellular ageing.

Organ theories

The organ theories are based on the contention that increments or decrements occur in organ functioning with increasing age. This theory contends that the immune system, brain and neuro-endocrine system are the organs principally affected.

Immunological theory

The immune theory[1,2] hinges on two main findings. Firstly, the functioning of the immune system declines qualitatively and quantitatively with age, with the thymus-dependent component (T lymphocytes) showing the greatest deterioration. This implies that the immune defence mechanisms will deteriorate with age, especially with regards to microbial pathogens.

Secondly, with the decline of the normal immune system, it becomes less able to discriminate between self and non-self, resulting in an increase in autoimmune diseases. This results in an increased incidence of chronic autoimmune diseases that are characteristically associated with ageing. The consequences of both manifestations include an increased vulnerability to disease and pathology with increasing age.

The efficacy of the immune system peaks at about puberty and then declines in old age to about 5–10% of its youthful value.[3] Such immune dysfunction with increasing age is generally manifested by a decline in the response of lymphoid cells to immunological stimuli.[1] This decline is primarily mediated by an age-associated deficit in the T cell arm of the immune system,[4] so that thymic involution may act as the master chronometer of the body.[1] Thus, there is increasing incidence of a number of diseases including cancer, maturity-onset diabetes and vascular disease. These may all reflect diminished immune capability.

This immune theory may however be criticized on a number of facets:

(1) The immune system as a cause of all age changes lacks universality, i.e. there are primitive organisms that lack an immune system, yet they still age.[5]
(2) The immune system is regulated by a variety of factors, especially the endocrine system,[6] i.e. the decline in the immune system may reflect neuro-endocrine malfunction.
(3) All cells probably undergo age changes that are genetically based, so that it is difficult to discern why the immune system should be more affected compared with other systems. The increased incidence of autoimmune diseases may in fact reflect antigenic changes in the target cells themselves as they age, rather than a decline in immune efficacy.

Thus, although the immune system decreases in efficacy with increasing age, there may also be other changes responsible for ageing.

Neuro-endocrine system theories

The neurological and endocrine systems influence all the tissues of the body. For instance, a disturbance in hypothalamic function may result in pituitary malfunction, the ramifications of which would affect all the major endocrine glands, e.g. menopausal steroid loss may lead to conditions necessary for osteoporosis. Certainly neuronal and endocrine cell loss with increasing age have been noted for many years but the effects of such losses on the ageing process remain controversial. Neuronal loss occurs selectively in the brain.[7] As a result, motor or sensory loss could reflect neuronal loss in a variety of regions, including cerebral cortex, caudata putamen, hippocampus, substantia nigra, etc. There only appears to be a 10% decrease in total brain weight with age,[7] and such a loss may not only reflect neuronal loss, but also fluid and/or ground substance loss. In addition, age related changes purported to reflect hormonal decline may in fact reflect changes in receptor concentrations[8] and end-organ functioning.[9]

As with the immune theory of ageing, the neuro-endocrine theory may be criticized on the basis that not all organisms that age have a complex neuro-endocrine system, and that the age related deficits in the neuro-endocrine system may reflect basic changes occurring in the genome of all cells as they age.

Physiological theories

Free radical theory

Free radicals are atoms or molecules bearing an unpaired electron. They are ordinarily very reactive due to the tendency for electrons to pair. Because the reaction of a free radical with a stable molecule produces another radical, chain reactions often result in which a single free radical initiates a process that consumes many stable molecules. The oxidation of polyunsaturated fatty acids, for example, readily occurs by a free radical chain reaction, giving rise to a host of aldehyde and hydrocarbon products.[10] Free radical reactions arise from:

(1) Exposure of cells and their organelles to ionizing radiation.
(2) Non-enzymatic reactions.
(3) Enzymatic reactions and oxygen reduction.

Because free radicals are highly reactive, all cells are susceptible to random damage caused by them. Such damage may include:

(1) Cumulative oxidative alterations in DNA, collagen and elastin.
(2) Oxidative mucopolysaccharide breakdown.
(3) Accumulation of metabolically inert substances by oxidative polymerization reactions.
(4) Changes in mitochondrial and lysosomal membrane characteristics.
(5) Capillary and arteriolar fibrosis, secondary to vessel injury by peroxidation products derived from serum and vessel-wall components.[11]

Free radical damage may be prevented by anti-oxidants, e.g. haem-containing peroxidases, superoxide transmutases and DNA repair mechanisms.

It is possible that ageing reflects the sum total of the deleterious free radical reactions proceeding continuously throughout the cells and tissues.[11] Indeed, free radicals have been included in the aetiology of a number of diseases including cancer, cardiovascular disease, immune depression and neuronal degenerative diseases[11] but since the role of anti-oxidants has yet to be fully formulated, the free-radical theory of ageing has yet to achieve universal acceptance.

Cross-linkage theory

This theory hinges on molecular changes in substances within the extracellular and intracellular compartments with age.[12] The theory holds that when two or more macromolecules become linked covalently or by a hydrogen bond, such linkages are said to be reversible and accumulate over time. Molecular aggregation and immobilization increases and the resulting inert or malfunctioning molecules accumulate and become increasingly inert, or malfunctioning molecules accumulate and become increasingly resistant to catabolic processes. For instance, DNA may become damaged, leading to mutation or cell death. Non-removable cross-linked aggregates may clog glandular processes, impeding the production or release of hormones and other cellular secretions. Cross-linking agents include aldehydes, alkylating agents, free radicals, antibodies and polyvalent metals.[13]

This theory may be criticized on the basis that many of the vital molecules that may be cross-linked undergo metabolic turnover, implying that only non-renewable cellular populations exhibit age changes. In addition, the factors resulting in cross-linkages have yet to be fully discerned.

Waste-product accumulation theory

A number of pigmented inclusion bodies, representing aggregated waste products that may impede cell function and cause age changes, have been noted in a variety of tissues, especially neurones.[14] The significance of such inclusions has yet to be discerned, although they may represent degenerated mitochondria[15] and lysosomal products.[16] These age-associated pigments are more frequently termed lipofuscin and probably result from auto-oxidative reactions of lipid components of lysosomes and other membranous intracellular organelles.[17] Lipofuscin granules contain a variety of substances, including:

(1) Proteins.
(2) Lipids.
(3) Carbohydrates.
(4) Cathepsin.
(5) Various enzymes, including alkaline phosphatase.
(6) Chromophores.[18]

Vitamin E deficiency increases lipofuscin deposition without accelerating other age changes; in addition, vitamin E administration does not prolong cell or tissue life or reduce lipofuscin accumulation.[19,20] Thus lipofuscin accumulation may play only a minor role in the mechanism of ageing. It is also unclear whether lipofuscin granules actually damage cells by impeding function.

Genome-based theories

There is a general belief that longevity is largely determined by genetic mechanisms:[21] in particular, a phenomenon, known as the Lansing effect, suggests that the progeny of older mothers have a shorter life expectation; an effect that may extend for several generations.[22]

Somatic mutation theory

This theory contends that the accumulation of a sufficient level of mutations in somatic cells will produce physiological decrements characteristic of ageing.[23] Surprisingly, few studies have been undertaken to confirm this widespread belief.

Error theory

This theory is really an extension of the somatic mutation theory, except that it contends that ageing reflects the accumulation of errors in DNA replication.[24] This theory again lacks basic support.

Programme theory

This theory contends that the life-span of a cell or tissue is programmed into the genome. It is supported by the fact that fibroblasts, grown in culture, can only undergo mitosis a finite number of times.[25] This theory assumes that initially well-ordered genetic programmes become progressively disordered, resulting in those changes recognized as ageing. This remains a theory; but there appears to be more widespread evidence in its favour compared with the other ageing theories.[26]

Oral tissues

The oral cavity is no different from the body as a whole, in that age changes reflect a gradual deterioration in oral health and well-being, albeit with great variability, both between individuals and between the different tissues (*Figures 12.1, 12.2*).

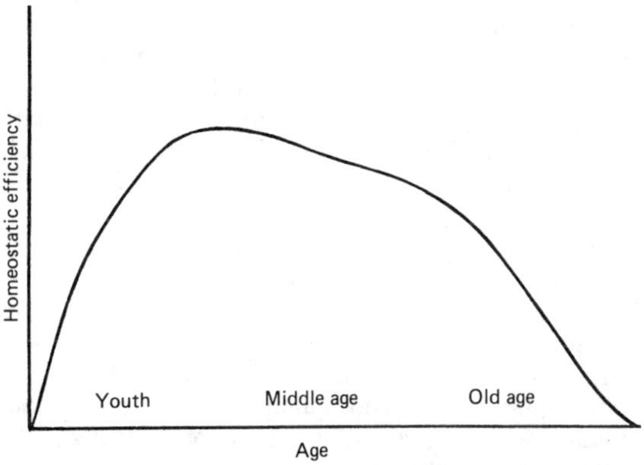

Figure 12.1 Effect of age on homeostatic efficiency.

Epithelium

Thinning and diminished keratinization are the two principal characteristics associated with advancing age in the oral epithelium.[27,28] In addition, a reduction in rete peg dimensions has been noted, presumably reflecting changes in the intervening basement membrane.[29] Whereas the oral epithelium shows an increase in cell density with increasing age,[30] whether this reflects an increase in mitotic activity,[31] no change in renewal time[30] or a reduction in the rate of renewal[32] has yet to be confirmed. There are no component blood vessels or lymphatics in epithelial tissues. These tissues are, however, metabolically active. Conceivably, therefore, some of the changes associated with age reflect disturbances in the underlying connective tissue reflected in the metabolism of the overlying epithelium.

Connective tissue

The increase in skin wrinkling with increasing age mainly reflects a loss of subcutaneous fat.[33] This does not apply to the gingiva, however, as there is no underlying subgingival adipose tissue. The underlying connective tissues do become coarser with increasing age[34] and this is associated with a reduction in the collagen turnover rate.[35]

In the periodontal ligament, a reduction in component cell number and degree of component collagenous fibre organization has been noted with increasing age,[36] together with a net loss of acid mucopolysaccharides.[37] In addition, a reduction in soluble collagen in the periodontal ligament has been noted,[38] but whether this reflects increased collagen cross-linking has yet to be discerned. It may reflect the fact that the periodontal fibroblasts

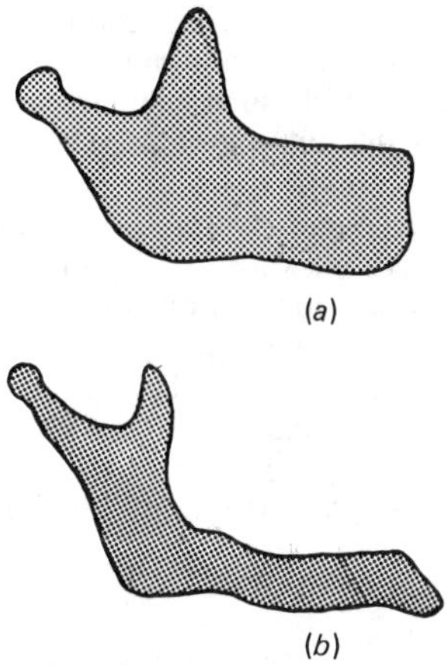

Figure 12.2 Change in mandibular form in young (*a*) and old (*b*) edentulous subjects.

synthesize type I, rather than type II collagen, with increasing age.[39] Other reported age changes include an increase in component elastic fibres[40] and a reduction in the number of epithelial rests of Malassez,[41] although the possible functional significance of such changes has yet to be investigated.

Cementum

Although there is continuous cementogenesis throughout life, the apical region of the root is primarily affected.[42] This may partly reflect continued passive eruption and migration of the teeth associated with continuous periodontal reattachment. Unlike bone, cementum undergoes only minor remodelling.[43] With increasing age, however, the cemental layer becomes not only increasingly acellular[44] but also increasingly irregular in surface outline.[36] Furthermore, continued cemental deposition results in slowly progressive reduction in the lumen of the apical foramina of tooth roots. The resultant progressive relative hypoxia of the pulp tissue is generally associated with a reduction in the pulpal cellular content. Again, to say that this is a natural consequence of advancing age presupposes that the factors influencing cementogenesis are well delineated.

Dentine–pulpal complex

With advancing age, the volume of the dentine increases at the expense of pulpal tissue. This may not be a reflection of age changes *per se* but the result of continued irritation of the dentine. Environmental stimuli that occur slowly, e.g. abrasion or attrition, are associated with an organized pulpal response that includes secondary dentine formation on the pulpal surface of dentine. This is associated with a reduction in the volume of the pulpal tissue and a diminution in the number of odontoblasts. With such changes, the reparative processes of the pulp tissue may become impaired. This reduction in the size of the pulp space results in odontoblastic overcrowding. As a result, some of the dentinal tubules lose their component odontoblastic processes. In addition, some of these dentinal tubules become obliterated, i.e. there may be dentinal tubular sclerosis. The net result is that the vitality of the dentine is reduced, but whether this reflects age changes *per se*, or the consequences of long-term low-grade irritation, remains conjectural.

Bone

With increasing age the lamina dura, the thin layer of cortical bone lining the alveolar socket, becomes thicker but more irregular.[37] In addition, there is an increase in the component number of interstitial lamellae.[36] Such changes are difficult to interpret, however, since the alveolar bone, in common with bone in other skeletal regions, constantly adapts to accommodate functional demands. If, with increasing age, less teeth are present in the oral cavity, then the occlusal forces acting on the remaining teeth may increase. This will be reflected by changes in alveolar bone morphology, i.e. the alveolar bone remodels to accommodate changes in function. On the other hand, masticatory forces probably decline with age,[45] which again would be expected to be associated with changes in alveolar bone morphology.

Junctional epithelium

In the healthy periodontium, the junctional epithelium is located close to the amelo-cemental junction, whereas with increasing age, the location of this epithelium migrates down the side of the tooth root. This may merely reflect the effects of continued periodontal breakdown associated with chronic periodontal disease,[46] but apical migration of the junctional epithelium with increasing age has been noted in the absence of plaque and gingival inflammation.[47] Other facts may therefore be associated with gingival recession, including continuous passive eruption[48] and mechanical trauma.[46] There is, however, a general consensus that continued periodontal destruction, consequent upon plaque accumulation, is the predominant aetiologic factor associated with continued gingival recession with advancing age.

Plaque

In the absence of efficient oral hygiene, dental plaque accumulates on the exposed tooth surfaces. If these exposed areas are enlarged due to gingival recession, then the potential surface for plaque accumulation will be increased.[49] In a study of plaque from young (20–24 years) and old (65–81 years) patients, no difference in dextran hydrolase, sucrase or amylase was noted between the two patient groups, although levan hydrolase activity was markedly higher in the younger age-group. This suggests a lower streptococcal plaque count in the older age-group.[49] In another study, the concentrations of IgA, IgM, and C3 (specific immune factors) and lactoferrin lysozyme and lactoperoxidase (non-specific immune factors), were all higher in the plaque of the older, compared with younger, age-groups of patients.[50] Although there are both quantitative and qualitative changes in the plaque with increasing age, their biological significance remains obscure.

Host response

Dental plaque accumulation in some patients may be associated with only mild gingivitis, but with severe periodontal recession in others, i.e. the response to plaque-derived irritants is a function of the host immune defence response. A number of studies have shown the efficacy of the host defence response in the oral cavity decreases with age.[51] Thus the susceptibility to periodontal disease is probably more important for the rate of periodontal destruction than the length of time the plaque is present (the age effect).

Wound healing

The rate of skin wound healing decreases with age.[49] This effect appears to be more pronounced in the connective than epithelial tissues.[44]

Conclusions

The ageing of a patient, or any part or region of a patient, may be regarded as the composite effect of ageing on the cells. It is, however, unreasonable to anticipate that all cells age in unison (*Figure 12.3*). Thus, some tissues age preferentially relative to others. For instance, the enamel is a relatively inert tissue, so that changes other than abrasion and attrition are unlikely with increasing age. By contrast, the oral mucosa may exhibit a variety of pathological changes reflecting continued trauma, in addition to infective and carcinogenic irritants. Detailed considerations of these facets are more appropriately contained in a pathology text. The main theme of this chapter is primarily to underline the paucity of knowledge concerning the true ageing changes in the oral cavity.

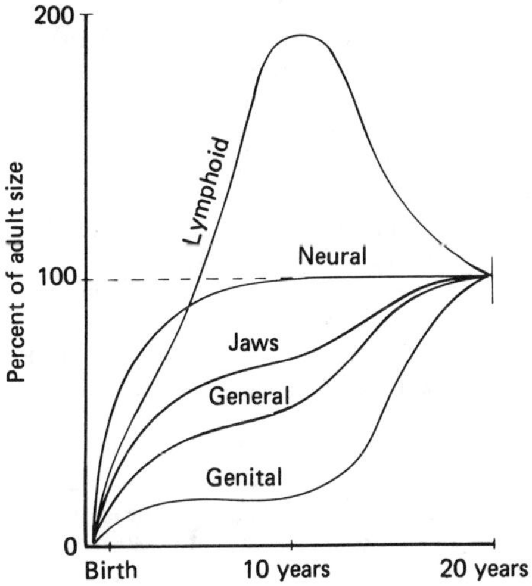

Figure 12.3 Growth changes in component body tissues.

Interestingly, although life expectancy has increased in the past century, such achievements as have been made simply allow more people to reach the limit of what appears to be a fixed life-span. If the three major causes of death in North America were eliminated, e.g. cancer, heart disease and stroke, only 10–20 years of additional life could be expected.

Review questions

1. Give an account of the theory of ageing that best fits the oral mucosa.
2. Contrast the age changes of bone with epithelium.
3. How does age affect wound healing?
4. Identify the genome-based theories of ageing.

References

1. WALFORD, R.L., WEIDRUCH, R.H., GOTTESMAN, S.R.S. and TAM, C.F. (1981) *Annual Review of Gerontology and Geriatrics*. New York: Springer
2. WEKSLER, M. (1981) The immune system and the ageing process in man. *Proc. Soc. Exp. Biol. Med.*, **165**, 200–205
3. WALFORD, R.L., JAWILD, S. and NAEIM, F. (1981) *The Immunological Theory of Aging*. Baltimore: Williams & Wilkins
4. KAY, M.M.B. (1979) An overview of immune aging. *Mech. Aging Dev.*, **9**, 39–59
5. HAYFLICK, L. (1985) Theories of biological ageing. *Exp. Gerontol.*, **20**, 145–159
6. MAKINODAN, T. and YUNIS, E. (1977) *Immunology and Aging*. New York: Plenum Press
7. BRODY, H. (1980) *Biological Mechanisms in Aging*. Washington: US Department of Health and Human Services
8. ROTH, G.S. (1980) *Biological Mechanisms in Aging*. Washington: US Department of Health and Human Services
9. ADELMAN, R.C. (1975) Disruptions in enzyme regulation during aging. *Basic Life Sci.*, **6**, 304–311
10. LAWRENCE, G.D. and COHEN, G. (1982) Ethane exhalation as an index of *in vivo* peroxidation. *Anal. Biochem.*, **122**, 283–290
11. HARMAN, D. (1981) The aging process. *Proc. Natl. Acad. Sci. USA*, **78**, 7124–7128
12. KOHN, R.R. (1978) *Principles of Mammalian Aging*. Englewood Cliffs, NJ: Prentice-Hall
13. ROCKSTEIN, M. (1974) *Theoretical Aspects of Aging*. New York: Academic Press
14. BONDAREFF, W. (1972) Age changes in the neuronal environment. *Science*, **176**, 1135–1136
15. HESS, A. (1955) Reaction of mammalian fetal tissues to injury. *Anat. Rec.*, **121**, 503–511
16. GEDIGK, P. and PIOCH, W. (1956) Uber die Speicherung von Schwermetallverbindungen in mesenchmalen Geweben. *Beitr. Path. Anat.*, **116**, 149–167
17. TAPPEL, A.L. (1973) Vitamin E and free radical peroxidation of lipids. *Ann. NY Acad. Sci.*, **203**, 12–28
18. TOTH, S.E. (1968) The origin of lipofuscin age pigments. *Exp. Gerontol.*, **3**, 19–30
19. NANDY, K. and BOURNE, G. (1966) Effect of centrophenoxine on the lipofuscin pigments in the neurones of senile guinea pigs. *Nature*, **210**, 313–314
20. STREHLER, B.L. (1969) Molecular biology of aging. *Naturwissenschaften*, **56**, 57–71
21. BIRREN, J.E. (1959) *Handbook of Aging and the Individual*. Chicago: University of Chicago Press
22. COMFORT, A. (1979) *The Biology of Senescence*. London: Churchill Livingstone
23. SZILARD, L. (1959) On the nature of the aging process. *Proc. Natl. Acad. Sci. USA*, **45**, 30–45
24. CUTLER, R. (1974) Evolution of longevity in primates. *J. Hum. Evol.*, **5**, 169–202
25. HAYFLICK, L. and MOOHEAD, P.S. (1961) The serial

cultivation of human diploid cell strains. *Exp. Cell Res.*, **25**, 585–621
26. SACHER, G.A. (1968) Mathematical analysis of the division delay produced by ionizing radiation. *Radiat. Res.*, **33**, 644–658
27. SHKLAR, G. (1966) The effects of aging upon the oral mucosa. *J. Invest. Dermatol.*, **47**, 115–120
28. PAPIC, M. and GLICKMAN, I. (1950) Keratinization of the human gingiva in the menstrual cycle and menopause. *Oral Surg.*, **3**, 504–516
29. LOE, H. and KARRING, T. (1972) The three-dimensional morphology of the epithelial-connective tissue interface of the gingiva as related to age and sex. *Scand. J. Dent. Res.*, **79**, 315–326
30. RYAN, E.J., TOTO, P.D. and GARGIULO, A.W. (1974) Aging in human attached gingival epithelium. *J. Dent. Res.*, **53**, 74–76
31. TOTO, P.D. and BORG, M. (1968) Effect of age changes on the permitotic index in the periodontium of mice. *J. Dent. Res.*, **47**, 70–73
32. LAVELLE, C.L.B. (1968) The effect of age on the proliferative activity of certain epithelial tissues. *J. Periodont. Res.*, **3**, 212–213
33. KANUNGO, M.S. (1980) *Biochemistry of Ageing.* London: Academic Press
34. WENTZ, F.M., MAIER, A.W. and ORBAN, B. (1952) Age changes and sex differences in the clinically 'normal' gingiva. *J. Periodontol.*, **23**, 13–25
35. CLAYCOMB, C.K., SUMMERS, G.W. and DVORAK, E.M. (1967) Oral collagen biosynthesis in the guinea pig. *J. Periodont. Res.*, **2**, 115–120
36. SEVERSON, J.A., MOFFETT, B.C., KOKICH, V. and SELIPSKY, H. (1978) A histological study of age changes in the adult human periodontal joint (ligament). *J. Periodontol.*, **49**, 189–200
37. LEVY, B.M., DREIZEN, S. and BERNICK, S. (1972) Effect of age on the marmoset periodontium. *J. Oral Pathol.*, **1**, 61–65
38. PAUNIO, K. (1969) Periodontal connective tissue. *Suom. Hammaslaak. Toim.*, **65**, 250–290
39. MAYNE, R., VAIL, M.S., MAYNE, P.M. and MILLER, E.J. (1976) Changes in type of collagen synthesized as clones of chick chondrocytes grow and eventually lose division capacity. *Proc. Natl. Acad. Sci. USA*, **73**, 1674–1678
40. VON HAIM, G. and BAUMGARTEL, R. (1968) A1; Ternsveranderungen in Periodont (Desmodont). *Dtsch. Zahn Z.*, **23**, 340–344
41. REEVE, C.M. and WENTZ, F.M. (1962) The prevalence, morphology and distribution of epithelial rests in the human periodontal ligament. *Oral Surg.*, **15**, 785–793
42. IVE, J.C., SHAPIRO, P.A. and IVEY, J.L. (1980) Age related changes in the periodontium of pigtail monkeys. *J. Periodont. Res.*, **15**, 420–428
43. TONNA, E.A. (1979) Explorations in the aging of skeletal dental tissues: an ultrastructural study of aging cementum. In *Geriatric Dentistry, Clinical Application of Selected Biomedical and Psychosocial Topics*, edited by C.J. Toga, K. Nandy and H.H. Chauncey. Lexington: Lexington Book
44. TONNA, E.A. (1976) Factors (aging) affecting bone and cementum. *J. Periodontol.*, **47**, 267–280
45. HERRING, S.W. (1977) Mastication and maturity. *J. Dent. Res.*, **56**, 1377–1382
46. LOE, H., ANERUD, A., BOYSEN, H. and SMITH, M. (1978) The natural history of periodontial disease in man. *J. Periodontol.*, **49**, 607–621
47. BEERTSEN, W., EVERTS, V., NIEHOF, A. and BRUINS, H. (1982) Loss of connective tissue attachment in the marginal periodontium of the mouse following blockage of eruption. *J. Periodont. Res.*, **17**, 640–658
48. GOTTLIEB, B. and ORBAN, B. (1936) Zahnfleisch Entzundung und Zahnlockerung. Berlin: Berlinische Verlagsanstalt
49. HOLM-PEDERSEN, AGERBAEK, N. and THEILADE, E. (1975) Experimental gingivitis in young and elderly individuals. *J. Clin. Periodontol.*, **2**, 14–24
50. COLE, M.F., DANA HSU, S., BAUM, B.J., BOWEN, W., SIERRA, L.I., AQUIRRE, M. and GILLESPIE, G. (1981) Specific and non-specific immune factors in dental plaque fluid and saliva from young and old populations. *Infect. Immun.*, **31**, 998–1002
51. CHURCH, H. and DOLBY, A.E. (1978) The effect of age on the cellular immune response to dento-gingival plaque extract. *J. Periodont. Res.*, **13**, 120–126

13

Stress and anxiety in dental treatment

Introduction

An all too small segment of the population visits the dentist regularly for routine dental assessment and treatment. The remainder, unfortunately, regard the dentist as a necessary evil, evoked only when the need becomes imperative. One study revealed that only 33% of the population attend a dentist regularly,[1] the remainder attending casually as only a last resort. Of the many factors associated with this apparent unconcern about regular dental care, dental fear and/or anxiety remain predominant.[2] In a study of the fears and anxieties that people hold in regard to illness, 89% of a sample were specifically fearful of dental treatment: a fear unrelated to educational level or general illness anxiety.[3] Thus many patients who attend a dentist are frankly afraid; this fear may manifest itself physiologically in a number of ways. More often than not, the patient will attempt to mask this anxiety, although occasional bouts of fainting provide the most blatant signs of fear. Anxiety may also be manifest by a host of other signs including:

(1) Sleep loss.
(2) Hunger.
(3) Pain.
(4) Excessive analgesic consumption.
(5) Sweating.
(6) Palpitations.
(7) Talkativeness, etc.

Often the treatment of such anxious patients also results in stress for the dentist and the dental team.

Physiology of stress

The body reacts in a number of ways when placed in a situation interpreted as adverse or threatening,[4] including anorexia,[5] over-eating,[6] gonadal functional disturbance,[7] disease,[8] decreased host defence reactions[9] and altered pain sensitivity.[10] The type of change that develops is related to both significance of the specific threatening situation to the individual and the individual's more general pattern of adaptation to day-to-day problems. This, in turn, is related to a patient's fears and phobias, developed mainly as a result of childhood experiences.[11]

The physiological responses to emotional stimulation are autonomic and controlled by a complex system involving the limbic structures, especially the amygdala, hypothalamus and reticular formation. Stimulation of the reticular formation induces cerebral arousal, alerting reactions,[12] panic and fear responses.[13] In such stressful situations there are increased systemic circulatory catecholamine levels, derived from increased sympathetic tone augmented by increased adrenal medullary secretion. This is the traditional 'fight or flight' reflex.[14] The results include:

(1) Vasodilatation of the skeletal muscle arterioles and coronary arteries.
(2) Increased cardiac output, associated with a raised blood pressure.
(3) Raised cerebral blood flow.
(4) Mobilization of sugar from hepatic glycogen stores.
(5) Increased cellular metabolism.
(6) Increased susceptibility of the cardiac ventricular muscle to extrasystole or ventricular fibrillation.

Such fight or flight reflexes also result in pituitary–adrenocortical activation, associated with increased 17-hydroxycorticosteroid output.[15] The results of increased glucocorticosteroid secretion include increased glucose production and utilization, mobilization of fat from storage depots and increased muscular efficiency.

Patients taking steroids, or whose adrenal cortices are either dormant or have undergone atrophy as a result of disease or therapy, are extremely susceptible to the damaging effects of a wide variety of stimuli that demand compensatory responses, including trauma, haemorrhage, fasting, anaesthetics and changes in environmental temperature. When such patients require dental treatment, it is important to ensure prior consultation with a physician.

The physical and emotional trauma associated with dental treatment primarily impinges upon hypothalamo–pituitary activity. In particular, trauma initiates the release of corticotrophin (ACTH), which enhances the production of adrenocortical hormones essential for accommodation to stressful situations. The secretion of ACTH is, however, dependent on a neurohormonal substance, corticotrophin-releasing factor (CRF), produced by the hypothalamus. This 41-amino-acid peptide stimulates the release of both ACTH and cortisol. It is believed that the episodes of ACTH secretion are preceded by hypothalamic CRF release, reaching the anterior hypophysis by the portal veins. While each ACTH secretory event causes discrete release of cortisol, because of cortisol's longer half-life and the increasing numbers of secretory episodes in the early morning hours, a diurnal pattern is present. CRF secretion appears to be primarily controlled by excitatory and inhibitory pathways originating in other areas of the central nervous system and, to a lesser extent, by the glucocorticoids.

The secretory responses are, however, complex and vary depending upon the nature of the stimulus.[16–18] Generally, acute trauma stimulates the secretion of corticotrophin (ACTH), B-endorphin/B-lipotrophin (B-LPH), prolactin and vasopressin.[19–21] The production of other pituitary hormones (e.g. growth hormone, thyrotrophin, the gonadotrophins and oxytocin) may be enhanced, depressed or unaffected.[22,23] Such pituitary responses to physical and emotional trauma occur as a result of changes in hypothalamic activity. In this regard, the hypothalamic connections with other parts of the central nervous system are of crucial importance.[24,25]

Classically, prolactin, vasopressin and ACTH are regarded as the stress hormones. The function of prolactin in this regard is obscure, although stimuli that raise the osmolarity of the extracellular fluids or reduce the blood pressure or volume (e.g. haemorrhage) result in vasopressin secretion. The regulation of osmolarity is very tightly controlled, with increases of as little as 1% being sufficient to cause vasopressin release and initiate antidiuresis. Hypovolaemia is also a potent stimulus of vasopressin release, in common with both nausea and hypoxia. Catecholamines and alcohol inhibit vasopressin secretion. Changes in osmolarity are detected by osmoreceptors, or possibly sodium ion receptors, in the hypothalamus. Reductions in blood volume or pressure are recognized by volume and stretch receptors in the atria and carotid sinuses and relayed by afferent neurones, via the brain stem nucleus tractus solitarium, to the hypothalamus.[26,27] Emotional trauma is also a powerful stimulus of vasopressin production, in addition to non-specific stimuli, e.g. pain and various drugs, especially anaesthetic agents. By contrast, ACTH is released in response to all noxious stimuli, with its secretion being the essential for adrenocortical steroid production. Thus physical and emotional stress of dental treatment may be reflected in the varied release of the different stress hormones.

Hypothalamo–pituitary–adrenocortical response

Physical stress results in increased ACTH, growth hormone and prolactin secretions coupled with inhibition of thyroid stimulating hormone, luteinizing hormone and follicular stimulating hormone. These hormonal changes may be considered as being beneficial to the organism, in that they:

(1) Increase vascular tone.
(2) Provide increased energy substrate.
(3) Slow down the basal metabolic rate.
(4) Shunt energy away from temporarily unneeded activities.

These changes in hormone secretion are probably due to alterations in the hypothalamo–pituitary–

adrenocortical axis. It is more likely, however, that the basic mechanisms are far more complex than the end-result of pituitary hormone secretion.

ACTH is formed in the adenohypophysis from a biologically inactive precursor molecule, pro-opiomelanocortin (POMC). This is then released into the bloodstream in response to corticotrophin-releasing factor(s) (CRF). CRF is produced in the hypothalamus and transported to the adenohypophysis via the hypothalamo–hypophyseal portal vessels.[28] The actual composition of CRF has yet to be defined, but probably comprises CRF-41 (a 41-residue peptide and vasopressin which act synergistically). The importance of vasopressin in the regulation of ACTH secretion has been emphasized repeatedly, and the general consensus contends that CRF activity is potentiated by vasopressin,[29,30] although adrenaline (epinephrine) may also be involved.[31] In addition, stress-induced release of ACTH may be partially effected by inhibition of the secretion of corticotrophin-release-inhibiting factor(s).[32] Substance P, which is present in the hypothalamus in large quantities, may inhibit spontaneous ACTH release.[33]

CRF secretion appears to be controlled primarily by excitatory and inhibitory nervous pathways originating from other parts of the CNS. These neuronal influences may be important not only in the regulation of the basal CRF secretion, but also in the initiation of the trauma-induced hypothalamo–pituitary–adrenocortical (HPA) function. The several regions of the brain involved include the amygdala, the hippocampus, the thalamus and the reticular formation.[34]

Other systems involved in the regulation of CRF secretion include:

(1) A central cholinergic pathway that stimulates CRF secretion.[35]
(2) Two distinct 5-hydroxytryptamine (5-HT) systems, one stimulatory and the other inhibitory of hypothalamo–pituitary–adrenocortical activity.
(3) Catecholamines.
(4) Opioid substances.

HPA activity is controlled to some extent by negative feedback mechanisms involving both ACTH and corticosteroids. Under non-stress conditions, the blood corticosteroids probably play an important part in the regulation of ACTH release. Corticosteroids inhibit ACTH secretion, probably by acting on specific receptors in the adenohypophysis, hypothalamus and other CNS sites. During stress, the corticosteroids appear to play an essential causal role in substrate mobilization required for hepatic glucogenesis (e.g. amino acids, glycerol, lactate), in addition to the compensatory responses to fluid loss caused by haemorrhage.[36] Glucocorticoids, at concentrations attained in the peripheral blood after trauma, exhibit marked immunosuppressive and anti-inflammatory properties. They inhibit the production or activity of numerous mediators involved in the physiological responses to anxiety, infection and metabolic disturbance, including prostaglandins and related compounds, kinins, histamine and lymphokines.

Thus corticosteroids suppress the body's normal defence mechanisms, conceivably preventing the normal responses to trauma proceeding to a stage of producing tissue damage and threatening homeostasis.

Haemostatic response

Acute stress, quite independently of trauma, produces a transient change in the haemostatic mechanism, which may be mediated by neurohumoral messages. These changes include thrombocytosis,[37] increased clotting activity[38] and increased plasminogen activator activity.[39]

It is not yet established whether the rise in these agents in the blood is the result of an active process or reflects passive circulatory changes which sweep platelets or plasminogen activator from the endothelium, to which they were loosely attached. The physiological benefit of these changes is not apparent, as normal individuals appear well equipped to confront most haemostatic challenges without such defence reinforcement. Possibly they reflect primitive responses to danger in anticipation of injury. It is clear, however, that all the arms of the haemostatic mechanism are acutely modified as a result of various kinds of stress, and these changes may be mediated by adrenergic pathways and/or the pituitary. None of these changes imply that platelet plug or fibrin formation or dissolution is actually occurring, just that the groundwork is laid down to allow these processes to occur should the appropriate stimulus appear. Trauma is associated with stress and these stress-induced changes will appear after injury. They will be superimposed on, and will often obscure, any platelet or clotting factor consumption resulting from local haemostatic mechanisms. These changes are, however, generally transient, lasting only hours.

In the days following many different types of injury, the haemostatic mechanism slowly evolves towards haemostatic security. The platelet count is raised to a variable, sometimes striking, degree[40] and platelet adhesiveness[41–43] and sensitivity to certain aggregating agents are also increased.[44] This implies that the platelets are therefore readied for any subsequent acute haemostatic emergency. Trauma is also followed by a period of sustained and striking increase in plasma fibrinogen level.[45] Although these changes do not indicate that the system is active, there is some indirect evidence that thrombin and fibrin formation are actually occurring at this time. Concurrent with these changes, the activity of the fibrinolytic system is also reduced. Such changes in the haemostatic mechanism towards security also increase the undesirable risk of thrombus and embolus formation.

Stress studies

An elevation of the heart rate is generally associated with anxiety states.[46] The blood pressure also tends to be raised but this is not necessarily a corollary.[47,48] Large increases in forearm blood flow accompany emotional stress,[49] in addition to increased palmar sweating and decreased salivary secretion.[50] In one study, increased salivary secretion was noted during dental treatment of aggressive patients, but significant reductions in defensive subjects.[51]

Anxiety, associated with anger and aggression, is usually linked with raised noradrenaline and adrenaline production[52] and free fatty acid mobilization.[15] This latter has been associated with increased coronary artery narrowing, reflecting atheromatous plaque deposition.[15] Anxiety, without fear or aggression, mainly causes raised adrenaline levels[53] which do not appear to be associated with pathological vascular changes.

In a number of heightened emotional states, e.g. hostility, apprehension and agitation, there is an associated increased plasma 17-hydroxycorticosteroid level.[54] A similar increase in corticosteroid levels has been noted in patients awaiting oral surgery.[55] Thus the stress produced by routine oral surgery or other forms of dentistry may not be insignificant. Patients who have undergone even quite minor oral or periodontal surgery may complain of feeling lifeless or fatigued the following day. It is not only the procedure that presents the challenge but the whole aura associated with the occasion. Often fear of the clinical environment, and even more the fear engendered by the imagination, results in many of the untoward reactions occurring in the dental surgery. Such effects may be augmented or exaggerated by others, including pain, stuffy rooms, concurrent illness, drugs and medications, and poor patient handling.

Subjective feelings of anxiety may often be translated to physiological manifestations, including:

(1) Changes in facial expression.
(2) Trembling.
(3) Palmar sweating.
(4) Cold extremities.
(5) Pallor.
(6) Nausea.
(7) Diarrhoea.
(8) Micturition frequency.
(9) Breathlessness.
(10) Palpitations.

Vasovagal reactions

A vasovagal reaction may be defined as 'the development of hypotension and brachycardia associated with the typical clinical manifestations of pallor, sweating and weakness'.

The most profound degree of vasovagal reaction results in fainting or syncope. The result is cerebral ischaemia and loss of consciousness due to an abrupt severe fall in blood pressure. Such episodes frequently affect young males,[56] especially when predisposed by a warm environment, anxiety, fear and pain. Whilst the upright position of the dental chair may be a contributory factor, syncope may still occur in the supine position.[57]

Physiologically, syncope is associated with an initial sudden increase in the blood pressure, probably associated with apprehension. This then stimulates the baroreceptors of the aortic arch and carotid sinuses to produce generalized inhibition of sympathetic tone. This leads to brachycardia and arteriolar dilatation, especially in the skeletal muscle. Such changes result in the following:

(1) Reduced cardiac output.
(2) Fall in total peripheral resistance.
(3) Hypotension.
(4) Syncope.[53]

Thus there is a generalized inhibition of sympathetic tone with a relative increase in vagal activity. Such a reaction is probably influenced by the cortical limbic system, which may be more sensitive in some patients than others.[58]

Arteriolar dilatation, resulting in systemic hypotension, may be associated with reduced cardiac filling.[59] The combined diminution in ventricular volume and increased ventricular wall tension may then trigger a depressor reflex initiated by intracardiac baroreceptors.[60]

Other forms of syncope may also occur in the dental chair. One is carotid sinus syncope induced by pressure over the carotid sinus in the neck.[61] This probably results from vagal inhibition and consequent fall in arterial pressure. The other, cough syncope, occurs during a spell of violent coughing, where high intrathoracic pressures are developed, associated with a reduction in the venous return to the heart.[62]

Hyperventilation

Overbreathing in anxious individuals usually starts insidiously but, as the rate and depth increases, increasing volumes of carbon dioxide are expired through the lungs. There is a consequent fall in the partial pressure of arterial carbon dioxide and a rise in blood pH, resulting in respiratory alkalosis which induces progressive cerebral arteriolar vasoconstriction.[44] Heart rate and cardiac output rise and there is a marked fall in peripheral vascular resistance. These effects occur in patients who have undergone sympathectomies or who have had brachial plexus blocks with local anaesthesia.[63] These reactions are therefore probably not mediated by the central nervous system but are the result of direct local vascular effects. During these episodes tetany often develops, with facial and lip stiffness, spasm of the hands and feet and increased motor nerve excitability. The effects appear to be associated with increased blood and tissue fluid calcium ion concentrations. Numbness and tingling of the extremities, together with the tetanic spasm, may further increase patient anxiety levels. Treatment requires increased carbon dioxide inhalation, usually by breathing into a bag or paper cup.

Arrhythmias

Many patients exhibit cardiac abnormalities when emotionally stressed, including extraventricular systoles.[64] In patients in the dental chair, most of such anomalies are nodal or mitral in origin and are of no clinical significance. More serious arrhythmias are more likely to occur in patients with pre-existing cardiac disease. The possible causative factors include:

(1) Excess carbon dioxide in the blood.
(2) Oxygen deficiency.
(3) Reflex sympathetic stimulation.
(4) Increased endogenous catecholamine secretion, rendering the myocardium more excitable.
(5) Atropine premedication to decrease saliva production.
(6) Vasoconstrictor components of local anaesthetic solutions, especially if injected directly into a vein.

Nausea and vomiting

Nausea is a subjective phenomenon, comprising a desire to vomit without attempted expulsive movements. Nausea may often be associated with a variety of signs and symptoms, including:

(1) Excessive saliva production.
(2) Sweating.
(3) Increase in heart rate.
(4) Variations in the rate, depth and regulation of respiration.

These symptoms are sometimes manifest in the anxious patient in addition to fear, pain, drugs or hypoxia. Nausea may also result from stimulation of the afferent nerves of the soft palate and pharynx, especially during dental impression taking. Vomiting may occur in association with general anaesthesia, resulting from drug reactions, respiratory obstruction, hypoxia and postoperative blood swallowing. If there is depression of the level of consciousness, such vomiting may result in laryngeal spasm. Alternatively, vomitus may enter the lungs to result in severe exudative oedema and bronchospasm, a condition termed Mendelson's syndrome. Bronchopneumonia or lung abscess may then follow.

Conclusions

The physiological processes underlying anxiety are exceedingly complex. In this short chapter, only a cursory overview has therefore been provided. The development of shock initiates a cascade of responses in an effort to re-establish homeostasis. Three of the most important hormonal and neurohormonal changes are the secretion of glucocorticoids, catecholamines and vasopressin. Regulation of adrenal function is more complex than originally thought. Haemorrhage is a potent stimulus for cortisol release, and both ACTH and ACTH-independent mechanisms have been described. The ACTH response to its releasing hormone, corticotrophin-releasing factor (CRF), is itself amplified by vasopressin, which appears to have intrinsic CRF properties. Nor-adrenaline and adrenaline levels increase many times above baseline within minutes of the onset of haemorrhagic shock; the enkephalins are co-released with the catecholamines, modifying their cardiovascular effects and producing analgesia. Hypovolaemia is also a potent stimulus for vasopressin secretion. Vasopressin is also released by pain, nausea and hypoxia, all of which are likely to be present in a patient with shock. Thus, the hormonal responses to shock are complex, often interacting with one another to stimulate or partially counteract their individual actions.

Review questions

1. Identify the main manifestations of stress towards dental treatment.
2. What is the haemostatic response to stress, and what is the physiological benefit to a patient?
3. Describe the physiological manifestations of a vasovagal attack.
4. How do the higher centres of the central nervous system influence a patient's reactions to stress?
5. What are the manifestations of cardiac arrhythmias?

References

1. TATTERSALL, W.R. (1964) General Dental Services Committee Report of the Ad Hoc Sub-Committee on Methods of Remuneration. *Br. Dent. J.*, **117**, 331–346
2. KEGELES, S.S. (1963) Some motives for seeking preventative dental care. *J. Am. Dent. Assoc.*, **67**, 90–98
3. ROBBINS, P.R. (1962) Some exploration into the nature of anxieties relating to illness. *Genet. Psychol. Monogr.*, **66**, 95–141
4. WOLFF, H.G., WOLF, S.G. and HARE, C.C. (1949) Life stress and bodily disease. *Proc. Ass. Res. Nerv. Ment. Dis.*, **29**, 1059
5. DONOHOE, T.B. (1984) Stress-induced anorexia. *Life Sci.*, **34**, 203–218
6. MORLEY, J.E. (1983) Minireview: stress-induced eating. *Life Sci.*, **32**, 2169–2182
7. COLLU, R. (1984) Effect of stress on the gonadal function. *J. Endocrinol. Invest.*, **7**, 529–537
8. KASL, E.V. (1984) Stress and health. *Annu. Rev. Publ. Health*, **5**, 319–341
9. DEAN, D.H. (1985) Immune response after oral surgical stress. *J. Oral Med.*, **40**, 183–184
10. CLARK, W.C. (1986) Altered pain and visual sensitivity in humans: the effects of acute and chronic stress. *Ann. NY Acad. Sci.*, **467**, 116–129
11. JACOBS, W.J. (1985) Stress-induced recovery of fears and phobias. *Psychol. Rev.*, **92**, 512–531
12. STEPHENS, S.S. (1951) *Handbook of Experimental Psychology*. New York: Wiley
13. SMYTHIES, J.R. (1967) Neurophysiology of anxiety. In *Studies of Anxiety. Br. J. Psychiat.*, **3**, 32–39
14. CANNON, W.B. (1929) *Bodily Changes in Pain, Hunger, Fear and Rage.* New York: Harper & Row
15. PRICE, D.B., THALER, M. and MASON, J.W. (1957) Pre-operative emotional states and adrenal cortical activity. *AMA Arch. Neurol. Psychiatr.*, **77**, 646–656
16. GLAVIN, G.B. (1985) Stress and brain noradrenaline. *Neurosci. Behav. Rev.*, **9**, 233–243
17. HERNANDEZ, D.E. (1986) Neuroendocrine mechanisms of stress ulceration. *Life Sci.*, **39**, 279–296
18. OEHME, P. (1985) Relation of substance P to catecholamine metabolism and stress. *Biomed. Biochim. Acta*, **44**, 1401–1409
19. AXELROD, J. and REISINE, T.D. (1984) Stress hormones: their interaction and regulation. *Science*, **224**, 452–459
20. COHEN, M.R., PICKAR, D. and DUBOIS, M. (1982) Clinical and experimental studies of stress and the endogenous opioid system. *Ann. NY Acad. Sci.*, **398**, 424–432
21. CALIGARIS, L. and TALEISNIK, S. (1983) Prolactin release induced by stress and the influence of oestrogen and progesterone treatments, sex and daily rhythm. *Acta Endocrinol.*, **102**, 505–510
22. RUISSEAU, P., TACHE, Y., BRAZEAU, P. and COLLU, R. (1978) Pattern of adenohypophyseal hormone changes induced by various stressors in female and male rats. *Neuroendocrinol.*, **27**, 257–271
23. GREENWOOD, R.C. and LANDON, J. (1966) Growth hormone secretion in response to stress in man. *Nature*, **210**, 540–541
24. SIEGEL, R.A., WEIDENFELD, J., FELDMAN, S., CONFORTI, N. and CHOWERS, I. (1981) Neural pathways mediating basal and stress induced secretion of luteinizing hormone, follicle stimulating hormone and testosterone in the rat. *Endocrinol.*, **108**, 2302–2307
25. GRAY, G.D., SMITH, E.R., DAMASSA, D.A., EHRENKRANTZ, J.R.L. and DAVIDSON, J.M. (1978) Neuroendocrine mechanisms mediating the suppression of circulating testosterone levels associated with chronic stress in male rats. *Neuroendocrinology*, **25**, 247–256
26. KWAAKAMI, M. and HIGUCHI, T. (1981) Effect of partial deafferentation of the hypothalamus on stress-induced LH suppression and prolactin release. *Neuroendocrinology*, **108**, 2302–2307
27. HANDLER, J.S. and ORLOFF, J. (1981) Antidiuretic hormone. *Ann. Rev. Physiol.*, **43**, 611–624
28. BIE, P. (1980) Osmoreceptors, vasopressin and the control of renal water excretion. *Physiol. Rev.*, **60**, 961–1048
29. DE GROOT, J. and HARRIS, G.W. (1950) Hypothalamic control of the anterior pituitary gland and blood lymphocytes. *J. Physiol.*, **111**, 335–346
30. GILLIES, G.E., LINTON, E.A. and LOWRY, P.J. (1982) Corticotrophin releasing activity of the new CRF is potentiated several times by vasopressin. *Nature*, **299**, 355–357
31. TURKELSON, C.M., THOMAS, C.R., ARIMURA, A., CHANG, D., CHANG, J.K. and SHIMIZU, M. (1982) *In vitro* potentiation of the activity of synthetic ovine corticotropin-releasing factor by arginine vasopressin. *Peptides*, **3**, 111–113
32. GIGUERE, V. and LABRIE, F. (1983) Additive effects of epinephrine and corticotrophin-releasing factor on adrenocorticotrophin release in rat anterior pituitary cells. *Biochem. Biophys. Res. Commun.*, **110**, 456–462
33. GILLIES, G.E., PURI, A., LINTON, E.A. and LOWRY, P.J. (1984) Comparative chromatography of hypothalamic-corticotrophin-releasing factors. *Neuroendocrinology*, **38**, 17–24
34. JONES, M.T., GILLMAN, B., HOLMES, M.C., HODGES, J.R. and BUCKINGHAM, J.C. (1978) Influence of substance P on hypothalamo-pituitary-adrenocortical activity in the rat. *J. Endocrinol.*, **76**, 183–184
35. KNIGGE, K.M. (1961) Adrenocortical response to stress in rat with lesions in hippocampus and amygdala. *Proc. Soc. Exp. Med. Biol.*, **108**, 18–21
36. HEDGE, G.A. and SMEELIK, P.G. (1968) Corticotrophin release: inhibition by intrahypothalamic implantation of atropine. *Science*, **159**, 891–892
37. ALBERTI, K.G. and JOHNSTON, D.G. (1977) Cortisol and catabolism: a new perspective. *Clin. Sci. Mol. Med.*, **52**, 333–336
38. SARAJAS, H.S.S., KONTTINEN, A. and FRICK, M.H. (1961) Thrombocytosis evoked by exercise. *Nature*, **192**, 721–722
39. BENNETT, B. and RATNOFF, O.D. (1972) Changes in antihemolytic factor procoagulant activity and AHF-

like antigen in normal pregnancy, and following exercise and pneumoencephalography. *J. Lab. Clin. Med.*, **80**, 256–263

40. BENNETT, N.B., OGSTON, C.M. and OGSTON, D. (1968) The effect of prolonged exercise on the components of the blood fibrinolytic enzyme system. *J. Physiol.*, **198**, 479–485
41. SHARNOFF, J.G., BAGG, J.F., BREEN, S.R. and ROGLIANO, A.G. (1960) The possible indication of postoperative thromboembolism by platelet counts and blood coagulation studies in the patient undergoing extensive surgery. *Surg. Gynecol. Obstet.*, **111**, 469–474
42. BENNETT, P.N. (1967) Postoperative changes in platelet adhesiveness. *J. Clin. Pathol.*, **20**, 708–709
43. BENNETT, N.B., OGSTON, C.M. and OGSTON, D. (1967) Studies on the blood fibrinolytic enzyme system following acute myocardial infarction. *Clin. Sci.*, **32**, 27–37
44. HARVEY, W.P. and LEVINE, S.A. (1952) Paroxysmal ventricular tachycardia due to emotion. *JAMA*, **150**, 479–480
45. LADER, M.H. and WING, L. (1966) *Physiological Measures, Sedative Drugs and Morbid Anxiety*. London: Oxford University Press
46. GOLDSTEIN, I.B. (1964) Physiological responses in anxious women. *Arch. Gen. Psychiat.*, **10**, 382
47. SHIP, I.I. (1960) The response of systolic and diastolic blood pressure to dental stress. *Oral Surg.*, **13**, 499–507
48. PECK, R.E. (1966) Observations on salivation and palmar sweating in anxiety and other psychiatric conditions. *Psychosomatics*, **7**, 343
49. BOGDONOFF, P.R., BOGDONOFF, M.M. and WOLF, S.G. (1961) Studies on salivary function in man. *J. Psychosom. Res.*, **5**, 170–174
50. MARTIN, B. (1961) The assessment of anxiety by physiological behavioural measures. *Psychol. Bull.*, **58**, 234–255
51. TAGGART, P. and CARRUTHERS, M. (1971) Endogenous hyperlipidemia induced by emotional stress of racing driving. *Lancet*, **i**, 363–366
52. EDMONDSON, H.D., ROSCOE, B. and VICKERS, M.D. (1972) Biochemical evidence of anxiety in dental patients. *Br. Med. J.*, **4**, 7–9
53. SHANNON, I.L., ISBELL, G.M. and PRIGMORE, J.R. (1962) Stress in dental patients. II. The serum free 17-hydroxycorticosteroid response in routinely appointed patients undergoing simple exodontia. *USAF School of Aerospace Medicine Report*, **62**, 27
54. HANNINGTON-KIFF, J.G. (1969) Fainting and collapse in dental practice. *Dent. Pract. Dent. Rec.*, **20**, 2–7
55. VERRILL, P.J. and AELLIG, W.H. (1970) Vasovagal faint in the supine position. *Br. Med. J.*, **4**, 348
56. GLICK, G. and YU, P.N. (1963) Haemodynamic changes during spontaneous vaso-vagal reactions. *Am. J. Med.*, **34**, 42–51
57. EPSTEIN, S.E., STAMPFER, M. and BEISER, G.D. (1968) Role of the capacitance and resistance vessels in vaso-vagal syncope. *Circulation*, **37**, 524–533
58. SHARPEY-SCHAFFER, E.P., HAYTER, C.J. and BARLOW, E.D. (1958) Mechanism of acute hypotension from fear to nausea. *Br. Med. J.*, **2**, 878–880
59. WEISS, S. and BAKER, J.P. (1933) The carotid sinus reflex in health and disease. *Medicine*, **12**, 297–354
60. CORSON, W.A. (1970) Cough syncope. *Minn. Med.*, **53**, 43
61. MEYER, J.S. and GOTOH, F. (1960) Metabolic and electroencephalographic effects of hyperventilation. *Arch. Neurol.*, **3**, 539–552
62. BURRUM, J.F., HICKMAN, J.B. and MCINTOSH, H.D. (1954) The effect of hypocapnia on arterial blood pressure. *Circulation*, **9**, 80–95
63. RYDER, W. (1970) The electrocardiogram in dental anaesthesia. *Anaesthesia*, **25**, 46–61
64. MENDELSON, C.L. (1946) Aspiration of the stomach contents into lungs during obstet anaesthesia. *Am. J. Obstet. Gynecol.*, **52**, 191–205

14

Saliva

Introduction

The saliva circulating in the mouth at any given time is termed whole saliva and comprises a mixture of secretions from the major and minor salivary glands. Each gland contributes unique ingredients that interact with the other oral contents. Some salivary components immediately attach to tooth surfaces, whereas others interact with the oral soft tissues, bacteria and food.[23] Over a 24 h period more than a litre of saliva is secreted, although both quantity and quality depend upon a variety of factors, including the time of day.[1] For instance, very little saliva is secreted during sleep, whereas abundant saliva flows at mealtimes, stimulated by sight and smell as well as taste. While the salivary digestive activities have long been known, the protective functions have greater dental significance. Thus, patients with decreased salivary flow exhibit rampant caries in addition to oral inflammatory lesions and infections.

The salivary components may be of value diagnostically in that they may be used to assay a variety of agents and drugs, including:

(1) Anti-epileptic drugs.
(2) Phenobarbital.
(3) Digoxin.
(4) Methadone.
(5) Pyschoactive drugs, e.g. diazepam, lithium carbonate.
(6) Amitriptyline.
(7) Steroids and other hormones, e.g. aldosterone and oestrogens.

In addition to the autonomic nervous system, a number of other factors can stimulate salivary secretion, e.g. insulin, thyroid hormone and mineralocorticosteroids. The salivary glands also produce traces of hormones that affect tissue growth and repair, i.e. salivary glands exhibit both exocrine and endocrine functions. Thus salivary glands represent complex organs producing a complex solution, saliva.

There is a widespread belief that salivary flow diminishes with age: this may hold true for only a portion of the population. Elderly people are, however, likely to be taking one or more daily medications, and since neural salivary control ultimately depends on neurotransmitters in contact with gland cells, saliva production can be affected by neuro-active drugs. For instance, atropine, certain tranquillizing and antidepressant drugs. Such long-term prescriptions that adversely affect saliva production may lead to a diminished ability to taste and enjoy food, difficulties in speech, mastication and swallowing and a significantly increased oral tissue vulnerability to injury or disease. Thus knowledge of the physiology of salivary secretion has both pathological and diagnostic significance.

Salivary glands

Gross morphology

There are three major salivary glands, which produce about 95% of total salivary volume, and numerous minor (accessory) salivary glands producing relatively miniscule amounts of saliva.

Parotid gland (Figure 14.1)

The parotid (literally 'next to the ears') glands provide 60–65% of total salivary volume. The glands are pyramidal in shape and engulfed by a dense fibrous capsule. This capsule may limit glandular expansion during inflammatory and other pathological changes, resulting in intense pain and discomfort. The capsule, together with the connective tissue septa that pass into the gland substance, provides support, augmented by a connective tissue matrix. The salivary glands therefore comprise both mesodermal (connective tissue) and epithelial (glandular cells) tissues, either of which may be subjected to pathological change.

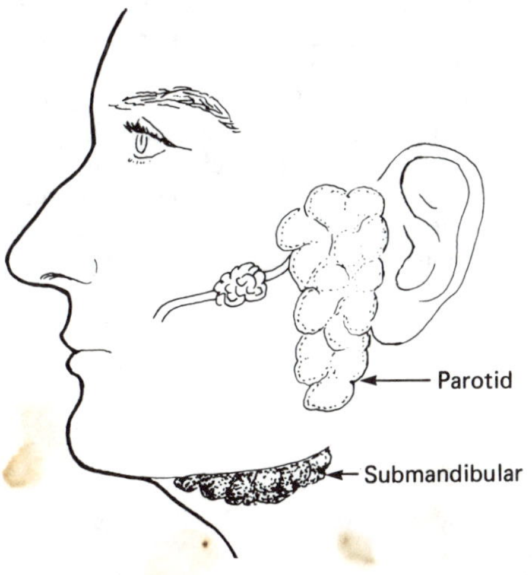

Figure 14.1 Major salivary glands. The parotid is located close to the posterior border of the mandibular ascending ramus, whereas the submandibular is located close to the mandibular inferior border.

The superficial surface of the parotid gland (the base of the pyramid) is defined by the zygomatic arch, the external auditory meatus, and just behind and below the angle of the mandible. The gland extends into the groove between the mandibular ramus and sternocleidomastoid muscle to reach the styloid process and associated muscles which separate the gland from the internal carotid artery and jugular vein. The external carotid artery enters the gland and divides into its terminal branches. The facial nerve also passes through the gland, dividing close to the anterior border. The main parotid duct (Stensen's duct) leaves the mesial angle of the gland to traverse over the masseter muscle and turn abruptly to enter the buccinator muscle prior to opening into the oral cavity in a small papilla close to the buccal surface of the maxillary first molar tooth. The duct is about 5 cm long and 3 mm in internal diameter, its walls comprising smooth muscle and fibrous tissue with an epithelial lining.

Submandibular gland

The submandibular glands produce about 20–30% of total salivary volume. The glands are irregular, walnut in shape, with a superficial inferior portion in contact with the skin and platysma muscle. Laterally, the gland is in contact with the mandibular body and medially with the extrinsic tongue and mylohyoid muscles. There may also be a small, deeper portion of the gland between the mylohyoid, hyoglossus and styloglossus muscles. This part of the gland extends forwards and inwards above the duct of the superficial portion to reach the posterior edge of the sublingual gland. After leaving the superficial part of the gland, the duct (Wharton's duct) passes beneath the deep part, between the mylohyoid and hyoglossus muscles, and between the sublingual gland and the genioglossus muscle to end at the summit of the sublingual papilla at the side of the lingual frenulum. This tortuous duct is approximately 5 cm long.

Sublingual gland

The sublingual glands produce 2–5% of total salivary volume. The glands lie immediately beneath the oral mucosal lining of the mouth floor, raising a small fold on either side of the tongue. The glands rest on the mylohyoid muscle, with the mandible lateral and the genioglossus muscle medial. This smallest of the major salivary glands has a series of small ducts (Bartholin's ducts) that open on to the surface of the sublingual folds on either side of the tongue.

Minor glands

Serous glands of von Ebner

These are small glands whose ducts open into the sulci of the circumvallate papillae.

Anterior lingual glands

These two irregular glandular groups lie on either side of the frenulum on the under-surface of the tongue, with several ducts piercing the overlying mucosa.

Lingual, buccal, labial and palatal glands

These glandular aggregates are scattered over the tongue surface, inside of the lips and cheeks, and palatal mucosa.

Blood supply

The blood supply to the parotid is derived from the facial and external carotid arteries, with a richer vascular supply to the ductal than acinar systems. In fact the blood flow is parallel, but in the opposite direction, to the salivary flow,[2] running along the glandular connective tissue septa. The facial and lingual arteries supply the submandibular gland, whereas the submental and sublingual arteries supply the sublingual gland. Venous drainage of all the glands is mainly through the external jugular vein. It appears that a portal vascular system exists within the gland with arterial blood flowing first to the ducts and then through capillaries which subsequently rejoin to form a portal vessel. This again splits to form capillaries around the acini.

Microscopic structure

Acinar region (*Figure 14.2*)

The structure of salivary glands is similar to other exocrine glands,[24,25] comprising a series of secretory units (acinar cells) clustered around a central lumen. These acini comprise the terminal or secretory end-piece of the gland, situated farthest from the oral cavity. They are supported by myoepithelial cells and a basement membrane. From each acinus the secretions pass to a series of interconnected ducts before passing out through the major salivary duct into the oral cavity.

Each acinus comprises a series of polygonal cells on a basement membrane centred around a central ductal lumen. The acinar cells of the sublingual and submandibular glands (and occasionally in the parotid) are said to comprise mucous cells. These cells contain large secretory vacuoles and areas of smooth parallel cisternae. Otherwise they have a similar form and appearance to serous cells. Serous cells comprise the majority of the acinar cells of the parotid and glands of von Ebner. Serous cells also occur in the anterior lingual and submandibular glands where they are located on the outer surface of mucous cell acini. Where serous cells predominate in an acinus, they are large, polygonal in shape, although when a gland is predominantly mucous, the serous cells have a crescent (demilune) or flattened shape. These serous cells are characterized by a nucleus lying towards the base membrane; this cellular region also contains an extensive endoplasmic reticulum. In the luminal region of the cell there are numerous granules and vacuoles whose size is determined by the functional cellular activity. The luminal region of the cell also appears to contain a few villi, whereas the lateral cell walls are interdigitated with those of adjacent cells, there being some intervening tight junctions in the apical regions.

It is generally believed that protein secretion starts with the synthesis of exportable protein at the attached ribosomes of the rough endoplasmic reticulum.[4] The protein is subsequently passed into a cisternal cavity of the reticulum, where it moves into the transitional zone. The elements then bud off to become Golgi vesicles. These vesicles transmit their contents to condensing vacuoles, which progressively fill and concentrate their content. The Golgi complex also processes the polysaccharide moieties into the forming secretory granules. Gradually, the immature granules become mature

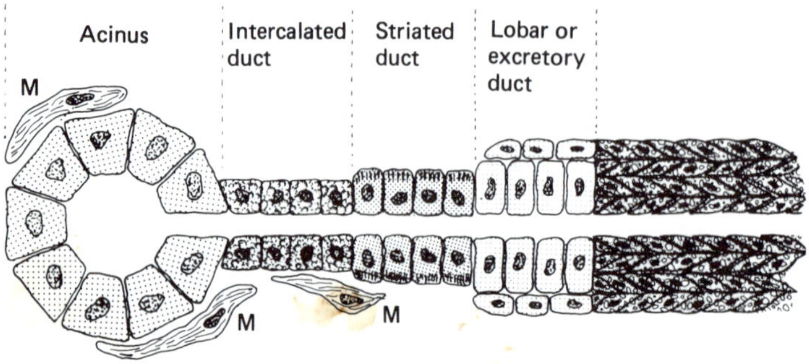

Figure 14.2 Diagrammatic illustration of a component of a major salivary gland. M, myoepithelial cell.

granules and reach an apical cellular location. The actual secretory mechanism, however, remains obscure. In mucous cells, masses of fused granules and mucus are discharged into the acinar lumen through breaks in the apical membrane. This apocrine process may be so extensive that the whole of the cellular contents are discharged.[5] Other studies have shown that the zymogen granules may fuse with the luminal membrane and discharge their contents, followed by luminal membranous withdrawal in the form of small smooth vesicles into the cellular cytoplasm.[6]

Ducts (Figure 14.3)

The secretions pass from the acinus to a short intercalated duct, whose lining cuboidal cells have a large central nucleus and many mitochondria but little endoplasmic reticulum. The cells have small cytoplasmic villi extending in towards the lumen. The duct lining cells are closely interdigitated one with another, but lack sufficient structural organization for electrolyte transport. They do, however, contain zymogen granules, which may contribute to subtle changes in salivary composition.

The intercalated ducts then pass abruptly into another short, but wide, striated duct. These latter are lined by columnar cells with marked cellular membrane interdigitations projecting towards the lumen. The cytoplasm in this region contains numerous linearly arranged mitochondria providing the striated appearance. The striated ducts actively resorb sodium ions from the primary acinar secretion, with the associated capillaries then transporting the ions away from the glands into the systemic circulation.

These striated ducts then pass abruptly into two-epithelial-cell-layered excretory ducts and, finally, to a stratified squamous epithelial-cell-lined terminal duct. Although these latter excretory ducts resorb electrolytes from the primary secretion, they are probably less efficient than the striated duct lining cells.

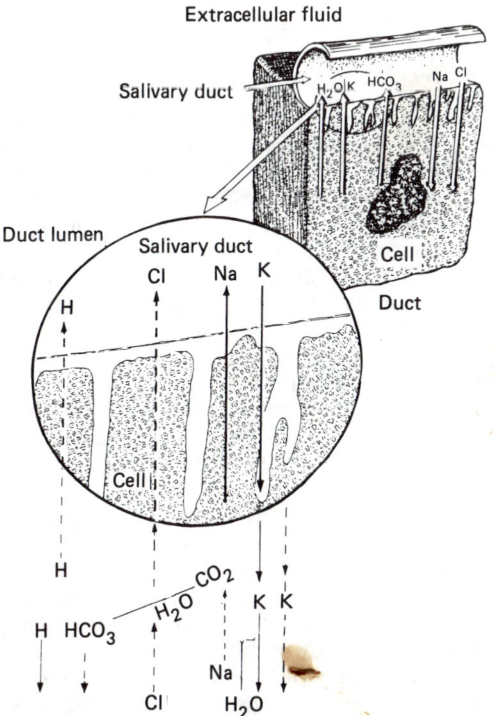

Figure 14.3 Diagrammatic illustration of ionic movements in salivary ducts.

Myoepithelial cells

These cells constrict the acini and ducts to facilitate salivary secretory flow. These stellate cells have long thin cytoplasmic processes that interdigitate around the acini and ducts. They generally contain longitudinally arranged myofibrils that immunochemically cross-react with antibodies to smooth muscle actomyosin.[26] They therefore resemble smooth muscle cells.

Mechanisms of salivary secretion

Acinar fluid formation

The acinar fluid consists of water, ions, small molecules and secretory products synthesized by the cells. This fluid is derived from the interstitial fluid, which in turn is derived from the blood in the adjacent capillaries. Molecules such as glucose, urea and amino acids diffuse freely through the capillary wall. As secretion is stimulated, however, the blood flow to the acinar region is increased, with the pressure gradient towards the acinus facilitating primary acinar fluid formation. Although the acinar cells are freely permeable to lipid-soluble substances and water, they are much less permeable to other substances, e.g. glucose. Thus, there must also be a form of active cellular transport for some substances, e.g. sodium and chloride ions. The acinar cells also synthesize salivary proteins, probably at the ribosomes. The proteins then pass into the cisternae of the endoplasmic reticulum, to be secreted from the cell surface by exocytosis. Stimulation of the salivary glands does not change the rate of protein synthesis, only the acinar cell discharge rate.

The role of the ducts

On passing through the ducts, the acinar fluid is transformed from an isotonic (or slightly hypertonic) fluid with analogous ionic concentrations to plasma, to a hypotonic fluid with low chloride and sodium ion concentrations. This function is essentially confined to the striated duct, facilitated by the marked interdigitations of the luminal cellular walls. Thus, there is active transport of sodium out of the fluid with active potassium transport in the opposite direction, passive chloride diffusion maintaining an electrochemical balance. Bicarbonate is also actively secreted into the fluid at this time. Partial salivary equilibration with plasma occurs in the excretory ducts, with the ion concentrations returning closer to those of plasma.

Salivary gland innervation

Salivary secretion results from neural, rather than hormonal, stimulation. Neural section not only results in the cessation of secretion but, ultimately, glandular atrophy. The liberal sympathetic innervation is derived from the superior cervical ganglion and follows the blood vessels into all the glands. They are then distributed to the acini and intercalated and striated ducts, but not the excretory ducts.

The parasympathetic secretomotor innervation to the parotid gland travels in a branch of the glossopharyngeal nerve which synapses in the otic ganglion. It subsequently passes with the auriculotemporal nerve to the gland. Both submandibular and sublingual glands derive their secretomotor innervation from the facial nerve, with the chorda tympani branch leaving the middle ear and passing as the chorda tympani to join the lingual nerve and synapse in the submandibular ganglion. Postganglionic branches then pass from this ganglion to the two glands. There are also other secretomotor pathways.[3] For example, section of the glossopharyngeal nerve decreases submandibular, sublingual and parotid secretions, while section of the chorda tympani results in parotid gland secretory depression. Secretomotor nerves to the submandibular and sublingual glands have also been found in the hypoglossal nerve and cervical branch of the facial nerve. The main parasympathetic nerve trunks pass to the main ducts and blood vessels, with small fibre plexuses forming around the striated and intercalated ducts and acinar surfaces, but not around the excretory ducts.

General sensory fibres appear to be carried to the parotid via the glossopharyngeal nerve and to the sublingual and sdubmandibular glands via the chorda tympani. Conceivably, these fibres comprise part of a feedback mechanism responding to glandular distension.

There appear to be no specialized sensory or secretomotor nerve endings within the glands, although there may be separation between acinar and myoepithelial innervations. Salivary secretory stimulation occurs primarily through cholinergic agents, although α-adrenergic agents may also be involved, together with calcium ions. Salivary stimulation appears to be mediated by an increase in the intracellular concentration of cyclic guanosine 3',5'-monophosphate (cGMP). β-adrenergic agents also cause salivary stimulation which is mediated by an increase in intracellular cyclic adenosine 3',5'-monophosphate (cAMP), although this does not require calcium ions. The secretion of electrolytes, water and proteinaceous substances (zymogen granules) is the net cyclic nucleotide effect on the acinar cells. The basal and luminal acinar membranes also become more permeable to sodium and potassium ions. In addition, stimulation results in a transient potassium ion efflux from the acinar cells to the lumen and interstitial fluid. This is associated with a net influx of sodium ions passively followed by water and chloride ions. Cholinergic or adrenergic stimulation also activates the sodium pump located near the tight junction between the acinar cells. Both cAMP and cGMP are also involved with protein secretion, with cAMP activating a protein kinase in the acinar cell, resulting in phosphorylation of another protein to effect zymogen granule membrane changes.

Salivary control

Afferent pathways

The rate of salivary gland secretion may be affected by three principal factors.

Local factors

Whenever the sensation of taste is stimulated, the salivary flow rate increases. The fibres carrying taste sensation pass along the chorda tympani in the lingual nerve (originating in the facial nerve) and the glossopharyngeal nerve. Glossopharyngeal nerve stimulation (supplying the posterior one-third of the tongue) results mainly in increased parotid salivary flow. Chorda tympani inputs and outputs appear similarly related.[2] Acid stimuli are the most effective salivary flow stimulants, salt and sweet less so, and bitter the least effective.

Olfactory irritants similarly cause increased salivary flow rates. There is, however, uncertainty as to whether non-irritating olfactory stimuli also have a similar effect or whether the salivary response is a conditioned reflex. Irritation (or touching) of the oral mucosa can also result in increased salivation; this feature is most pronounced following new denture or orthodontic appliance insertion. In these latter instances, increased salivation is usually temporary, although it may initially alarm the patient. Unilateral proprioceptive stimulation in the periodontal ligament, muscles of mastication or temporomandibular joint predominantly leads to ipsilateral increased salivary secretion.[2]

Emotional (psychic) stimuli

The sight of food, talking about food, or the noise of food preparation are sufficient to activate the conditioned reflexes leading to increased salivation.[1] By contrast, discussion or thought about disliked foods may result in diminished salivary secretion. This indicates that salivation can be influenced by the higher centres, e.g. fear or rage, although the details of such controls have yet to be defined.

Stimulation from other organs

Oesophageal irritation causes reflex salivation, although gastric irritation leads to increased salivation as a component of the nausea/vomiting reflex. Thus, oesophageal carcinoma may be associated with marked salivation, whose subsequent swallowing may induce severe pain.

Central control

The afferent stimuli are finally integrated in the cell bodies of preganglionic secretomotor neurones. The cell bodies of the sympathetic nervous system appear to lie in the lateral columns of the first five thoracic nerves, with the salivary spinal reflex centres being influenced by the medulla and higher centres, e.g. hypothalamus. The nuclei of the facial and glossopharyngeal nerves contain the cell bodies of the parasympathetic system. This area, the nucleus salivatorius, comprises a neuronal cluster in the reticular formation extending from the facial nucleus to the nucleus ambiguus. The nucleus salivatorius has been subdivided into two components:

(1) *Nucleus salivatorius superior:* stimulation causes secretion from the ipsilateral submandibular gland.
(2) *Nucleus salivatorius inferior:* stimulation causes secretion from the ipsilateral parotid gland.

This functional delineation is not discrete, however, in that stimulation of any area may result in secretion of all the glands from both sides.

Other higher centres also influence salivary secretion (e.g. sleep, rage, fear and conditioned reflexes). For instance, stimuli from the cerebral cortical area at the lower end of the fissure of Rolando, the junction of the frontal and anterior sigmoidal gyri and the amygdaloid nuclei influence the rate of salivary secretion.

Efferent pathway

The control of salivation is mainly under parasympathetic control, although there may also be a sympathetic component.[9]

Passing through the facial nerve, parasympathetic fibres pass via the chorda tympani to reach the lingual nerve and then, synapsing in the small ganglia around the submandibular and sublingual nerves, short postganglionic fibres pass into the glands.

The glossopharyngeal fibres pass through the tympanic and lesser superficial petrosal nerves to reach the otic ganglion where they synapse with the postganglionic fibres of the auriculotemporal nerve which supplies the parotid gland.

Autonomic control

The sympathetic fibres synapse in the superior cervical ganglion, with postganglionic fibres then passing to all the salivary glands.

The parasympathetic postganglionic neurotransmitter is acetylcholine, whereas that of the sympathetic postganglionic terminals is norepinephrine (noradrenaline). In addition to salivary secretion, the autonomic nervous system also exerts control over the glandular vasculature, excretory duct activity and myoepithelial cells. Neural control of salivary gland function is therefore complex.

Salivary composition[7,8]

Although saliva in the acini is isotonic or slightly hypotonic, it is always hypotonic after passage through the duct system. The duct cells are active in the reabsorption of sodium (followed passively by chloride ions) as well as potassium and bicarbonate secretion. Some water may be added to the secretions by the duct cells, although they are relatively impermeable to water. In fact, more than 99% of saliva is water, so that it is not surprising that saliva is a water metabolic cycle component.

Proteins

Although plasma cells and duct cells may provide a minor contribution to the salivary protein content, the acinar cells are primarily responsible. The quantity of salivary protein increases with the flow rate: the average for the parotid being 2.3 ± 1.7 g/litre, submandibular 1.2 ± 0.8 g/litre and sublingual 2.6 ± 0.70 g/litre.

Serum proteins

The serum proteins present in saliva may amount to 20% including IgG, IgM, IgA in addition to albumin and some α- and β-globulins.[27–30] Although serum albumin estimations range from 1–10% of total protein, the concentrations decrease with increased flow rates. The salivary γ-globulins are in different forms and concentrations from those in the blood. In fact, these γ-globulins are probably synthesized within the glands themselves; a feature that may also apply to some of the salivary albumin.

Secretory IgA is synthesized by plasma cells within the glands in addition to the mucosal epithelial cells. Secretory IgA is therefore different from plasma IgA, due to a non-lymphoid-derived glycoprotein designated as the secretory component. This makes the secretory IgA more resistant to enzymic proteolysis. Secretory IgA comprises 90% of the total parotid IgA and 85% of whole saliva IgA, 30–35% of which is derived from the minor glands. This secretory IgA exhibits three possible functions:

(1) Inhibition of bacterial colonization, probably by agglutination.
(2) Binding to specific bacterial antigens involved with adherence.
(3) Affecting specific enzymes essential for bacterial metabolism.

Proteins synthesized within the glands

A number of proteins analogous to those found in blood may be detected in saliva, including:

(1) Factor VII (pro-activator).
(2) Factor IX (Christmas factor).
(3) Factor VIII (antihaemophiliac globulin).
(4) A platelet factor.

Salivary enzymes

Amylase

Approximately 30% of the protein found in saliva is α-amylase, with submandibular amylase activity being only about 20% of that in the parotid; there is very little amylase activity in the sublingual and minor glandular secretions.[31] α-Amylase (ptyalin) is calcium-dependent and is activated by chloride ions. This enzyme hydrolyses cooked starch to maltose, the primary action being the disruption of the α 1,4 glycosidic linkages. The enzymic activity is, however, limited since the enzyme is readily inactivated by a pH of 4 or less. Amylase activity may still continue in the centre of a bolus if protected from the acidic gastric environment. α-Amylase is probably synthesized as the glycosylated form and modified by the removal of carbohydrate or sequential deamination after transcription or secretion. The concentration of α-amylase increases with the rate of salivary secretion.

Lysozyme

Lysozyme is present in all major body fluids but occurs at high concentrations in saliva, in addition to lacrimal fluid and nasal and bronchial secretions.[16] The concentration of lysozyme is greater in submandibular saliva than that of the parotid.[32] Lysozyme acts on the B(1–4) bond between *N*-acetyl-muramic acid and *N*-acetyl-glucosamine in the Gram-positive bacterial cell wall component peptidoglycan[17] leading to its subsequent disruption and microbial death. Lysozyme may in fact be lytic only in environments which flux in pH and ionic strength.[18] Lysozyme may also be bactericidal in the absence of lysis,[19] in addition to inhibiting mucosal colonization by microbial aggregation.[20]

Acid phosphatase, cholinesterase, ribonuclease

These enzymes are present in similar concentrations in parotid and submandibular saliva, with phosphatase having an optimum pH of 4.0.

Lipase

A specific lipase occurs in parotid saliva.

Peroxidase

An antibacterial peroxidase system occurs in parotid saliva, in addition to milk and tears, and comprises lactoperoxidase, thiocyanate and hydrogen peroxide. This system inhibits growth and acid production of a variety of micro-organisms, including streptococci, lactobacilli, fungi and enteric bacteria. Although lactoperoxidase and thiocyanate are normal salivary constituents,[21] hydrogen peroxidase is generated by a number of oral micro-organisms.[22] Lactoperoxidase catalyses thiocyanate oxidation by hydrogen peroxide, resulting in the formation of a number of substances, including hypothiocyanite which oxidizes bacterial enzymes containing sensitive thiol groups. Lactoperoxidase also retains activity when adsorbed on hydroxyapatite and salivary sediment, thereby protecting the enamel surface.

Kallikrein

Kallikrein splits serum β-globulin into bradykinin, which then passes back into the gland and into the blood vessels. Kallikrein may therefore cause functional vasodilatation to supply an actively secreting gland.

Miscellaneous enzymes

A vast enzymic array has been detected in saliva, including:

proteases	phosphatases
amino-peptidases	sulphatase
carboxypeptidases	acid and alkaline ribonucleases
lipases	glycolytic pathway enzymes:
urease	succinic dehydrogenase
glucuronidase	malate dehydrogenase
hyaluronidase	lactate dehydrogenase
neuraminidase	glutamate dehydrogenase
esterases	β-hydroxybutyrate
cholinesterase	dehydrogenase.

Mucoproteins and glycoproteins

The majority of salivary proteins contain a large proportion of carbohydrate in their molecules, including galactose, mannose, hexosamine and fucose.[33] Proline, glycine and glutamic acid comprise the major amino acid components. These negatively charged proteins probably interact with the positively charged calcium on hydroxyapatite surfaces. They also probably contribute to the enamel pellicle, in addition to contributing to enamel remineralization and preventing tooth surface bacterial colonization.

Blood group substances

The carbohydrate–protein complexes present on the cell-membranes of red blood corpuscles are characterized by the presence or absence of two antigens A and B that differ in their terminal sugar chains. Approximately 80% of the population exhibit the antigens corresponding to their blood groups (A,B,AB) or the glyoprotein H substance, which lacks the terminal polysaccharide chains. Other blood group antigens (e.g. the Lewis antigen family) have also been described in saliva. In fact, the Lewis antigen is found in body fluids and adsorbs to the surface of red blood corpuscles; its presence in saliva does not necessarily indicate a salivary origin. 'Non-secretors' may have Lewis (a) antigen in their saliva, whereas 'secretors' have either Lewis (a) or Lewis (b) antigens.

Hormones

Two hormone-like substances have been described in saliva: parotin, which facilitates calcification and helps to maintain serum calcium levels, and a nerve growth factor that affects growth and development of sympathetic nerve fibres.

Carbohydrates

In addition to carbohydrates bound to proteins, parotid saliva also contains glucose at a similar concentration to blood. In addition to glucose, submandibular saliva also contains hexose and fucose, with small amounts of hexosamine and sialic acid.

Lipids

Saliva contains small quantities of diglycerides, triglycerides, cholesterol and cholesterol esters and phospholipids, in addition to corticosteroids (mainly cortisone). These lipids may play a role in salivary protein binding, bacterial adsorption to apatite and plaque microbial aggregation.

Nitrogen-containing compounds

Nine different amino acids have been found in parotid saliva, 12 in submandibular and 18 in whole saliva. Many of these are probably derived from microbial protein degradation. Salivary urea and uric acid concentrations appear directly correlated with those of the blood. Citrate and lactate arise from carbohydrate metabolism, with lactate in particular increasing after food intake. Most of the water-soluble vitamins have been found in saliva.

Lactoferrin

Lactoferrin is an iron-binding protein synthesized by glandular epithelial cells and polymorphonuclear leucocytes. The bactericidal effect of lactoferrin is blocked by secretory IgA and by prior saturation with iron. Conceivably, lactoferrin functions with other antimicrobial agents, e.g. lysozyme and lactoperoxidase to monitor the oral microbial flora.

Inorganic substances

The ions found in all physiological fluids are also present in saliva, albeit at concentrations modified by salivary secretion.[34,35]

Sodium

Sodium ions are present in acinar fluid at similar concentrations to extracellular fluid, although there is some resorption in the striated ducts. Resting saliva contains only traces of sodium ions, although the concentration increases with salivary secretion (i.e. there is less time available for reabsorption in rapid salivary secretion).

Potassium

Except for the terminal duct, potassium is pumped into salivary secretions, so that the concentration is partly dependent upon the secretion rate.

Chloride

The chloride concentration in acinar secretions mirrors that of plasma, whereas subsequently chloride is passively reabsorbed along with sodium in the striated duct. Also, as the salivary flow rate increases, bicarbonate is produced and actively transported into saliva: this also leads to increased chloride reabsorption.

Bicarbonate

The level of bicarbonate in resting saliva is low but markedly increases with glandular metabolic activity. Bicarbonate is the principal salivary buffer. The efficacy of this buffer on dental plaque may be compromised by its thickness and composition.

Hydrogen ion

Salivary pH is low in resting secretions, but rises up to pH 8.0 in fast-flowing saliva, largely reflecting the bicarbonate content.

Iodine

Salivary glands actively transport iodine into saliva, so the concentration is generally higher than that of plasma. Interestingly, salivary glands also tend to concentrate radio-active iodine used for thyroid assays.

Fluoride

The fluoride content of saliva is less than that of serum, and is directly correlated with dietary intake.[36] The fluoride concentration of dental plaque, however, is much greater than that of saliva, the additional fluoride probably being derived from the enamel surface.

Thiocyanate

The thiocyanate is present in saliva at higher concentrations than in serum, and may complex with the bacteriostatic lactoperoxidase system.

Calcium

The calcium content of submandibular saliva is approximately double that of parotid saliva. This probably contributes to the marked prevalence of calculus on the lingual aspect of the mandibular incisors. The concentration of calcium in whole saliva decreases with increasing salivary flow. This probably results from the increased parotid contribution in rapid salivary flow rates.

The principal salivary calcium phosphate salts include dicalcium phosphate dihydrate, octacalcium phosphate, tricalcium phosphate and hydroxyapatite. Homeostasis between these various salts is assisted by two salivary acidic peptides (one rich in tyrosine and another rich in proline). These acidic peptides maintain saliva as a supersaturated calcium and phosphate solution, tending to prevent enamel demineralization in addition to facilitating enamel remineralization. Calculus formation probably reflects interference with this process.

Phosphate

Almost all salivary phosphate is inorganic; the concentration decreases with increased flow rates.

In general:

(1) Total protein, amylase and sodium bicarbonate concentrations increase with increasing salivary flow rates.
(2) Potassium and, possibly, fluoride concentrations do not change with increasing salivary flow rates.
(3) Phosphate, urea, amino acids, uric acid, ammonia, serum albumin and magnesium concentrations decrease with increasing salivary flow rates.
(4) Chloride, calcium and protein-bound carbohydrate concentrations fall at first and then slowly increase with increasing salivary flow rates.

Factors affecting salivary flow rate

Diurnal variation

As with many bodily functions, salivary flow rates exhibit diurnal variations.[9] In general, protein concentrations tend to be high in the afternoon. By contrast, sodium and chloride concentrations are high in the early hours of the morning, while potassium is high in the early afternoon. Whereas calcium and phosphate concentrations appear to remain stable during the day, the calcium concentration increases at night.

Duration of stimulus

If the salivary glands are stimulated for longer than three minutes, the concentration of many components is reduced, although after a short period, bicarbonate, calcium and protein concentrations begin to rise again. Magnesium, phosphate and potassium concentrations, however, plateau after an initial fall. Chloride concentrations fall during periods of stimulation, whereas sodium and iodide concentrations are unaffected by the duration of stimulation after the first few minutes.

Nature of the stimulus

Variations in salivary composition may reflect differing proportions of the major secretions (e.g. larger parotid contributions) or differences in stimulus-susceptibility of the various glands.

Dietary factors

Functional salivary glandular activity is influenced by mechanical and/or gustatory factors, e.g. copious salivary flow results from the smell of food or new denture insertion.

Plasma concentrations

Amino acid, calcium, glucose, potassium, urea and uric acid salivary concentrations are correlated with those in plasma, along with those of chloride and sodium, in addition to those of sex hormones and cortisol.

Hormonal influences[10]

Aldosterone

Aldosterone results in increased sodium reabsorption in the striated ducts.

Antidiuretic hormone

Antidiuretic hormone facilitates water reabsorption by the striated duct cells.

Other hormones

Both testosterone and thyroxine result in increased salivary secretion.

Salivary secretion increases during pregnancy, but is reduced at menopause resulting in a dry mouth (xerostomia).

Local hormones

Bradykinin, and its predecessor kallidin, result in increased salivary secretion reflecting increased acinar vasodilatation.

Functions of saliva

Digestive functions

Amylase is the main digestive enzyme of saliva, with a critical pH of 6.8, i.e. close to oral pH. When food passes to the stomach, with pH below 4.0, continued, albeit temporary, amylase activity may still occur in the food bolus prior to its gastric juice penetration. Amylase activity may also provide a useful function by digesting starch from the interproximal tooth contact areas.

Water balance

Vomiting or hyperpnoea (panting) may result in dehydration with loss of water through the oral cavity. As saliva is derived from extracellular fluid, factors that influence extracellular fluid will also affect salivary volume. Thus, vasopressin (antidiuretic hormone) secretion will result in increased water resorption through the striated salivary duct walls.

Xerostomia (dry mouth) is the principal manifestation of salivary deficiency, and may result from a variety of factors, including old age, and the administration of many drugs, especially tranquillizers, mood-elevators, amphetamines, antihistamines, in addition to cardiac and antihypertensive medications (*Table 14.1*).

Salivary gland diseases

Salivary glands may be affected by the whole range of disease processes, including inflammatory, infective and neoplastic diseases. In addition, some specific disease processes affect the salivary glands, e.g. Mikulicz's disease. Sjögren's syndrome.

Systemic disease

Salivary glands do not function in isolation from the remainder of the body but are affected by a whole host of systemic diseases, including hyperthyroidism, pernicious anaemia, multiple sclerosis, vitamin deficiencies and poorly controlled diabetes mellitus.

Emotional states

Emotional states, e.g. anxiety and depression, are known to affect salivary gland function. These effects illustrate the overriding control of the higher central nervous system centres on salivary function.

When xerostomia is present, the mouth feels dry, the tongue may stick to the palatal mucosa, teeth or buccal mucosa. The patient may also complain about a painful tongue (glossitis), in addition to altered taste and loose dentures. Without meticulous oral hygiene, patients often develop rapid cervical carious lesions and acute periodontal infections.

Sialorrhoea (ptyalism) is excessive salivary flow, most commonly seen following the insertion of new prosthodontic or orthodontic applicances. Increased salivary flow rates may also occur during the first trimester of pregnancy, during orgasm, as well as in some disease states, including Parkinson's disease, cerebral palsy and epilepsy, and in some psychological disorders. Excessive salivation may be one of the manifestations of primary herpetic and other

Table 14.1 Medications associated with xerostomia (dry mouth)

Medicament(s)	*Use(s)*
Acetazolamide	Diuretic
Amitriptyline	Tricyclic antidepressant
Amphetamines	CNS stimulant
Atropine and diphenoxylate	Antidiarrhoeal
Belladonna	Anticholinergic, antispasmodic
Chlordiazepoxide and clindinium bromide	Antidiarrhoeal
Chlorisondamine	Antihypertensive
Chlorothiazide	Diuretic
Chlorpromazine	Antipsychotic
Clidinium bromide and chlordiazepoxide	Antidiarrhoeal
Clonidine	Antihypertensive
Desipramine	Tricyclic antidepressant
Dicyclomine	Anticholinergic, antispasmodic
Diphenoxylate and atropine	Antidiarrhoeal
Doxepin	Tricyclic antidepressant
Ephedrine (in various combinations)	Bronchodilator
Ethacrynic acid	Diuretic
Fenfluramine	Anorexic
Fluphenazine	Antipsychotic
Furosemide	Diuretic
Glycopyrrolate	Anticholinergic
Guanethidine and hydrochlorothizide	Antihypertensive
Haloperidol	Antipsychotic
Hexocyclium	Peptic ulcer
Hydrochlorothiazide	Diuretic
Hydrochlorothiazide and guanethidine	Antihypertensive
Hydrochlorothiazide and triamterene	Antihypertensive
Imipramine	Tricyclic antidepressant
Isocarboxazid	Antidepressant
Isopropamide	Peptic ulcer
Mazindol	Anorexic
Methadone	Analgesic
Methyclothiazide	Diuretic
Methyldopa	Antihypertensive
Methylphenidate	CNS stimulant
Nortriptyline	Tricyclic antidepressant
Pargyline	Antidepressant
Perphenazine	Antipsychotic
Phenelzine	Antidepressant
Phenmetrazine	CNS stimulant
Phentermine	Anorexic
Prochlorperazine	Antipsychotic
Promazine	Antipsychotic
Propantheline	Anticholinergic, antispasmodic
Protriptyline	Tricyclic antidepressant
Pseudoepehedrine (in various combinations)	Bronchodilator
Spironolactone	Diuretic
Tetracyclines	Antibiotic
Thioridazine	Antipsychotic
Thiothixene	Antipsychotic
Tranylcypromine	Antidepressant
Triamterene and hydrochlorothiazide	Antihypertensive
Trifluoperazine	Antipsychotic
Triflupromazine	Antipsychotic

infections, but usually disappears on resolution of the problem.

Excretory functions

Saliva provides an important excretory route for several blood components, including urea, uric acid, ammonia and thiocyanate, the majority being subsequently reabsorbed in the gut. Toxic blood levels of heavy metals may also reflect salivary lead, mercury and bismuth secretion, subsequently leading to characteristic oral soft tissue deposits.

Solvent function

By facilitating comminution and digestion, the dissolution of foodstuffs is probably one of the major salivary functions.

Protective functions

In addition to protecting the oral tissues from dehydration, saliva has a major function in mechanical food and microbial debris lavage. Salivary mucus tends to take a relatively constant course along specific routes to the oesophagus,[11,12] with the salivary flow rate, tongue movements and swallowing reflexes all involved in this mechanism. Based on studies of patients with xerostomia (dry mouth), it has been shown that this process of mechanical lavage is probably responsible for the low incidence of primary oral infections and inflammatory lesions in normal patients.

The lubricating role of glycoprotein and mucoproteins not only facilitates food bolus deglutination, but also facilitates tongue movements in speech, i.e. xerostomia may be associated with choking.

Several component compounds provide specific defence mechanisms of saliva, including:

(1) Salivary lysozyme which acts by breaking the 1–4 link between *N*-acetyl-muramic acid and *N*-acetyl-glucosamine, two of the main bacterial cell wall mucopeptides. Salivary lysozyme enters the mouth from a number of sources, including the major and minor salivary glands,[13] the tissue exudate that flows from the gingival crevice[14] and from leucocytes within saliva. The commensal oral flora appears to be unaffected by high lysozyme concentrations.[15] Thus, apart from preventing non-commensal micro-organisms colonizing the mouth, the role of salivary lysozyme remains obscure.

(2) Human saliva contains secretory IgA, with small amounts of IgG and IgM. Most of the IgM and secretory IgA are of salivary gland origin, whereas IgG and a small proportion of IgA and IgM are derived from the gingival exudate. IgA probably facilitates microbial aggregation, thereby facilitating salivary mechanical lavage. IgA may also complex with protein covering the oral epithelium to provide a protective immunoglobulin coating. Certainly, oral bacteria coated with IgA are more easily phagocytosed by leucocytes than bacteria coated with IgG or IgM. IgA cannot fix complement, however, so there is no evidence for a direct bacteriolytic effect.

(3) Peroxidases which act as antibacterial enzymes.

(4) Globulin and thiocyanate which exhibit antibacterial properties.

(5) Component salivary leucocytes which exhibit antibacterial properties.

(6) The component supersaturation with calcium apatite which in addition to the bicarbonate buffer inhibits enamel decalcification.

Salivary anti-caries activity

There is general agreement that saliva may be one of the innate mechanisms against dental caries, although the detailed mechanics of such activity has yet to be elucidated. At present, a number of potential mechanisms appear to be involved:

(1) Increased salivary flow could increase carbohydrate clearance from the oral cavity.

(2) Salivary components could reduce the acid formed by carbohydrate fermentation in the dental plaque, either by promotion of less acidogenic plaque micro-organisms, or micro-organisms that form weaker acids on carbohydrate fermentation.

(3) Salivary bicarbonate could buffer acids formed during carbohydrate fermentation in the dental plaque.

(4) The rate of glycolysis could be increased by salivary urea, bicarbonate or sialin, so that plaque carbohydrate would be metabolized faster, thereby reducing the duration of enamel exposure to critical pH levels.

(5) Salivary components could increase enamel resistance to acid decalcification, due to its component fluoride activity.

(6) Salivary components could diffuse into plaque, resulting in increased plaque fluid saturation with respect to hydroxyapatite or fluorapatite.

(7) Salivary components (e.g. calcium, phosphate, hydroxyl and fluoride ions) could promote subsurface remineralization of carious lesions.

(8) Saliva could promote microbial clearance from the oral cavity, thereby decreasing plaque formation.

(9) Salivary components might increase acquired pellicle thickness prior to plaque microbial colonization.

Conclusions

The secretion of saliva not only varies in rate between different individuals but also in its composition. Rather than providing just lubrication for the oral tissues, it is important for the metabolic health of the mouth as a whole. The significance of the various salivary components, however, has yet to be fully defined, although it is known to be intimately involved in the host defence mechanisms of the oral cavity.

Review questions

1. What is the location of the minor salivary glands?
2. How is saliva initially formed?
3. What are the principal functions of saliva?
4. What are the main types of enzymes in saliva?
5. How is the flow of saliva controlled?

References

1. DAWES, C. (1969) The effects of flow rate and duration of stimulation on the concentration of protein and the main electrolytes in human parotid saliva. *Arch. Oral Biol.*, **14**, 277–294
2. BURGEN, A.S.V. and SCHNEYER, C.A. (1967) *Secretory Mechanisms of the Salivary Glands*. New York: Academic Press
3. EMMELIN, N. and ZOTTERMAN, Y. (1972) *Oral Physiology*. Oxford: Pergamon
4. CASTLE, J.D., JAMIESON, J.D. and PALADE, G.E. (1972) Radioautographic analysis of the secretory process in the parotid acinar cell of the rabbit. *J. Cell Biol.*, **53**, 290
5. TANDLER, B. (1972) Microstructure of salivary glands In *Proceedings of Symposium on Salivary Glands and their Secretions*, edited by N.H. Rowe. Ann Arbor: University of Michigan Press
6. AMSTERDAM, A., OHAD, I. and SCHRAMM, M. (1969) Dynamic changes in the ultrastructure of the acinar cell of the rat parotid gland during the secretory cycle. *J. Cell Biol.*, **41**, 753
7. SCHNEYER, L.V. and SCHNEYER, C.A. (1967) *Secretory Mechanisms of the Salivary Glands*. New York: Academic Press
8. DAWES, C. and WOOD, C.M. (1973) The composition of human lip mucous gland secretions to the volume of whole saliva in man. *Arch. Oral Biol.*, **18**, 337–342
9. FERGUSON, D.B. and FORT, A. (1974) Circadian rhythms in human resting submandibular saliva flow rate and composition. *Arch. Oral Biol.*, **19**, 47–55
10. CHAUNCEY, H.H., FELLER, R.P. and HENRIQUES, B.L. (1966) Comparative electrolyte composition of parotid, submandibular and sublingual secretions. *J. Dent. Res.*, **45**, 1230
11. BLOOMFIELD, A.L. (1921) Dissemination of bacteria in the upper respiratory passages. I. The circulation of foreign particles in the mouth. *Annu. Rev. Tuberc.*, **5**, 903–914
12. BLOOMFIELD, A.L. (1922) Dissemination of bacteria in the upper air passages. II. The circulation of bacteria in the mouth. *Johns Hopkins Hosp. Bull.*, **33**, 145–149
13. HOERMAN, K.C., ENGLANDER, H.R. and SHKLAR, I.L. (1956) Lysozyme–its characteristics in human parotid and submaxillo-lingual saliva. *Proc. Soc. Exp. Biol. NY*, **92**, 875–878
14. BRANDTZAEG, P. and MANN, W.V. (1964) A comparative study of the lysozyme activity of human gingival pocket fluid, serum and saliva. *Acta Odontol. Scand.*, **22**, 441–455
15. GIBBONS, R.J., DE STOPPELLAR, J.D. and HARDEN, L. (1966) Lysozyme insensitivity of bacteria indigenous to the oral cavity in man. *J. Dent. Res.*, **45**, 877–881
16. FLEMING, A. and ALLISON, V.D. (1922) Further observations on a bacteriolytic element found in tissues and secretion. *Proc. R. Soc. B*, **94**, 142–151
17. SALTON, M.R.J. (1961) The anatomy of the bacterial surface. *Bacteriol. Rev.*, **25**, 77–99
18. METCALF, R.H. and DIEBEL, R.H. (1969) Differential lytic response of enterococci associated with addition order of lysozyme and anions. *J. Bacteriol.*, **99**, 674–680
19. EPSTEIN, L.A. and CHAIN, E. (1940) Some observations of the preparation and properties of the substrate of lysozyme. *Br. J. Exp. Pathol.*, **21**, 339–354
20. KRUSE, H. and HURST, A. (1972) Preparation of spheroplasts from *Streptococcus lactis*. *Can. J. Microbiol.*, **18**, 825–831
21. BRANDTZAEG, P. (1966) Local factors of resistance in the gingival area. *J. Periodont. Res.*, **11**, 19–42
22. HAMON, C.B. and KLEBANOFF, S.J. (1973) A peroxidase-mediated *Streptococcus mitis* dependent antimicrobial system in saliva. *J. Exp. Med.*, **137**, 438–450
23. KLINEBERG, I., ELLISON, S.A. and MANDEL, I.D. (1979) *Saliva and Dental Caries. Microbiol. Abst. (sp. suppl.)*
24. THORN, N.A. and PETERSEN, O.H. (1974) *Secretory Mechanisms of Exocrine Glands*. Copenhagen: Munksgaard International
25. JAMIESON, J.D. (1972) Biology of the secretory process in exocrine cells. In *Symposium on Salivary Glands and their Secretion*, edited by N.H. Rowe. Ann Arbor: University of Michigan Press
26. ARCHER, F.L. and KAO, V.C.Y. (1968) Immunohistochemical identification of actomyosin in myoepithelium of human tissues. *Lab. Invest.*, **18**, 669–674
27. BRANDTZAEG, P. (1974) Mucosal and glandular distribution of immunoglobulin components: differential localization of free and bound secretory component in secretory epithelial cells. *J. Immunol.*, **112**, 1553–1559
28. BRANDTZAEG, P., FJELLANGER, I. and GJERULDSEN, S.T. (1970) Human secretory immunoglobulins. I. Salivary secretions from individuals with normal or low levels of serum immunoglobulins. *Scand. J. Haematol.*, **12**, 1–83
29. ARNOLD, R.R., PRUITT, K.M. and COLE, M.F. (1979)

Salivary antibacterial mechanisms in immunodeficiency. In *Saliva and Dental Caries*, edited by I. Klineberg, S.A. Ellison and I.D. Mandel. *Microbiol. Abs. (sp. suppl.)*

30. CRAWFORD, J.M., TAUBMAN, M.A. and SMITH, D.J. (1975) Minor salivary glands as a major source of secretory immunoglobulin A in the human oral cavity. *Science*, **190**, 1206–1209
31. MERRITT, A.D. and KARN, R.C. (1977) The human a-amylases. *Adv. Hum. Genet.*, **8**, 135–234
32. COLE, M.F., ARNOLD, R.R. and MESTECKY, J. (1976) Studies with human lactoferrin and *S. mutans*. In *Microbial Aspects of Dental Caries*, edited by H.M. Stiles, W.J. Loesche and T.C. O'Brien. Washington: Information Retrieval
33. YOSIZAWA Z. (1972) *Glycoproteins: their Composition, Structure and Function*. Amsterdam: Elsevier/North-Holland
34. THAYSEN, J.H., THORN, N.A. and SCHWARTZ, I.L. (1954) Excretion of sodium, potassium, chloride and carbon dioxide in human parotid saliva. *Am. J. Physiol.*, **178**, 155–159
35. VOGEL, J.J., NOUJOKS, R. and BRUDEROLD, F. (1965) The effective concentrations of calcium and inorganic orthophosphate in salivary secretions. *Arch. Oral Biol.*, **10**, 523–534
36. SHANNON, I.L., FELLER, R.P. and CHAUNCEY, H.H. (1976) Fluoride in human parotid saliva. *J. Dent. Res.*, **55**, 506–509

15

Calcium metabolism and bone

Introduction

Bone is a highly organized complex tissue. It is characterized by abundant extracellular matrix in which three principal bone cell families are found, each existing at a number of different stages of development and maturation. Each of these cellular families exist in a delicate state of equilibrium with each other, although external factors, e.g. hormones, drugs and mechanical forces, may disturb or change these cellular equilibria.[1] The extracellular matrix contains collagen and other proteins, proteoglycans and mineral. The metabolic activity of bone matrix and its component cells resides in a constant state of flux, controlled by a large number of humoral and other agents.[2] In the adult, bone removal and replacement occur continuously but these processes are tightly controlled, so that in fact there is remarkable constancy in the total bone present throughout the majority of adult life. Bone loss, associated with ageing or with disease, leads to osteoporosis and fractures and reflects disturbances in the maintenance of skeletal balance.[3]

Bone mineral

Bone mineral accounts for approximately 70% of the dry weight of cortical bone.[4] This proportion is higher in calcified cartilage and much higher in enamel but lower in trabecular bone. In fully mineralized bone, the calcium content is about 0.6 g/cm^3. The mineral in bone, calcified cartilage, dentine, enamel and ectopic calcific deposits mainly comprises very small hydroxyapatite crystals, although the crystals are much larger in enamel. In addition, a small amount may occur in the amorphous phase and other crystal forms. In lamellar bone, at least 80% of the mineral lies within the collagen fibres, with the crystals orientated with their long axis roughly parallel to the fibrils. In incompletely calcified bone, the mineral shows a periodicity of 70 nm, similar to that of collagen. This may reflect the initial mineral deposition occurring in the holes between the heads and tails of adjacent collagen molecules. In more heavily calcified collagen, this periodicity becomes obscured as the mineral is deposited in other sites close to and outside the fibrils. In woven bone, calcified cartilage and ectopic calcification, most of the crystals lie outside the fibrils in a more disordered manner.

Hydroxyapatite forms the major mineral phase and comprises part of the family of apatite minerals characterized by specific X-ray diffraction patterns and very small crystal sizes. Biological minerals are not pure hydroxyapatite, however, as the mineral may contain many other constituents, including carbonate, citrate, sodium and magnesium. Thus, 70% of the body's citrate, 60% of the magnesium and 50% of the sodium reside in the skeleton and many other elements are present in trace quantities. The significance of these trace elements has yet to be firmly established.

Calcium salt heterogeneity

The low Ca/P ratio in biological minerals may reflect the presence of calcium salts other than hydroxyapatite. These include tricalcium phosphate hydrate, octocalcium phosphate, dicalcium phosphate dihydrate (brushite) and amorphous calcium phosphate.

Ion substitution

Ions in the apatite can undergo substitution, either within the lattice or on the surface. In view of the complexity of the fluid surrounding these crystals, this process of substitution may involve a number of substances. For instance, calcium may be replaced by hydrogen or sodium ions, strontium, radium, magnesium or lead cations. Phosphate may be substituted by carbonate, and hydroxyl ions by fluoride. This latter results in the formation of fluorapatite which has a lower solubility than hydroxyapatite. This is the basis for the dental use of fluoride for caries prevention.

Surface binding

The small size of biological apatite crystals results in a large crystal surface per unit volume. This surface is able to bind charged materials by surface adsorption and by inclusion in the hydration shell (aqueous layer) around the crystals.

The materials that bind in this way include bicarbonate, calcium, citrate, magnesium, phosphate, potassium, proteins (e.g. osteocalcin, osteonectin), pyrophosphate and sodium. Even if only a small portion of the crystal surface is exposed to extracellular fluid, the total area involved is still very large. This accounts for the rapid uptake and release of many compounds to the plasma. These absorption reactions occur very quickly when the hydration layer of the crystal surface is involved, although slower exchange reactions reflect the role of bone as an ion bank.

Since bone mineral is in close contact with extracellular fluid, the clacium and phosphate concentration of the latter should be related to bone mineral solubility.[5] The plasma calcium and phosphate ion concentrations are, in fact, far higher than expected from the solubility of pure hydroxyapatites. This may reflect:

(1) The higher solubility associated with small crystal size.
(2) The presence of more soluble calcium salts.
(3) Altered surface properties due to other ions, e.g. carbonate.
(4) More soluble salts (e.g. amorphous calcium phosphate) which may persist if their conversion to less soluble crystalline forms is retarded by other bone substances, e.g. albumin citrate, glycosaminoglycans, magnesium, osteocalcin, pyrophosphate.
(5) Effective separation of the mineral phase from extracellular fluid by living cells generating ionic gradients.

Bone cells[6]

Osteoblasts

Osteoblasts synthesize the extracellular matrix components and prime the matrix for its subsequent mineralization. These appear to be derived from two main sources:[7] the periosteal lining cells in cortical bones and the stromal cells in the bone marrow in trabecular bone.

The major type of protein synthesized by osteoblasts is Type I collagen. This undergoes its final stages of maturation to produce fibrils in the extracellular compartments, with the release of procollagen peptides into the circulation. Osteoblasts also produce glycosaminoglycans (mainly chondroitin 4-sulphate) and specific proteoglycans. Other osteoblastic products include the glycosaminoglycans, proteoglycans, osteocalcin, osteonectin and sialoproteins.[8] Proteins (e.g. albumin) may also enter bone from plasma. Analogous cell types (e.g. ameloblasts) produce specific enamel proteins, e.g. the amelogenins, whereas the odontoblasts produce collagen, proteoglycans, glycoproteins and specific phosphoproteins.[9]

Osteocytes

Osteocytes are derived from osteoblasts and lie in concentric layers in bone matrix. These cells are in contact with each other through a network of canaliculi which also connect them to osteoblasts on the bone surface. Such intimate intercommunications facilitate osteocytic control of mineral exchange between bone and plasma.

Osteoclasts

Osteoclasts are large multinucleated cells lying on the surface of bone in varyingly shaped Howship's lacunae. They are probably only responsible for resorption of calcified bone or cartilage; this resorption occurring on their ruffled surfaces. Osteoclasts appear to be derived from macrophage-like bone marrow stem cells with a different lineage from osteoblasts.[10,11] The mechanisms by which osteoclasts resorb bone have yet to be determined but may include the following processes:

(1) Secretion of calcium-chelating organic anions (e.g. citrate) facilitating solubilization of the mineral phase.
(2) Local lactate and/or acid production.
(3) Specific transport mechanisms, e.g. sodium and hydrogen ion exchange.
(4) Transcellular calcium transport.

Bone matrix components are probably degraded by extracellular proteinases, e.g. collagenase, proteoglycanase and lysosomal acid hydrolases, including proteolytic cathepsins.

Bone calcification[2,4,12,13]

Calcium may be deposited both inside cells and in the extracellular compartment. Within the cells, the calcific deposits are initially in the form of amorphous granules in the mitochondria. These calcium phosphate packets may then be translocated from the mitochondrial sites to the extracellular mineralization zone. In the extracellular matrix, precipitation is first seen in association with matrix vesicles. It appears to begin on the membrane and extend to extravesicular clusters. These then coalesce into a continuous extracellular mass of heavily calcified tissue within and around the collagen fibrils. Where precipitation first begins on the collagen fibrils, specific sites corresponding to the 'hole' regions are initially involved. As mineralization progresses, axial periodicity of the collagen is first accentuated. This suggests that growth follows a specific fibril controlled pattern. Conceivably, the matrix vesicle mechanism of mineralization may predominate in woven bone and cartilage. By contrast, collagenous mineralization induction may be more important in lamellar bone.

Mineralization does not begin until several days following matrix formation. Once started, it proceeds rapidly, with about 66% of the final amount of mineral being deposited within a few hours. This primary mineralization process reflects increasing numbers of crystals. The subsequent secondary mineralization phase occurs over longer periods of months. The entire mineralization process is accompanied by water and non-collagenous protein loss.

In pure solutions, increasing the ionic concentration to a critical point will result in the induction of homogeneous nuclei formation; these are large enough to grow spontaneously and will not subsequently dissolve. In biological conditions, however, heterogeneous nucleation occurs on the surface of foreign particles. This facilitates spontaneous crystal growth at lower supersaturation levels. The best nucleating agents are the crystals of the precipitated compound itself. These include new crystal formation by secondary nucleation. After nucleation, the crystals grow until a critical size is reached. Thus a relatively high degree of supersaturation is necessary to initiate precipitation in the absence of nucleating agents. Solutions of lower ionic concentration can, however, remain in a supersaturated, metastable state for long periods of time, without precipitation. Once the crystallization has started, metastable solutions will sustain crystal growth. As crystallization progresses, crystals will mature to the thermodynamically most stable form. This may involve:

(1) Filling in the lattice structure.
(2) Transformation to other crystal forms.
(3) Crystal aggregation, modulated by local environmental inhibitors and promotors.

Calcification theories

The mechanisms of calcification have yet to be defined although a number of theories have been formulated. In fact, there may be no one mechanism of calcification.

Nucleation theory

This proposes that organic matrix components facilitate precipitation by acting as heterogenous nucleating agents. Glycosaminoglycans were once thought to be such nuclei but collagen is now considered to be a more likely candidate. Conceivably, this may include specific phosphorylation sites, or other bone specific proteins, which can bind to both collagen and mineral, e.g. the phosphoproteins including osteonectin.[8,14] Phospholipids may also act as nucleating agents, e.g. acidic phospholipids (phosphatidylserine, phosphatidylinositol) are usually present in calcified tissues and can form calcium–acidic–phospholipid–phosphate complexes.[4,15,16] The nucleating effect of matrix vesicles may also depend on their phospholipid membrane complexes. In addition, phosphoproteins may serve as potential nucleating proteins.

Booster theory

This theory proposes the existence of a mechanism to boost the local calcium and phosphate ion product to a point where precipitation occurs. Conceivably, this might involve alkaline phosphatase catalysis of phosphate ester hydrolysis, thereby increasing the local inorganic phosphate concentration. Alkaline phosphatase, however, occurs in many tissues that do not calcify. Alternatively, calcium or phosphate concentrations may be increased locally by a membrane transport system. Certainly, mitochondria can accumulate calcium against concentration gradients. Conceivably, matrix vesicles might also act in this way, although whether they are capable of concentrating calcium or phosphate against concentration gradients remains obscure.[17]

Matrix vesicles[12]

Small round vesicular extracellular matrix vesicles about 100 nm diameter are involved in the initiation of calcification.[12,18] They are probably derived from cell processes originating from the plasma membrane. These vesicles comprise the major sites for extracellular alkaline phosphatase, in addition to nucleoside triphosphate pyrophosphatase.[19,20] The lipid components of matrix vesicles could also be important for facilitating transmembrane calcium and phosphate transport.

What actually triggers matrix vesicle formation remains obscure.[12] Intracellular calcium phosphate deposits close to the plasma membrane occur at times of vesiculation. Such precipitates may promote plasma membrane shedding. Alternatively, matrix vesicle formation may be linked to an increase in the production of superoxide radicals and lipid peroxidation products in mineralization.[21] Since matrix vesicles appear to be associated with hydroxyapatite deposits, they may comprise a mechanism for initial hydroxyapatite deposition, although further research is required to confirm this supposition.

Mechanisms of calcification

The first mineral phase to form is probably amorphous calcium phosphate, octocalcium phosphate or brushite,[4] depending upon local environmental conditions, e.g. pH, other ions, the degree of supersaturation. This initial phase is probably subsequently transformed to hydroxyapatite. Pyrophosphate may play an important role in these initial stages of calcification. The first steps may involve the production of an amorphous phase of calcium pyrophosphate in addition to calcium phosphate, with inorganic pyrophosphate promoting initial amorphous calcium phosphate precipitation but inhibiting its subsequent transformation to crystalline hydroxyapatite.[22] In the presence of low nucleoside triphosphate concentrations, matrix vesicles can generate inorganic pyrophosphate very efficiently. The associated matrix vesicle alkaline phosphatase probably functions as the major enzyme for destroying inorganic pyrophosphate. Thus the balance between these two enzyme systems may regulate local inorganic pyrophosphate concentrations.

Mineralization inhibitors

Collagens and other potential nucleating agents occur in tissues that do not calcify. Thus there may be some mechanism that inhibits tissue mineralization. Collagen molecules may be packed more closely together in soft tissues than they are in bone: this may impede phosphate ion access to intrafibrillar nucleation sites. Soft tissues may be protected by inhibitors which are selectively removed at calcification sites.

Pyrophosphate, and other compounds with P–O–P bonds, can inhibit crystallization, even at low concentrations. Alkaline phosphatase may therefore serve to destroy pyrophosphate, and related inhibitors, to allow mineralization to occur. Other potential inhibitors include citrate, magnesium, proteins (e.g. albumin) and polyanions (e.g. glycosaminoglycans), although there is scant information regarding their metabolic role. Some of the inhibitors may be matrix components produced and acting locally, e.g. proteoglycans in varying aggregated forms. These mechanisms require much further evaluation before definitive statements may be made regarding their efficacy.

Disordered skeletal mineralization *(Table 15.1)*

Numerous disorders affect bone,[3,23] with hypomineralization of bone, cartilage and teeth predominating. In addition, calcification may also occur in sites outside the usual skeleton:

(1) Dystrophic calcification (where there is a pathological change in the tissue itself).
(2) Metastatic calcification (where calcification is secondary to an increase in the concentration of the precipitating ions in tissue fluids, e.g. hypercalcaemia).

The mineral phases in all types of ectopic calcification are calcium phosphate, although calcium carbonate may occur as well as mixed salts containing calcium, magnesium, phosphate and carbonate. Such ectopic calcifications tend to occur at certain select sites[13] (e.g. calcification of the basal ganglia in hypoparathyroidism), although the

Table 15.1 Sites of pathological calcification

Muscle and related tissues
Periarticular
Haematomas
Paraspinal ligaments
Dystrophic calcification
Costal cartilage, arteries and veins in ageing
Blood vessels in specific disorders, e.g. Monkeberg's medial calcinosis
Heart valves after rheumatic fever
Bursae and tendons
Skin – scleroderma
Around joints, e.g. in renal failure with secondary hyperparathyroidism
Kidney
Lymph nodes, e.g. tuberculosis lesions
Metastatic calcification due to hypercalcaemia (e.g. in primary hyperparathyroidism) or hyperphosphataemia (e.g. chronic renal failure)
Blood vessels (especially arteries)
Kidney
Cornea
Brain
Gastric mucosa
Lungs
Other metabolic disorders
Oxalosis
Renal tubular acidosis
Joint disease
Chondrocalcinosis
Hydroxyapatite deposition in osteoarthrosis
Urinary tract stones
Calcium oxalate, calcium phosphate or a mixture

reasons remain obscure. Most body tissue fluids are in a metastable state and require only a nucleating agent for the initiation of mineralization. Since the relevant ion concentrations are generally above the solubility product for most calcium salts, reverse calcification does not usually occur after removal of the primary causative agent.

Hormonal control of extracellular calcium *(Table 15.2)*

Plasma calcium is maintained with remarkable constancy despite wide calcium intake differences. Approximately half this total is ionized, the remainder being mainly bound to blood albumin. Since this concentration is much greater than the critical intracellular concentration, any major extracellular fluid concentration change would be associated with gross metabolic disturbances that would eventually lead to death. Thus a redundant set of interlocking mechanisms has evolved to allow man to survive major dietary calcium intake fluctuations. These mechanisms mainly centre on the endocrine system.

Parathyroid hormone[24]

Parathyroid hormone functions to conserve calcium and eliminate phosphorus. The main factor controlling parathyroid hormone secretion is plasma

Table 15.2 Agents that act on osteoblasts or osteoclasts

Hormones	*Agents*
Activators of bone resorption	
Parathyroid hormone	Prostaglandins e.g. PGE_2
$1,25(OH)_2$ vitamin D	Interleukin 1
Thyroxine	Transforming growth factors
	Colony stimulating factors
	Tumour necrosis factor
	Lymphotoxin
	Epidermal growth factor
Inhibitors of bone resorption	
Calcitonins	Gamma-interferon
Oestrogens	
Activators of bone formation	
Vitamin D metabolites	Insulin-like growth factors
Insulin	Various growth factors not yet fully characterized
Insuline-like growth factors	Prostaglandins
Oestrogens (?)	
Anabolic steroids	
Thyroxine	
Inhibitors of bone formation or mineralization	
Glucocorticoids	Transforming growth factors

calcium.[25] This hinges on an exquisitely calcium-sensitive adenylate-cyclase, with hypercalcaemia stimulating the cyclase, followed by cyclic AMP generation, protein phosphorylation and peptide parathyroid hormone secretion.

Parathyroid hormone adenylate cyclase requires magnesium, as severe hypomagnesaemia grossly impairs parathyroid hormone secretion. There are receptors in the parathyroid glands for the active hormonal form of vitamin D (1,25-dihydroxycholecalciferol).

Thyroid-derived calcitonin also stimulates the secretion of parathyroid hormone. When calcitonin secretion is grossly elevated, as in medullary thyroid carcinoma, further elevation of calcitonin secretion may be accompanied by an increased plasma parathyroid hormonal level. Such a physiological increase in parathyroid hormone secretion appears to depend in the short term on liberation of the very limited peptide parathyroid hormone stores. There appear to be two major mechanisms in the control of parathyroid hormonal secretion: in the long term, parathyroid glandular hyperplasia or atrophy; in the short term, calcium-dependent intracellular hormonal degradation.

These mechanisms operate by enhancement or inhibition of the degradative pathways by hypercalcaemia or hypocalcaemia respectively. Chronic hypocalcaemia leads to hyperplasia of the parathyroid glands. By contrast, acute hypocalcaemia is followed by an immediate secretion increase due to stored hormone liberation, combined with inhibition of intracellular peptide degradation. Once the parathyroid glands have greatly enlarged, an elevated parathyroid hormone secretion will persist, even in the presence of marked hypocalcaemia.

There are three main sites of parathyroid hormone activity.

Kidney

The action of parathyroid hormone on the kidney includes:

(1) Marked enhancement of phosphate excretion.
(2) Increased calcium resorption.
(3) Acceleration of the conversion of 25-hydroxycholecalciferol to its active metabolic form 1,25-dihydroxycholecalciferol.[26]

The combination of these effects on the kidney leads to enhancement of plasma calcium, and reflects the activity of two second messengers, cyclic AMP and intracellular calcium.[27,28]

Bone

Parathyroid hormone indirectly enhances osteoclastic activity in the skeleton. In fact, parathyroid hormone stimulates osteoblasts, which then secrete a local osteoclastic activator factor, probably prostaglandins, interleukin 1 and leukotrienes. This then results in increased osteoclastic activity. In addition, parathyroid hormone may have an anabolic effect on bone, so that the net bone mass is increased.[29] The cellular mechanisms involved presumably resemble those in the kidney, with the increase in cyclic AMP acting as a second messenger, perhaps associated with an increase in intracellular calcium.

Intestinal tract[30]

Enhancement of calcium and phosphorus absorption, associated with parathyroid hormone, is probably indirectly associated with the increased renal production of 1,25-dihydroxycholecalciferol (calcitriol).

Parathyroid hormonal pathophysiology

Primary hyperparathyroidism is a fairly common disorder. It is reflected as an increased number of parathyroid gland cells occurring in one or several glands. These cells are, however, not less responsive than normal cells to the inhibitory effects of hypercalcaemia. Rather, the increased cell number produces an excessive total secretion of parathyroid hormone since there is an irreducible minimum of parathyroid hormone secretion by each cell, regardless of plasma calcium level. In hyperparathyroidism, there is:

(1) Hypercalcaemia.
(2) Hypophosphataemia.
(3) Hyperphosphaturia.
(4) Increased urinary cyclic AMP levels.

Thus, it is the increased number of parathyroid gland cells that are responsible for the changes in plasma calcium concentration, rather than any qualitative change in their calcium sensitivity. By contrast, the hypercalcaemia of malignant disease results from direct skeletal destruction by malignant cells or osteoclastic activation by factors liberated from tumour cells.

Chronic renal failure is almost always associated with some degree of parathyroid hyperplasia. This is due to the hyperplastic drive directed at the glands by the combination of low plasma calcium with low plasma calcitriol.

Vitamin D

In normal conditions, the inclusion of Vitamin D in the diet is not required for full health: rather, Vitamin D is synthesized in the skin and functions as a precursor to an extremely potent seco-steroid calcium-regulating hormone. Vitamin D_3 (cholecalciferol) is a steroid derivative, whereas 7-dehydrocholesterol is the immediate precursor present in the skin. Vitamin D_3 is inactive by itself. Before it can produce its characteristic effects on calcium metabolism, therefore, Vitamin D_3 must undergo two successive hydroxylations. The first stage is 25-hydroxylation (in the liver and other tissues) to produce the major circulating form. The critical hydroxylation in the production of biological activity takes place in the kidney. This compound is much more potent than its precursor and is responsible for all the biological effects of Vitamin D_3 on calcium metabolism. A second, poorly active renal steroid is also formed, 24,25-dihydroxycholecalciferol, but this may be an escape route, when further 1,25-dihydroxycholecalciferol production is not required.

The most active metabolite of Vitamin D_3 (1,25-dihydroxycholecalciferol or calcitriol) is formed in the distal part of the convoluted tubule. The secretion of this metabolite is affected by a number of mineral and hormonal factors.

Mineral

Hypocalcaemia stimulates the production of calcitriol even without hormonal intervention, whereas hyperphosphataemia has the reverse effect.[31] They probably play quite an important part in Vitamin D regulation and may sometimes override the actions of other regulators (e.g. parathyroid hormone).

Hormonal

Parathyroid hormone

Parathyroid hormone stimulates the production of calcitriol in the presence of hypocalcaemia and serves to potentiate the action of calcium deficiency. When parathyroid hormone secretion coincides with hypercalcaemia, however, this stimulating effect of parathyroid hormone can be overcome. Thus, not all cases of hyperparathyroidism are associated with increased calcitriol secretion. Growth hormone and prolactin both have a stimulating effect on calcitriol production, and may in fact be the major physiological hormonal regulators.

Growth hormone and prolactin

During growth, pregnancy and lactation, where demands for calcium are high, 1,25-dihydroxycholecalciferol production is increased and plasma levels tend to be elevated.

Calcitonin[32]

Calcitonin directly stimulates calcitriol production at a site in the proximal tubule adjacent to, but distinct from, that acted upon by parathyroid hormone.[34] Whereas such an action may not have physiological significance, the elevated calcitonin levels associated with growth, pregnancy and lactation may have some role, together with growth hormone and prolactin.

Vitamin D metabolites

Vitamin D metabolites, especially calcitriol, exert a direct inhibitory effect on calcitriol production. They represent an important regulatory control mechanism minimizing excess, unwanted calcitriol production and maximizing its production when the circulating levels of Vitamin D metabolites are low.

Vitamin D action

Calcitriol passes through the cell membranes to bind with high affinity nuclear receptors, which then associate with specific chromatin regions to induce many other actions. Such receptors may be found in the gut, kidney, bone and lactating breast, in addition to immune cells and nerve cells. In some of the immune system cells, calcitriol induces differentiation. It is therefore possible that calcitriol has two types of effect:

(1) Increasing calcium transport in the calcium-transporting organs, especially the gut.
(2) Multiple permissive effects on a wide range of body cells.

Another class of high affinity receptor also occurs within the glands producing the peptides that regulate Vitamin D_3 metabolism. Such receptors are found in the parathyroid gland, thyroid C cells and the pituitary and presumably represent part of feedback loops. As a result, occupation of calcitriol receptors in the parathyroid glands inhibits parathyroid hyperplasia, diminishing parathyroid production in the long term. Similarly, occupation of the receptors in the C cells stimulates calcitonin production, minimizing the hypercalcaemia consequent upon the actions of 1,25-dihydroxycholecalciferol on the skeleton.

Classically, Vitamin D deficiency leads to rickets in children or osteomalacia in adults (under-mineralization of the protein bone matrix). The major action of Vitamin D in enhancing mineralization is indirect, since mineralization of rachitic or osteomalacic bone can occur in the absence of Vitamin D, e.g. by infusion or provision of adequate dietary calcium. Rickets is healed by enhancing calcium absorption from the gut rather than by a direct action on bone.

There is no doubt also that Vitamin D enhances bone osteoclastic activity and this activity is responsible for the hypercalcaemia induced by toxic doses of Vitamin D or its metabolites. Thus rickets and osteomalacia are the consequences of inadequate supplies of the active Vitamin D component, calcitriol. These diseases are characterized by impairment of bone matrix mineralization.

The common cause of rickets is dietary deficiency due to insufficient exposure of the skin to sunlight. Familial forms of rickets may also occur, due to: renal defects involving phosphorus loss; lack of renal calcitriol production with low plasma levels; deficiency or lack of receptors, so that rickets occurs despite high plasma calcitriol levels.

In renal osteodystrophy, inadequate production of calcitriol by damaged kidneys results in bone disease, calcium malabsorption and parathyroid hyperplasia.

Table 15.3 Agents affecting skeletal mineralization

Agent	*Mode of action*
Promoters	
Vitamin D metabolites (e.g. 1,25$(OH)_2$ Vitamin D_3)	Promote mineralization of cartilage bone as a result of increased intestinal absorption; also have direct effect on skeletal cell proliferation and differentiation
Fluoride	Fluoride may activate osteoblastic activity as well as affect the composition of mineral phase by producing fluoropatite. Large oral doses of fluoride lead to poorly mineralized bone
Inhibitors	
Bisphosphonates	Bisphosphonates (diphosphonates) impair bone mineralization at high doses, probably by directly interfering with crystal growth
Aluminium salts	Oral ingestion of aluminium salts, e.g. $Al(OH)_2$ or $Al_2(CO_2)_2$, binds to dietary phosphate leading to impaired bone mineralization
Strontium	Inhibits production of active vitamin D metabolites (1,25$(OH)_2D_2$)
Others	
Lead	Lead (Pb) ions deposit with bone mineral
Tetracyclines	Tetracycline antibiotics have a high affinity for calcium ions and bone mineral. They deposit in developing teeth leading to discoloration in bone

Table 15.4 Examples of major causes of defective skeletal mineralization producing rickets and/or osteomalacia

Vitamin D deficiency
- Dietary deficiency
- Deficient endogenous synthesis due to insufficient ultraviolet irradiation
- Gastrointestinal disorders with malabsorption

Disorders of vitamin D metabolism
- Hereditary 'pseudo vitamin D deficiency' or 'vitamin D dependency'
  - Type I due to renal 1 hydroxylase deficiency
  - Type II due to steroid receptor defect for 1,25$(OH)_2D_3$
- Other
  - Anticonvulsants (phenytoin)
  - Hepatobiliary diseases
  - Lead intoxication
  - Renal insufficiency
  - Acidosis
  - Hypoparathyroidism
  - Parenteral alimentation

Acidosis
- Distal renal tubular acidosis (classic or Type II)
  - Primary
  - Secondary
  - Ureterosigmoidostomy
  - Drug-induced

Chronic renal failure
- 1,25$(OH)_2$ vitamin D_3 deficiency
- Uraemia

Phosphate depletion
- Dietary
- Impaired renal tubular phosphate reabsorption
  - Hereditary
  - Acquired

Generalized renal tubular disorders (Fanconi syndrome)
- Primary renal
- Associated with systemic metabolic abnormality
- Systemic disorder with associated renal disease
  - Hereditary, e.g. Wilson's disease
  - Acquired, e.g. neurofibromatosis, multiple myeloma

Intoxications
- Lead
- Outdated tetracycline

Primary mineralization defects
- Hereditary
  - Hypophosphatasia
- Acquired
  - Fluoride treatment

Calcium deficiency
- Extreme dietary deficiency

States of rapid bone formation with or without a relative defect in bone resorption
- Osteopetrosis
- Defective matrix synthesis

Calcitonin

Essentially calcitonin is a hormone produced by the C cells of the thyroid gland, although precursors may also occur in the central nervous system and perivascular nerves.[34] The major factor controlling calcitonin secretion is the plasma calcium level. Specific receptors are present in C cells.[35] This suggests that the action of calcitriol in elevating calcitonin secretion involves a direct action of the seco-steroid on the C cells. It is suggested that gastrin and cholecystokinin produce an acute increase in calcitonin secretion after a meal, thus conserving skeletal calcium.

Calcitonin acts in a variety of ways.

(1) Calcitonin acts directly on the osteoclast producing an immediate inhibition of bone resorbing activity.[36,37]
(2) When given therapeutically, calcitonin also results in a reduction in osteoclastic cell number over a long time.
(3) Calcitonin acts on the kidney, enhancing 1,25-dihydroxycholecalciferol production and increasing mineral excretion.[33]
(4) Calcitonin possesses a central analgesic action.[38]

It seems that calcitonin is the treatment of choice in Paget's disease and can result in healing of advancing osteolytic lesions. Calcitonin may also provide temporary effective treatment of hypercalcaemia associated with advanced malignancy.

Thus the mechanism of bone mineralization and calcium metabolism are both complex and interrelated. This is illustrated by the variety of factors that influence skeletal mineralization (*Tables 15.3, 15.4*). A great deal more research is, however, required before these mechanisms are fully comprehended. As a result, the descriptions provided by this chapter may be rejected at some time in the future.

Conclusions

It is difficult to discuss calcium and bone metabolism as distinct entities. This only goes to emphasize the marked degree of interaction between bone as a skeletal unit and bone as a reservoir of calcium: it is impossible to separate the two features. The reader is therefore encouraged to read this chapter and the next (Chapter 16) together.

Review questions

1. What features prevent calcification in non-skeletal tissues?
2. Contrast the activity of calcitonin with vitamin D.
3. How do osteoclasts and osteoblasts contribute to calcium metabolism?
4. What theory of calcification can you support?
5. What forms of disordered calcification can you describe?

References

1. OWEN, M. (1985) Lineage of osteogenic cells and their relationship to the stromal system. *Bone Mineral Res.*, **3**, 1–26
2. VAUGHAN, J. (1981) *The Physiology of Bone*, 3rd edn. Oxford: Oxford Scientific Publications
3. REVELL, P.A. (1986) *Pathology of Bone*. Berlin: Springer-Verlag
4. POSNER, A.S. (1985) The mineral of bone. *Clin. Orthop.*, **200**, 87–99
5. NEUMAN, M.W. (1982) Blood: bone equilibrium. *Calcif. Tissue Int.*, **34**, 117–120
6. NIJWEIDE, P.J., BURGER, E.H. and FEYEN, J.H.R. (1986) Cells of bone: proliferation, differentiation and hormonal regulation. *Physiol. Rev.*, **66**, 855–886
7. RODAN, G.A. and RODAN, S.B. (1984) Expression of the osteoblastic phenotype. *Bone Mineral Res.*, **2**, 244–285
8. FISHER, L.W. and TERMINE, J.D. (1985) Noncollagenous proteins influencing the local mechanisms of calcification. *Clin. Orthop.*, **200**, 362–385
9. VEISS, A. (1985) Phosphoproteins of dentine and bone. In *The Chemistry and Biology of Mineralized Tissues*. Birmingham, Ala.: Ebsco Media
10. HORTON, H.A., PRINGLE, J.A.S. and CHAMBERS, T.J. (1985) Identification of human osteoclasts with monoclonal antibodies. *N. Engl. J. Med.*, **312**, 923–924
11. HORTON, M.A., RIMMER, E.E.F., LEWIS, D., PRINGLE, J.A.S. and CHAMBERS, T.J. (1984) Cell surface characterization of the human osteoclast: phenotypic relationship to other bone-marrow derived cell types. *J. Pathol.*, **144**, 282–294
12. ANDERSON, H.C. (1985) Matrix vesicle calcification: review and update. *Bone Mineral Res.*, **3**, 109–149
13. RUSSELL, R.G.G. and KANIS, J.A. (1984) Ectopic calcification and ossification. In *Metabolic Bone and Stone Disease*, edited by B.E.C. Nordin. Edinburgh: Churchill Livingstone
14. GLIMCHER, M. (1984) Recent studies of the mineral phase in bone and its possible linkage to the organic matrix by protein bound phosphate bonds. *Philos. Trans. R. Soc. Lond. (Biol.)*, **304**, 479–506
15. YAARI, A.M. and SHAPIRO, I.M. (1982) Effect of phosphate on phosphatidylserine-mediated calcium transport. *Calcif. Tissue Int.*, **34**, 43–48
16. YAARI, A.M., BOSKEY, A.L. and SHAPIRO, I.M. (1984) Phosphate modulation of calcium transport by a calcium-phospholipid-phosphate complex of calcifying tissues. *Calcif. Tissue Int.*, **36**, 317–319
17. REGISTER, T.C. and WUTHIER, R.E. (1984) Effect of vanadate, a potent alkaline phosphatase inhibitor on Ca and P uptake by matrix vesicle enriched fractions from chicken epiphyseal cartilage. *J. Biol. Chem.*, **259**, 3511–3518
18. ALI, S.Y. (1984) Isolation of matrix vesicles from calcifying cartilage. In *Methods of Calcified Tissue Preparation*, edited by G.R. Dickson. Amsterdam: Elsevier

19. HSU, H.T. (1983) Purification and partial characterization of ATP pyrophosphohydrolase from fetal bovine epiphyseal cartilage. *J. Biol. Chem.,* **258**, 3463–3468

20. CASWELL, A.M. and RUSSELL, R.G.G. (1985) Identification of ecto-nucleoside triphosphate pyrophophatase in human articular chondrocytes in monolayer culture. *Biochim. Biophys. Acta,* **847**, 40–47

21. SHAPIRO, I.M., MATSUMOTO, H. and GOLUB, E.E. (1985) Does superoxide control the formation of matrix vesicles in growth cartilage? In *Proceedings of Cell Mediated Calcification and Matrix Vesicles Conference*. Amsterdam: Elsevier

22. CHENG, P-T. and PRITZKER, K.P.H. (1983) Pyrophosphate, phosphate ion interaction: effects on calcium pyrophosphate and calcium hydroxyapatite crystal formation in aqueous solutions. *J. Rheumatol.*, **10**, 769–777

23. NORDIN, B.E.C. (1984) *Metabolic Bone and Stone Disease.* Edinburgh: Churchill Livingstone

24. WONG, G.L. (1986) Skeletal effects of parathyroid hormone. *Bone Mineral Res.*, **4**, 103–132

25. HABENER, J.F., ROSENBLATT, M. and POTTS, J.T. (1984) Parathyroid hormone: biochemical aspects of biosynthesis, secretion, action and metabolism. *Physiol. Rev.*, **64**, 985–1053

26. AVIOLI, L.V. and KRANE, S.M. (1978) *Metabolic Bone Disease*, Vol 2. New York: Academic Press

27. CHASE, L.R. and AURBACH, G.D. (1967) Parathyroid function and the renal excretion of 3, 5-adenylic acid. *Proc. Nat. Acad. Sci. USA*, **58**, 518–525

28. CHASE, L.R. and AURBACH, G.D. (1968) Renal adenyl cyclase: anatomically separate sites for parathyroid hormone and vasopressin. *Science*, **159**, 545–547

29. PARSONS, J.A. and ZANELLI, J.M. (1980) Physiological role of the parathyroid glands. In *Handbuch der inneren Medizin, Klinische Osteologic*, edited by F. Kuhlencordt and H. Barteheimer. Heidelberg: Springer

30. WASSERMAN, R.H. and CHANDLER, J.S. (1985) Molecular mechanism of intestinal calcium absorption. *Bone Mineral Res.*, **3**, 181–212

31. HAUSSLET, M.R., BAYLINK, D.J. and HUGHES, M.R. (1976) The assay of 1, 25-dihydroxyvitamin D_3: physiologic and pathologic modulation of circulating hormone levels. *Clin. Endocrinol.*, **5**, 151S–165S

32. TALLMAGE, R.V., COOPER, C.W. and TOVERUD, S.U. (1983) The physiological significance of calcitonin. *Bone Mineral Res.*, **1**, 74–142

33. KWASHIMA, H., TORIKAI, S. and KUROKAWA, K. (1981) Calcitonin selectively stimulates 25-hydroxyvitamin D_3-1-hydroxylase in proximal straight tubule of rat kidney. *Nature*, **291**, 327–329

34. FOSTER, G.V., MACINTYRE, I. and PEARSE, A.G.E. (1964) Calcitonin production and the mitochondrion rich cells of the dog thyroid. *Nature*, **203**, 1029–1030

35. FREAKE, H.C. and MACINTYRE, I. (1982) Specific binding of 1, 25-dihydroxycholecalciferol in human medullary thyroid carcinoma. *Biochem. J.*, **206**, 181–184

36. CHAMBERS, T.J., MCSHEEHY, P.M.J., THOMSON, B.M. and FULLER, K. (1985) The effect of calcium-regulating hormones and prostaglandins on bone resorption by osteoclasts disaggregated from neonatal rabbit bones. *Endocrinology*, **116**, 234–239

37. CHAMBERS, T.J., FULLER, K., SHEEHY, P.M.J. and PRINGL, J.A.S. (1985) The effect of calcium-regulating hormones on bone resorption by isolated human osteoclastoma cells. *J. Pathol.*, **145**, 297–305

38. BRAGA, P., FERRI, S., SANTAGOSTINO, A., OLGIATI, V.R. and PECILE, A. (1978) Lack of opiate receptor involvement in centrally induced calcitonin analgesia. *Life Sci.*, **22**, 971–978

16

Bone

Introduction

Bone is of vital importance to the dentist. For instance, orthodontics involves tooth movement within the jaw, orthognathic surgery centres on the modification of craniofacial morphology and periodontal disease essentially comprises local pathological alveolar bone changes. In addition to trauma, the jaws are frequently involved in local infections, e.g. periapical abscesses, whereas tumours and cystic lesions may also occur within the craniofacial tissues.

What is bone?

Functions

Bone is essentially a specialized form of connective tissue[1–7] exhibiting a variety of functions:

(1) Protection.
(2) Site of muscle origin and insertion.
(3) Rigidity.
(4) Haemopoiesis.
(5) Labile mineral pool

Thus, as well as providing skeletal units, bones and bone tissues are intimately associated with the maintenance of homeostasis of the body as a whole.

Bone morphology

Morphologically, bones may be categorized into a number of groups.

(1) Tubular, e.g. the femur.
(2) Cuboidal, e.g. the carpus.
(3) Flat, e.g. the frontal bone.
(4) Irregular, e.g. the vertebrae.

Each bone generally comprises a delimiting shell (or cortex) whose thickness varies not only from bone to bone but also from region to region within a given bone. The interior of the bone is occupied by varying amounts of cancellous tissue whose component trabeculae, as well as the proportion of cancellous to cortical bone, vary, primarily depending upon the mechanical requirements of the bone as a whole. In the spaces between the cancellous trabecular bone (the medullary spaces), there are blood vessels, nerves, fat and haemopoietic tissue.

In the adult, most of the haemopoietic function is confined to the axial skeleton and proximal part of the appendicular skeleton, although this may change with profound blood loss, e.g. persistent severe menstrual loss. The entire skeleton serves the haemopoietic function in the infant, however, although the extent is slowly reduced during the completion of growth and development. Thus, at the macroscopic level, the bones of the skeleton demonstrate a marked degree of heterogeneity.

Except at the musculotendinous insertions and at their articular surfaces, the bones are covered by a thin tough fibrous membrane (the periosteum) whereas at the articular and musculotendinous insertion regions, this tissue imperceptibly blends with the surface fibres of those tissues. The inner layer of the periosteum, the cambium layer, has bone-forming potential. This layer provides a source of new bone during growth and functions in both a resorptive and additive capacity during remodelling. In the adult, the bone-forming potential of the periosteum may be reactivated in trauma, infection or in association with tumours, although at all times there is a fine balance between bone formation and resorption for the maintenance of skeletal integrity. In the child, the periosteum is only loosely attached to the underlying bone, whereas in the adult, it is firmly attached, especially in the region of the palatal mucosa. Numerous capillary blood vessels penetrate the periosteum to augment the vascularization of bone, in addition to providing nutrients to this vital tissue. On disruption of this tissue as a result of inflammatory exudate accumulation, e.g. a dental abscess, the viability of both periosteum and bone may be compromised.

The macro- and microstructure of the bony skeleton in the adult exhibits a close correlation between morphology and mechanical needs, in addition to metabolic functions associated with calcium, phosphorus and magnesium metabolism. The component osteons (haversian systems) of cortical bone are, from a mechanical viewpoint, more compacted than those in trabeculae, i.e. in cancellous bone the trabeculae are arranged so as to resist the mechanical forces and these mechanical factors are mirrored by the structures at a microscopic level. Thus, bones reflect the intricate interactions between metabolic and mechanical forces.

The jaws

In the jaws, there is also a distinction between basal and alveolar bone. For instance, the mandibular body or ramus grows and develops in conjunction with the inferior alveolar nerves and vessels, whereas the alveolar bone grows in response to tooth eruption, adapts and remodels according to the dental needs, and undergoes resorption following tooth loss. Thus in ectodermal dysplasia, a group of genetic disorders associated with deciduous and permanent tooth anodontia, the alveolar bone fails to develop, despite normal basal jaw growth. Such dissociation between alveolar and basal bone has implications in the orthodontic treatment of craniofacial disproportion.

The alveolar bone may be considered the region of the jaws that forms and supports the tooth sockets. This comprises a thin cortical plate, termed the lamina dura, in which the principal periodontal fibres are inserted. In addition, the supporting alveolar bone invests the alveolus proper and comprises trabeculae that support the alveoli with a surrounding cortical layer. This is much thinner in the maxilla than the mandible. In some regions of the jaws, e.g. the mandibular incisor region, the trabecular region of the alveolus may in fact be very thin. In such regions, one or more tooth roots may be partially or totally denuded of bone (fenestrations or dehiscences) and these may have significance if associated with alveolar bone loss due to chronic periodontal disease or if they occur in an area in which fixed bridge or denture abutments are contemplated.

The visible differences between bone, cartilage and tendons depend on the variable composition of their matrices. Dense fibrous connective tissue comprising tendons is formed from well-orientated collagen bundles that function in tension. Bone and cartilage, by contrast, have to resist compression and shearing forces as well as tension and are therefore composed of a composite of different materials. These composites comprise mineral and proteoglycan to resist compressive forces and collagen for strength in tension and bending movements. Thus, variations in the type of collagen or state of aggregation of the proteoglycans will also affect the mechanical properties of a bone. Bone is therefore heterogeneous at all levels of structure.

Microscopic structure

Cancellous (spongy bone) essentially comprises trabeculae containing osteocytes located within intercommunicating lacunae. The basic structure of cortical (compact) bone is the haversian system, consisting of a central vascular canal surrounded by 8–10 concentric lamellae or layers, each demarcated by modified matrix termed cement lines. Each lamella contains a number of osteocytes that communicate with the vasculature of the haversian canals by a number of perpendicularly orientated canaliculi. These Volkmann's canals then connect the central vascular canals with the endosteal and periosteal surfaces. The haversian systems comprise dynamic structures, with old haversian systems being continually resorbed and replaced by new ones. The remnants of the old haversian system, located between the adjacent haversian systems, remain as interstitial lamellae. The first-formed lamellae are those on the periphery of the haversian system. They are generally more highly calcified than those of more recent origin.

Bone therefore comprises two phases: the osseous matrix, consisting of both organic and inorganic components, and the cellular component, essentially comprising osteoblasts, osteocytes and osteoclasts.

Bone cells

The skeleton is not merely a collection of inanimate mechanical structures but is constantly undergoing remodelling and growth, primarily resulting from osteoblast, osteocyte and osteoclast cellular activity.

Osteoblasts[8]

The osteoblasts are the cells responsible for the synthesis of the bone matrix, comprising both collagen fibres and ground substance. They form a continuous layer over the bone surface, which, if disrupted, may be associated with bone necrosis. Active osteoblasts are plump and cuboidal with a marked basophilic cytoplasm, whereas inactive cells appear flat and inconspicuous. There is general agreement that proteins synthesized by the ribosomes of the rough endoplasmic reticulum of the osteoblasts are released into the cisternae and then packaged into secretory granules by the Golgi apparatus. The limiting membranes of these organelles then fuse with the plasmalemma of the osteoblast, thereby discharging their contents into the extracellular milieu. The resulting organic matrix (osteoid) then undergoes mineralization to form bone. Where bone is actively forming, the cells are seen to line a thin layer of unmineralized bone matrix – the osteoid seam. This osteoid seam results from mineralization, following the formation of organic bone matrix; these two processes do not occur simultaneously.

Osteoblasts have a high alkaline phosphatase content which is considered to function in the process of calcification; their activity in protein synthesis is correlated with the prominent rough endoplasmic reticulum and Golgi apparatus. The surface of osteoblasts, especially that adjacent to the bone matrix, exhibits numerous fine cytoplasmic processes which make contact with the processes of the osteocytes. The functional activity of these cells is influenced by a variety of factors, including parathyroid hormone (which decreases collagen synthesis) and cortisol (which inhibits the maturation of pre-osteoblasts to osteoblasts). In fact, many factors decrease osteoblastic activity, whereas there are very few stimulatory factors.

Osteocytes

Generally, osteocytes are considered to comprise osteoblasts that have become incorporated within bone matrix. Using radioactive tracers, osteocytes have been shown to become incorporated within bone matrix in a few days in areas of active bone formation, whereas in other areas 2–3 months may elapse prior to incorporation. In immature woven bone, these cells are large, plump, closely packed together and exhibit rudimentary cytoplasmic processes. In mature lamellar bone, they are flattened and widely separated with fine cytoplasmic interconnecting processes connecting with both adjacent osteocytes and the central haversian canals. Rather than comprising a quiescent cellular population, the osteocytes are believed to be intimately associated with the rapid adjustment of serum calcium ions, in addition to possessing osteolytic capabilities associated with local bone remodelling. Osteocytic osteolysis may be responsible for short-term remodelling activity, whereas osteoclastic resorption is more closely associated with long-term bone remodelling. Upon resorption of mature lamellar bone by osteoclastic activity, the osteocytes may be released from their bony lacunae. Whether they subsequently undergo necrosis or transformation into primitive osteoprogenitor cells remains unclear.

Osteoclasts[9,10]

The osteoclasts are typically large, multinucleated cells lying in shallow crypts (Howship's lacunae) on the bone surface. In addition to a high acid phosphatase content, the cells contain many lysosomal dense bodies, a well developed Golgi apparatus and many mitochondria. The mitochondria contain electron-dense matrix vesicles, composed of calcium phosphate, which are considered to be associated with the regulation of intracellular calcium.

Adjacent to the bone, osteoclasts have a brush border formed by multiple infoldings of the plasma membrane. The bone in juxtaposition to the brush border is in a state of partial demineralization in which collagen fibres and free, randomly arranged, crystals of hydroxyapatite may be detected. The prominence of this osteoclastic brush border seems to be related to the degree of active bone resorption that is occurring. Calcitonin has been associated with involution of this osteoclastic region, whereas thyroid hormone has been associated with its increased prominence. In addition, there is evidence that monocytes may also be capable of resorbing bone, again with a brush border characteristic of resorbing cells.

The process of bone resorption is considered to involve a number of mechanisms:

(1) Release of lysosomal hydrolytic enzymes, resulting from the fusion of lysosomal membranes

with the plasmalemma of the brush border, leading to enzymic release into the extracellular milieu.

(2) Action of endocytosis, whereby pinocytotic vesicles traverse the brush border to fuse with the primary lysosomes to form secondary lysosomes.

(3) Release of acids of metabolic origin into the microcompartment delineated by the resorbing bone.

Lowering of the pH, enzymatic attack and endocytosis therefore appear to be involved in demineralization and osteolysis.

The relationship between osteoblasts and osteoclasts remains enigmatic. One theory contends that there is a common stem cell that can differentiate into an osteoblast or an osteoclast. Another theory holds that the mesenchymal cell can differentiate into a pre-osteoclast; later the osteoclast can differentiate into pre-osteoblasts and then osteoblasts and finally osteocytes. A third view is that the osteoblasts and osteoclasts are two distinct cell lines. The osteoblast has a common stem cell with other collagen-producing cells (fibroblasts and chondroblasts) and arise locally from fixed non-migratory mesenchymal cells. The osteoclast is closely related to the macrophage and blood monocyte, possibly being associated with a common local stem cell.

Bone dynamics

In normal bone there is a balance between bone formation and resorption, with little change in total mass except for the almost imperceptible decrease that occurs with age. On the other hand, the bones are in a constant state of flux, with bone trabeculae being constantly formed and modified in response to changing mechanical requirements. Remodelling of cortical bone involves the formation of new osteonal systems. Conceivably, a resorption cavity is produced by an osteoclastic front, the cutting zone, which advances into the existing cortical bone. The cutting zone is followed by proliferating mesenchymal cells which differentiate into connective tissue and blood vessels; this, in turn, is followed by the production of lamellar bone to fill the cavity with new concentric lamellae. The remains of the old osteonal system then become interstitial lamellae.

Bone not only arranges its trabecular pattern but also gains or loses tissue as a whole in response to stress. The mechanism(s) responsible for bone formation or resorption in response to mechanical stimuli remain obscure but may be correlated with chemical and/or electromagnetic forces.

Periosteum

The periosteum comprises a dense sheath of connective tissue that invests bone, with the exception of the articular cartilage. Of the two component layers, the outermost comprises dense fibrous connective tissue containing a number of blood vessels, whereas the inner cambium layer has a looser consistency containing collagen fibres that enter the osseous tissue as Sharpey's fibres. These serve to anchor the periosteum on to the bone surface.

The endosteum comprises a layer of delicate reticular tissue that lines the medullary cavity. Whereas the periosteum contains progenitor cells important for bone remodelling and resorption, the endosteal layer contains progenitor cells that subserve both haemopoietic and osteogenic functions. In addition, both periosteal and endosteal layers may provide a limiting membrane controlling the egress and ingress of ions.[11]

Bone mineral

Bone mineral resembles chemically precipitated hydroxyapatites. As in synthetic systems, an unstable amorphous precursor is the first bone mineral to be deposited, but this is quickly converted to a poorly crystallized hydroxyapatite form. The most distinctive features of bone apatite are small crystal size, lack of chemical perfection and internal chemical disorder. These properties result in bone mineral being insoluble enough for stability, yet reactive enough for mineral homeostasis and normal bone resorption. Above a certain minimal crystal size, the solubility of the mineral is independent of size. Below this critical size, the crystal is so small that the weaker bonding of the surface ions to the total crystal becomes important.

The inorganic phase of bone occupies approximately 70% by weight. Although the percentage by weight of collagen decreases as osteoid materializes, volumetrically the amount of collagen in osteoid is analogous to that in mature bone. The mineral phase of bone consists largely of calcium, phosphate, carbonate and citrate ions, with 80–90% being located within the collagen fibrils. The basic crystalline unit of bone is the hydroxyapatite crystal.

Hydroxyapatite is a basic calcium phosphate, found in both bone and tooth mineral. The simplest grouping of atoms which can define the mineral hydroxyapatite is $Ca_{10}(PO_4)_6(OH)_6$. The ions in this hydroxyapatite structure may be replaced by a variety of similar ions from solution under physiological conditions. For instance, Sr^{2+} and Pb^{2+} may substitute for Ca^{2+} or F^- for OH^-. The ability of bone to remove lead from body fluids is an asset, although the long term storage of radioactive strontium is cause for worry. When F^- substitutes for OH^-, the solubility of an apatite is lowered, with an increase in average crystal size. About one part per million of fluorine in drinking water stabilizes tooth apatite against caries, and oral doses of fluorine, in conjunction with calcium and vitamin D, have been used in the treatment of osteoporosis.

Hydroxyapatite, precipitated from solution under conditions similar to the physiological state, results in needle-like crystals that can be detected only by electron microscopy. Such crystals are carbonate-containing and characterized by internal disorder. High pressure and/or temperature is required to obtain large pure apatite crystals. When hydroxyapatite is precipitated from supersaturated calcium phosphate solutions at or above pH 7, an unstable amorphous calcium phosphate precursor results. Amorphous calcium phosphate appears as microscopic spheres 30–100 nm diameter, comprising randomly packed apatite clusters each of about 0.95 nm diameter. In water, the amorphous calcium phosphate dissolves and renucleates as hydroxyapatite crystals. Pyrophosphate, diphosphonates or adenosine triphosphate can delay or prevent the transformation of amorphous calcium phosphate to hydroxyapatite. The earliest bone mineral deposited is an amorphous calcium phosphate, whereas stable amorphous calcium phosphate granules may also be found in the mitochondria of certain cells, especially those involved in tissue mineralization.

Thus bone mineral resembles chemically precipitated hydroxyapatites. Bone crystals never exceed 40–50 nm in their largest dimension and, although small on first formation, they increase with maturity associated with increased chemical homogeneity. With ripening, the bone crystal approaches, but never reaches, the perfect hydroxyapatite formula. Bone mineral has a high surface area per unit weight and the surface is chemically reactive with its environment. Studies of surface bonding suggest that a chemical linkage probably exists between the mineral in bone and certain free polar groups of collagen.[12] The average size of crystals in bone affected by pathological processes, e.g. Paget's disease, is associated with smaller bone crystals than in the nearby unaffected bone, reflecting the high resorption and redeposition of Pagetic bone. Also fluorine stabilizes bone crystals by reducing their solubility and increasing the average crystal size.

At one time, a large proportion of mature bone was considered to comprise amorphous calcium phosphate but more recent studies have shown that initial bone deposition occurs in the amorphous phase. Mature bone actually comprises a poorly crystallized, carbonate-containing, highly disordered hydroxyapatite, which contains trace elements of other metals, e.g. zinc and magnesium.

Organic phase[13]

The organic matrix of bone is first deposited as osteoid by osteoblasts, and only later becomes calcified. Collagen is the basic constituent of the organic phase of bone (95%), the remainder comprising mucopolysaccharides containing chondroitin 4- and 6-sulphates. These chondroitin sulphates primarily comprise alternating residues of glucuronic acid and *N*-acetylgalactosamine. The basic unit of collagen is the tropocollagen molecule, an oligomeric protein comprising three left-handed helices twisted around each other to form a right-handed super-helix. Each tropocollagen molecules has a diameter of 1.5 nm and a length of 280 nm. The 64 nm periodicity seen in collagen fibres results from a quarter-length overlap of the component tropocollagen molecules. The amino acid sequence of the individual subunits of the tropocollagen molecule is often Gly–X–Y, indicating that a glycinyl residue occupies every third position in the chain. Nearly every fourth of the residues are amino acids proline and hydroxyproline, although hydroxylysine may also be present. The hydroxylysine residues are important for their cross-linkages between adjacent tropocollagen molecules. The collagen of bone is Type I, i.e. similar to that of dentine, skin and tendons, although these last generally fail to calcify under physiological conditions.

Osteogenesis[14–22]

The production of osteoid, the non-mineralized phase of bone matrix, consists predominantly of collagen together with a ground substance of acidic mucopolysaccharides. The osteoblasts are primarily thought to be involved in this function. The mRNA coding for the procollagen molecules is transferred by ribosomes of the rough endoplasmic reticulum. The resulting procollagen is segregated in the cisternae of the rough endoplasmic reticulum and then packaged into secretory vesicles by the Golgi apparatus. These vesicles then make their way to the proximal region of the osteoblast by means of microtubules. Subsequently, the limiting membrane of the secretory vesicle fuses with the plasmalemma so that the vesicular contents are discharged into the extracellular milieu.

The procollagen molecules first formed in the osteoblasts have a high molecular weight, due to the presence of non-helical telopeptides at the amino and carboxyl terminals: these are termed registration peptides, since their presence facilitates the registration of the tropocollagen molecules to form the precise quarter-staggered array that yields the characteristic 64 nm periodicity. Either preceding or concomitant with registration of the tropocollagen molecules, the non-helical and non-enzymatically protected telopeptides are cleaved by procollagen peptidases.

Maturation of the resultant collagen fibres essentially entails the formation of cross-links between adjacent peptide chains of the same tropocollagen molecule and between adjacent tropocollagen molecules. This involves oxidation of specific lysine or hydroxylysine residues by the copper-requiring system, lysyl oxidase. The aldehyde derivatives of lysine and hydroxylysine so formed may then react spontaneously in one of three ways:

(1) A hydroxylysine and histidine residue may be added to an aldol condensation product to form a histidino-hydroxymerodesmosine.
(2) An aldehyde derivative may react with an unmodified lysine or hydroxylysine residue to form a Schiff base.
(3) An aldehyde derivative may react with a second aldehyde derivative to form an aldol condensation product.

Mineralization

There is no unified theory of bone mineralization. Any mineralization theory must account for several factors. Firstly, the calcium and phosphate ion concentration of serum and extracellular fluid exists in a metastable solution. Thus any mineralization model must allow for a local increase in the concentration of these ions resulting from a cellular process, e.g. the release of amorphous calcium phosphate from osteoclasts or nucleating sites, effecting an increase in the local concentrations of calcium and phosphate ions by their binding in close proximity.

Secondly, Type I collagen of bone is similar to that of skin and tendon, yet the last two tissues only infrequently undergo calcification. Conceivably, this is a reflection of alterations in the physical parameters of various forms of type I collagen, e.g. solubility.

Thirdly, certain substances present in extracellular fluid and serum are capable of inhibiting apatite crystal formation *in vitro*. For instance, pyrophosphate forms complexes with calcium ions, thereby lowering the available ion concentration. Although once considered to play an active role in calcification, the acidic mucopolysaccharides of bone matrix (chondroitin 4- and 6-sulphates) may form inhibitors in normal and ectopic calcification.

The theories of intra- or intercellular tissue mineralization fall into three main categories.

(1) Mechanisms that would locally raise the calcium and phosphate solution ion product to levels at which mineral would precipitate spontaneously.
(2) Mechanisms or substances that would create nucleating sites or remove barriers to these sites.
(3) Mechanisms or substances that prevent mineral formation and must be removed or rendered inactive to permit calcification.

The initial mineral deposits in the organic matrix of bone appear to occur at discrete sites in, or on, the collagen fibrils.[34] It is currently thought that collagen itself is not an apatite nucleator but that other tissues closely associated with collagen serve this function, e.g. phosphoproteins.[35] The phosphoproteins may play a structural and/or regulatory role in the calcifying organic matrix by providing an epitaxial substrate for apatite nucleation. Although phosphoproteins may induce apatite formation, they are probably more involved in controlling the size, shape and orientation of the bone crystals. In fact, a number of proteins have been suggested as nucleators in the initiation of bone apatite, including γ-carboxyglutamic acid (GLA)-containing proteins and lipids.

In 1923, the enzyme alkaline phosphatase was considered to hydrolyze phosphate esters to produce an excess of free inorganic phosphate, elevating the calcium and phosphate ion product at specific calcification centres to the degree necessary to produce apatite precipitation. Alkaline phosphatase has been shown to be present in mineralizing extracellular vesicles and is used as a marker of active tissue mineralization.[2]

There are also calcium-binding proteins in areas of tissue mineralization. Such compounds may be associated with raising the solution calcium phosphate product or acting as a nucleating centre where phosphates can bind to the calcium and produce a mineral deposit. Phosphoproteins and those containing a large amount of γ-carboxyglutamate are the principal calcium-binding proteins, although certain lipid complexes and proteolipids (e.g. phosphatidylserine and phosphatidylinositol) may act as transporters of calcium and/or nucleators of apatite. The overall concentration of lipid in the metaphysis of a long bone increases sharply from the zone of calcification, decreasing rapidly after calcification.[23]

Collagen is considered to be the principal nucleator of bone mineral. *In vitro* experiments have shown that only native collagen exhibiting the 64 nm periodicity in the long fibril axis direction will act as a nucleator of hydroxyapatite.[24] X-ray diffraction studies have shown that bone mineral is first deposited in holes distributed along the collagen fibrils and subsequently followed by bone apatite deposition on or near these fibrils. There is strong *in vitro* evidence that collagen can nucleate hydroxyapatite from metastable calcium phosphate solution and the close association of mineral and collagen during osteogenesis suggests a positive role for this fibrous protein. Conceivably, the galactose groups in the collagen molecule act as the nucleating centres.

It has been noted that the phosphate ion appears prior to the requirement for calcium. Conceivably, the phosphorylated groups that are actually attached to negatively charged peptides of bone collagen bind the newly formed apatite crystals to the organic matrix.

Calcium–phospholipid–phosphate complexes occur in mineralizing as opposed to non-mineralizing areas of bone. Such substances may originate from cell membranes and/or extracellular matrix vesicle membranes and provide efficient nucleators of hydroxyapatite.

Mineralized tissues are, therefore, not simply the end-product of precipitations of inorganic crystals from supersaturated solution in micro-environments that happen to be composed of organic molecules. They are in fact organic, matrix-induced processes[27] under the constant control of viable cells. The hallmarks of biomineralization processes are the precise timing, localization and at times orientation of mineral deposition within a given tissue. In general, cells first produce the biosynthetic precursors to their extracellular organic matrix, then assemble and probably modify the composite matrix for subsequent mineralization. A variety of non-collagenous proteins may therefore be critical to the ultimate biomineralized state before the appearance of the mineralized phase. Because many of these proteins bind to hydroxyapatite, their final location in the mineralized matrix is usually associated with crystal surfaces, even though their real biological function may well have been executed earlier within the cells or in the non-mineralized matrix. The amorphous mineral precursor is generally nucleated heterogeneously, possibly on adjacent sequences of carboxyl, sulphate or phosphate groups associated with proteins. After a crystal has been nucleated, other proteins may bind stereospecifically to certain crystal planes or surfaces and limit growth on that face while allowing others to grow at a rate limited only by the solution activity of the precipitating ions. This process regulates the final shape and/or orientation of the crystal relative to those made in free solution.[28] Alternatively, non-collagenous proteins may bind preferentially to a growing amorphous precursor precipitate or other intermediate mineral form, thereby altering the chemical potential of the surfaces of the early forms.[29] Then, as this early mineral is changed to a more thermodynamically stable form, the proteins may no longer interact stereospecifically with the new mineral surface and would be chemically inert or simply diffuse away. The new stable crystal could then grow and replicate at the free solution rate. Thus, a cell may use an intrinsic crystal property of an early metastable mineral to direct the character, location and shape of its final, stable mineral product. Alternatively, non-collagenous proteins may be associated with secondary crystal growth. A principal corollary of such stereospecific protein control of mineral nucleation is that accidental mineral deposition becomes extremely improbable. Also, controlled mineralization involving non-collagenous protein assemblies is unlikely to be duplicated by random associations of the constituent proteins at other sites in the body.

Subsequent growth of a bone crystal may involve cellular control of the local environment to help or hinder the diffusion of ions at certain crystal faces.[30] Such matrix-associated changes in diffusional rates or local ion activity is most likely to occur during slow growth of large biocrystals, e.g. enamel.

Other calcium-binding proteins, including those found in serum, may affect biomineralization by competing with solution ions for the crystal surfaces, even if only in a non-specific manner. Alkaline phosphatase is capable of inactivating the inhibitory action of diphosphometabolites previously bound to amorphous calcium phosphate,[31] so that this enzyme may be important in the removal of low molecular weight crystal growth inhibitors in some types of mineralization.

The cessation of crystal growth and replication in the presence of an extracellular fluid metastable in calcium and phosphate occurs at the periosteal and endosteal bone surfaces and locally around each living cell adjacent to or within the mineralized matrix, e.g. trabecular lining cells. The mineral phase in bone is always kept several micrometres distant from living cells. With cell death, the mineral often invades the cellular space. Such control may be associated with poisoning of the growth surface with inhibitors, or modification of the crystal surface.

Phosphate-containing proteins have been known to be present in bone for a number of years,[32] with the acidic glycoprotein osteonectin being the best known.[33] Osteonectin binds strongly to hydroxyapatite and denatured collagen. Osteonectin has both high- and low-affinity binding sites for calcium and appears to be produced by osteoblasts for nucleating and orientating apatite crystal growth along collagen fibrils.

Conceivably, cell mitochondria store bone mineral in a reactive amorphous state for passage to the matrix vesicles, the latter's membranes subsequently providing nucleators for mineralization.[25] Thus, although calcium phosphate solution may be supersaturated with hydroxyapatite, the presence of proteoglycan aggregate molecules may delay and/or prevent apatite precipitation. Indeed, the enormous proteoglycan aggregate molecules may be enzymatically cleaved to produce much smaller subunits as the calcification region is approached, i.e. it appears that the proteoglycan inhibitor is probably cleaved enzymatically and removed prior to mineralization. Thus alkaline phosphatase, in addition to other enzymes, calcium-binding protein, collagen, lipids, cellular mitochondria, extracellular vesicles and the proteoglycans are probably all involved in mineralization of bone, although whether they act co-operatively or independently has yet to be elucidated.

Non-collagenous proteins undergo degradation at the time when the mineral content of bone rises from an initial 70% to 95% of its adult values.[18] At present, there is debate as to whether the surfaces of the crystallites in bone must be cleaned of all binding proteins before the final mineral content of bone can be reached, or whether the early rapid 70% of final mineralization in bone may reflect mineralization of one micro-environment (e.g. the collagen fibrils) while the later, more complete mineralization may reflect mineral deposition of a second independent environment.

Mechanical properties of bone[26]

As previously emphasized, bone is not a homogeneous tissue, but varies at both the macro- and microscopic level. This is reflected in the physical properties of bone which vary both between and within different skeletal units. The tensile strengths of haversian systems depend upon a number of factors. For instance, the tensile properties are superior when the collagen fibres are predominantly arranged parallel to the axis of tension compared with other collagenous orientations. Haversian systems with a high level of calcification are stiffer than those with a low level of calcification, although there are scant differences in tensile strength. This suggests that the tensile strength of a bone is dependent on the orientation and number of component collagen fibres. The compressive properties of haversian systems are also dependent on the arrangement of the component collagen fibres. For instance, maximum compressive strength and stiffness occur with circumferential collagenous arrangements relative to the haversian system and least with a longitudinal collagenous orientation. Thus, circumferential collagenous fibre arrangement results in superior compressive but inferior tensile properties, whereas longitudinal collagen fibres impart superior tensile but inferior compressive properties to a bone. Fully calcified haversian systems have a greater compressive strength and elastic modulus than those with a minimal degree of calcification.

Conclusions

The physiological mechanisms underlying both bone formation and resorption are changing very rapidly, reflecting the remarkable advances in research. There is, however, scant information concerning the interaction between osteoblasts and osteoclasts, or between osteocytes and osteoblasts. As a result, the detailed mechanisms for the control of bone cell functions have yet to be formulated. Unfortunately, alveolar bone has yet to be targeted for detailed research investigation, so it is not known whether it shares the structures and functions of the skeleton as a whole or is unique.

Review questions

1. What is the physiological relationship between osteoblasts and osteocytes?
2. Are osteoblasts derived from the same stem cell as osteoclasts?
3. What are the primary functions of bone?
4. What are the principal mechanisms for bone mineralization?
5. How might the arrangement of bone trabeculae accomodate changes in functional demands?

References

1. FROST, H.M. (1972, 1973) *Orthopaedic Lectures*, Vols. 2 & 3. Springfield: C.C. Thomas
2. MURRAY, P.D.F. (1936) *Bones – A Study of the Development and Structure of the Vertebrate Skeleton.* Cambridge: Cambridge University Press
3. THOMPSON D'ARCY, W. (1961) *On Growth and Form.* Cambridge: Cambridge University Press
4. VAUGHAN, J.M. (1975) *The Physiology of Bone.* Oxford: Clarendon Press
5. BASSETT, C.A.L. (1978) Pulsing electromagnetic fields. In *A New Approach to Surgical Problems in Metabolic Surgery*, edited by H. Buchwald and R. Varcho. New York: Grune & Stratton
6. NEUMAN, W.F. and NEWMAN, M.W. (1958) *The Chemical Dynamics of Bone Mineral.* Chicago: University of Chicago
7. WEINSTOCK, M. and LEBLOND, C.P. (1974) Formation of collagen. *Fed. Proc.*, **33**, 1205–1218
8. HALL, B.K. (1975) The origin and fate of osteoclasts. *Anat. Rec.*, **183**, 1–12
9. HALL, B.K. (1971) Histiogenesis and morphogenesis of bone. *Clin. Orthop.*, **74**, 249–268
10. HANCOX, N.M. (1972) The osteoclast. In *The Biochemistry and Physiology of Bone*, edited by G.H. Bourne. London: Academic Press
11. IRVING, J.T. (1958) A histological strain for newly calcified tissues. *Nature*, **181**, 704–705
12. POSNER, A.S. and BEEBE, R.A. (1975) The surface chemistry of bone mineral and related calcium phosphates. *Semin. Arthritis Rheum.*, **4**, 267–291
13. GLIMCHER, M.J. (1960) Specificity of the molecular structure of organic matrices in mineralization. In *Calcification in Biological Systems*, edited by R.F. Sognaes. Washington: American Association for the Advancement of Science.
14. SOBEL, A.E. and BURGER, M. (1954) Calcification. *Proc. Soc. Exp. Biol. Med.*, **87**, 7–13

15. ROBINSON, R. (1923) The possible significance of hexose phosphonic esters in ossification. *Biochem. J.*, **17**, 286–293
16. BAYLINK, D., WERGEDAL, J. and THOMPSON, E. (1972) Loss of protein polysaccharides at sites where bone mineralization is initated. *J. Histochem. Cytochem.*, **20**, 279–292
17. IRVING, J.T. (1978) Theories of mineralization of bones and teeth. In *Textbook of Oral Biology*, edited by J.H. Shaw, E.A. Sweeney, C.C. Cappuccino and S.M. Meller. Philadelphia: W.B. Saunders
18. HIRSCHMAN, A. and DZIENWIATKOWSKI, D. (1966) Protein-polysaccharide loss during endochondral ossification. *Science*, **154**, 393–395
19. FLEISCH, H., RUSSELL, R.G.G. and FRANCIS, M.D. (1969) Diphosphonates inhibit hydroxyapatite dissolution *in vitro* and bone resorption in tissue culture and *in vivo*. *Science*, **165**, 1262–1264
20. FLEISCH, H. and RUSSELL, R.G.G. (1970) Pyrophosphate and polyphosphate. In *International Encyclopedia of Pharmacology and Therapeutics, Sect. 51. Pharmacology of the Endocrine System and Related Drugs, Vol. 1*, edited by H. Rasmussen. Oxford: Pergamon
21. KIMMICH, G.A. and RASMUSSEN, H. (1969) Regulation of pyruvate carboxylase activity of calcium in intact rat liver mitochondria. *J. Biol. Chem.*, **244**, 190–199
22. ALI, S.Y., SAJDERA, S.W. and ANDERSON, H.C. (1970) Isolation and characterization of calcifying matrix vesicles from epiphyseal cartilage. *Proc. Natl. Acad. Sci. USA*, **67**, 1513–1520
23. WUTHIER, R.E. (1973) Enzymatic lipid, and electrolyte composition of epiphyseal cartilage subcellular fractions. *J. Dent. Res.*, **52**, 175
24. GLIMCHER, M.K., KATZ, E.P. and TRAVIS, D.F. (1965) The solubilization and reconstitution of bone collagen. *J. Ultrastruct. Res.*, **13**, 261–274
25. LEHNINGER, A.L. (1970) Mitochondria and calcium transport. *Biochem. J.*, **119**, 129–138
26. ASCENZI, A. and BONUCCI, E. (1968) The compressive properties of single osteons. *Anat. Rec.*, **161(B)**, 377–391
27. LOWENSTAM, H.A. (1981) Minerals formed by organisms. *Science*, **211**, 1126
28. ADDADI, L. and WEINER, S. (1985) Interactions between acidic proteins and crystals: stereochemical requirements in biomineralization. *Proc. Natl. Acad. Sci. USA*, **82**, 4110
29. EANES, E.D. and TERMINE, J.D. (1983) Calcium in mineralized tissues. In *Calcium in Biology*, edited by T.G. Spiro. New York: Wiley
30. NEUMAN, W.F. (1980) Bone mineral and calcification. In *Fundamental and Clinical Bone Physiology*, edited by M.R. Urist. Philadelphia: J.B. Lippincott
31. TERMINE, J.D. and CONN, K.M. (1976) Inhibition of apatite formation by phosphorylated metabolites and macromolecules. *Calcif. Tissue Res.*, **22**, 149
32. SPECTOR, A.R. and GLIMCHER, M.J. (1973) The identification of O-phosphoserine in the soluble anionic phosphoproteins of bone. *Biochim. Biophys. Acta*, **303**, 360
33. TERMINE, J.D., KLEINMAN, H.K., WHITSON, S.W., CONN, K.M., MCGARVEY, M.L. and MARTIN, G.R. (1981) Osteonectin, a bone-specific protein linking mineral to collagen. *Cell*, **26**, 99
34. GLIMCHER, M.J. (1976) Composition, structure and organization of bone and other mineralized tissues and the mechanisms of calcification. In *Handbook of Physiology – Endocrinology*, edited by R.O. Greep and E.B. Astwood. Baltimore: Williams & Wilkins
35. BOSKEY, A.L. and POSNER, A.L. (1983) Calcification and structure of hard tissue. In *Structure–Property Relationship in Biomaterials, Vol 3*, edited by G.W. Hastings and P. Ducheyne. Boca Raton: CRC Press

17

Growth and development of the craniofacial skeleton

Introduction

Approximately 7% of all live births in the United States have some mental or physical defect evident at birth or later. Craniofacial defects are among the most common, e.g. cleft lip and cleft palate which affect 1:600 white infants. The incidence is higher among orientals, native Americans and Eskimos but lower among blacks. Other craniofacial malformations include jaw deformities, dental anomalies, ossification defects of the facial and cranial bones, too wide or narrow spacing between the eyes, facial asymmetry and fetal alcohol syndrome. Indeed, congenital malformations now loom as significant causes of infant mortality and morbidity, partly reflecting the declining incidence of infections compared with previous decades, as well as more accurate birth defect detection. High percentages of malformations also occur among embryos or fetuses lost in the first trimester or in later miscarriages and stillbirths. A small proportion of craniofacial malformations can be traced to specific genetic or chromosomal disorders, and others to potent environmental factors, e.g. malnutrition, exposure to radiation, alcohol or drugs (*Table 17.1*), and problems in pregnancy and/or delivery. For the most part, the causes of craniofacial malformations remain obscure, although their effects may be profound for the patient, family and society.

Pregnant women are increasingly aware of the need to maintain healthy diets, avoid unnecessary medications and seek medical care throughout pregnancy. They know of the risk to the fetus of certain diseases and infections and are alerted to the latest findings of toxicologists and scientists studying environmental factors. In the past decade, the dangers to fetuses of certain anti-epileptic drugs and alcohol have been identified, e.g. fetal alcohol syndrome is characterized by wide spacing of the eyes, microcephaly and lower-than-normal intelligence. In addition, the importance of proper nutrition has been emphasized by studies that have suggested that vitamin supplementation may decrease the risk of malformation in some pregnancies. For instance, the outbreak of rubella (German measles) infection in 1964 resulted in 20 000 children developing severe congenital malformations, whereas the rate of rubella-caused malformations has

Table 17.1 Teratogens and dentofacial development

Teratogen	*Effect*
Accutane 13-*cis*-retinoic acid	Hemifacial microsomia, Treacher Collins syndrome
Aminopterin	Anencephaly
Aspirin	Cleft lip and palate
Cigarette smoke (hypoxia)	Cleft lip and palate
Cytomegalovirus	Microcephaly, hydrocephaly, microphthalmia
Dilantin	Cleft lip and palate
Ethyl alcohol	Central mid-face discrepancy
6-Mercaptopurine	Cleft palate
Rubella virus	Microphthalmia, cataracts, deafness
Thalidomide	Hemifacial microsomia
Toxoplasma	Microcephaly, hydrocephaly, microphthalmia
Valium	Cleft lip and palate
Vitamin D excess	Premature suture closure
X-radiation	Microcephaly

dropped to a little over 1:100 000 live births since the development of the rubella vaccine.

Genetic factors obviously contribute to the shaping of the face and oral structures. Although evolutionary forces are said to be responsible for the high frequency of malocclusion observed in many populations, changes with respect to dental occlusion appear to have occurred too rapidly to be explained by evolutionary changes alone. Environmental factors have therefore been implicated as important influences, including nutritional deficiencies, teratogens and other prenatal exogenous factors. Postnatally, dietary factors, facial trauma, abnormal breathing patterns and postural or oral habits (e.g. thumb sucking) are just a few of the myriad factors linked with craniofacial malformations.

Undoubtedly, skull development and growth hinges on the interaction between genetic and environmental factors. Research into the mechanisms of craniofacial anomalies has focused on the period of gestation, since at this period genetic misinformation is first expressed and/or the effect of teratogenic agents occurs. The embryonic period (2–8 weeks gestation) is characterized by cell, tissue and organ differentiation and this is then followed by the fetal growth period (3–10 lunar months). While congenital anomalies commonly arise during the fetal period, in fact they are the progressive expression of a disorder in the zygote or embryo. Postnatally, further growth and development may result in the exacerbation of such disorders or, less commonly, their masking due to compensatory growth changes.

Craniofacial form

Comparison of neonate and adult skulls demonstrates the differential effects of development and growth. The cranial vault dominates fetal, neonatal and early childhood skulls. Cranial development, in fact, peaks early, with 65% of its ultimate growth present at birth and 95% by 10 years of age. By contrast, facial growth begins more slowly and continues longer, with 40–50% present at birth and only 65% by 10 years of age.

The head is divisible into three regions.[1]

(1) The upper face is primarily derived from the frontonasal process and follows the neural growth pattern.
(2) The mid-face comprises the orbits, nose and maxilla, and so follows neural (ocular globes), cranial base (nasal capsule) and branchial arch (maxillary processes) growth patterns.
(3) The lower face essentially comprises the mandible, which follows the somatic growth pattern.

Although these three cranial regions follow different growth patterns, they are not discrete entities. Thus maldevelopment of one region variably affects that of others. This hinders evaluation of the factors influencing craniofacial form. Indeed, craniofacial development and growth is exceedingly complex and only a few of the underlying mechanisms are just beginning to be resolved. In general, the braincase (calvarium) and facial skeleton (viscerocranium) tend to grow more in anteroposterior length than height or width: a feature that accounts for the value of lateral cephalographs for the evaluation of cranial form.

The growth mechanisms by which the changes in skull proportions are achieved are essentially similar to those of the skeleton as a whole. Because of its rigidly mineralized matrix, bone can only grow by surface accretion. The osteocytes, trapped within their lacunae, cannot divide and form additional matrix. This inability to grow interstitially sets bone clearly apart from cartilage and other connective tissues. As bone can only grow by surface addition, there must also be surface resorption. Without such a mechanism, bones would become progressively distorted with growth. The combined processes of surface addition and resorption are termed remodelling. Generally, when the external surface of a region of bone is depository, its internal surface will be resorptive, and vice versa.[2] In addition to the cranial remodelling changes at the surface, there is another portion of the skull, the chondrocranium (comprising the cranial base, otic and nasal capsules), where cartilaginous growth occurs, subsequently to be replaced by bone. As will be evident later, the chondrocranium plays an important role in craniofacial development and growth.

Facial embryology[3,4]

There is a ten-fold increase in head size between the fourth to eighth week of gestation. This illustrates both the rapidity of cranial development at this period and accounts for the catastrophic consequences of maldevelopment that may be apparent at later stages of development.

The process of overt facial differentiation begins during the 3–4th week of gestation with dorsal neural crest tissue migration into the adjacent mesenchyme. The neural crest cells stream around the developing eyes to enter the anterior frontonasal process and posterior branchial arches. This neural crest mesenchymal invasion produces five embryonic facial processes:[5] the frontonasal process; bilateral maxillary processes and bilateral mandibular processes.

The ectodermal furrows between these processes are obliterated as they fill with proliferating mesenchyme and neural crest tissue. Impairment of neural crest cell migration, and/or mesenchymal growth, results in craniofacial anomalies associated with facial clefts.[5] Thus at the completion of neural crest cell migration in the fourth week of embryonic life, the cells contribute to almost all of the loose mesenchymal tissue in the facial region that later differentiates into skeletal and connective tissues, including the jaws and teeth (*Figure 17.1*). Severe facial asymmetry in some patients may be related to unequal neural crest migration to each side of the face. Certainly diminished neural crest migration has been implicated in Treacher Collins syndrome (mandibulofacial dysostosis), where both maxilla and mandible are underdeveloped due to a generalized lack of mesenchymal tissue. It appears that the neural crest cells with the longest migration path are most susceptible to maldevelopment, whereas those going to the central area tend to complete their migratory movement. At this time, the main divisions of the central nervous system are established: the forebrain; the midbrain; the hindbrain and the spinal cord.

Invagination of the nasal placodes surrounded by the elevated medial and lateral nasal swellings dominates the face of the 5-week-old fetus. The eyes appear as elevations on the lateral face and the furrow between the two mandibular processes fills with mesenchyme, unifying the lower jaw and lip. Mandibular symphyseal clefts result from failure of this migratory proliferation. The first branchial groove, below the mandibular processes, also fills centrally with mesenchyme, the most lateral aspect becoming the external auditory meatus. In this regard, malformation or mal-location of the external auditory meatus often serves as a marker for craniofacial anomalies. At this time, the development of the nervous system proceeds with trifurcation of the forebrain into the median diencephalon and the paired hemispheres, as well as hindbrain segmentation into the myelencephalon and metencephalon.

In the sixth week, the oropharynx is opened with the rupture of the stomodeum. The medial nasal swellings merge into a single globular process, which in turn differentiates into the soft tissue nose, central upper lip and premaxilla. These structures comprise the primary palate, with cleft lip and/or palate reflecting their maldevelopment. The maxillary processes continue to enlarge and approach both medial and lateral nasal processes, with the furrow between the maxillary and nasal processes

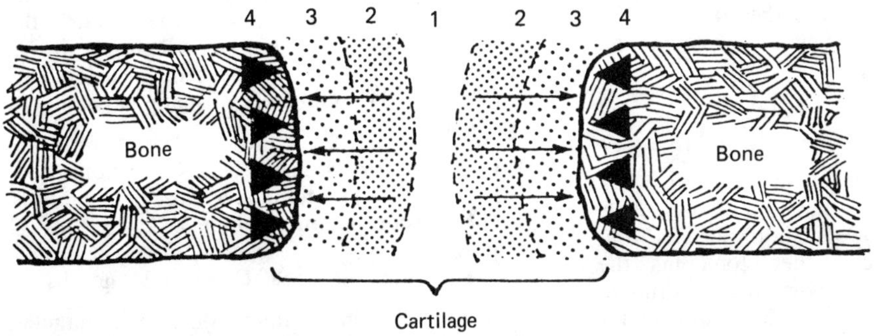

Figure 17.1 The layers of a cranial suture. 1, middle (cellular) zone; 2, capsular zone; 3, cambial zone; 4, edge of cranial bone

deepening to form the naso-optic groove and subsequent nasolacrimal duct. The relative mesial migration of the eyes and nares results from a reduced growth rate in the frontonasal process coupled with increased lateral head expansion. If these differential growth rates are disturbed, orbital hypertelorism (increased spacing between the eyes) may result. Facial clefting may reflect disordered medial and lateral nasal process fusion, mesencymal proliferation superficial to the nasolacrimal canal and lateral maxillary and mandibular process fusion. At this time, there is rapid expansion of the oral cavity, with the external auditory meatus assuming a posterolateral location.

By the eighth week of gestation, the face assumes more human characteristics. Subsequent changes include relative mesial migration of the eyes, formation of the eyelids, continued reduction of the oral opening, formation of the lips, enlargement of the cheeks and definition of the auricle and external auditory meatus. The eyelids fuse at 9–10 fetal weeks and reopen at 25–26 weeks. The nasal bridge develops at 8–12 weeks. From the end of the first trimester until term there is an absolute increase in the size of all body parts. There is, however, a general reduction in head prominence, with a reduction in the forehead/face ratio and a broadening of the middle and lower portions of the face. Craniofacial development is therefore complex, so that it is a marvel that craniofacial anomalies are not more frequent.

Cranial growth

The skull comprises two main components:

(1) The neurocranium (braincase) that includes the desmocranium, formed by intramembranous ossification, and the cranial base, formed predominantly by endochondral ossification.
(2) The viscerocranium (facial skeleton).

The dominance of the neurocranium over the facial skeleton at birth and early childhood reflects early brain development. The accelerated neural growth rate slows after the second year, when the viscerocranium commences its major development.

Neurocranium

Neurocranial ossification begins in the 7–8th week of gestation and continues until childhood. This process begins as discrete ossification centres within the most superficial aspect of the ectomeninx (the outer layer encasing the embryonic brain). Prior to ossification, collagen fibres in the dura mater organize into discrete bundles that prefigure the cranial suture system and adhere to the sutures as they develop. The braincase contours are influenced by this dural fibre system, with premature sutural fusion (craniosynostosis) being a manifestation of disordered dural collagen. A particular form of craniosynostosis, termed Cruzon's syndrome, arises due to prenatal fusion of the superior and posterior sutures of the maxilla along the wall of the orbit. Such premature sutural fusion prevents the maxilla from translating downwards and forwards resulting in midface underdevelopment.

With calverial ossification, syndesmotic articulations develop from the mesenchyme between the ossification centres, while the periosteum develops from the superficial mesenchyme. The non-ossified intrabony articulations, present at birth, are termed sutures when small and fontanelles when large.

During the early stages of development, the margins of the component cranial vault dermal bones grow towards one another through the ectomeninx covering the brain. Two zones can be distinguished in each approaching bone territory:

(1) A cambial zone comprised of fine, radially arranged collagen bundles, numerous osteoprogenitor cells and a layer of osteoblasts.
(2) A woven bone zone produced by the activity of the osteoblastic layer.

Between the approaching bone territories, the fibres of the ectomeninx run at right angles to the advancing plates of woven bone. As the bone margins advance, they split the ectomeninx into outer pericranial and inner dural layers. Just before the cambial layer of the two approaching territories meet, a third capsular layer becomes defined at the leading edge of each territory. The adjacent territories then unite with each other to form the definitive sutures. These layers persist for some time after the bone territories have met, during which time the cells of the cambial layer undergo frequent mitosis and woven bone trabeculae are rapidly formed at the bone edges, the rate of bone formation greatly exceeding that on the non-sutural surfaces. Later, the cambial zones are much reduced in thickness with a reduction in osteoblastic cell layer activity. The cambial layers are progressively reduced during adulthood, with bone uniting the adjacent bony surfaces. The essential growth sites in a suture are therefore the two cambial layers (*see Figure 17.1*).[6] The fontanelles usually close shortly after birth.

(1) The posterior fontanelle closes at 2 months.
(2) The anterolateral fontanelle closes at 3 months.
(3) The posterolateral fontanelle closes at 12 months.
(4) The anterior fontanelle closes at 24 months.

Premature fusion of either sutures or fontanelles is significant, not only for normal brain growth and development, but for the development of the midface and lower face. The sutural system is arranged in the three planes of space.

(1) The coronal plane: the frontoparietal and occipitoparietal sutures.
(2) The sagittal plane: the interparietal and interfrontal sutures.
(3) The transverse plane: the squamoparietal, squamo-occipital, sphenoparietal and sphenofrontal sutures.

The greatest growth increments are generally in the sutures of the coronal plane.

Intracranial hydrostatic pressure appears to be the major stimulus for neurocranial growth (*Figure 17.2*). The expanding cranial volume (due to increasing volume of the brain and associated intracranial fluid) displaces the neurocranial plates outward. The calvarium therefore grows by bone deposition at the sutures in response to increased tension, i.e. sutural growth occurs in response to osseous displacement rather than causes it. Whereas sutural growth predominates up to four years of age, surface apposition and resorption accounts for subsequent neurocranial growth and contour changes. Subsequently, the development of the two cranial vault surfaces diverge.

(1) The inner calvarial table reflects the growth of the intracranial contents, and is generally resorptive in nature.
(2) The outer table is progressively deformed by muscular attachments and is generally depository in nature, apart from the pneumatization of the paranasal sinuses.

In fact the endocranial calvarial surface is principally depository, with such resorption as does occur being limited to areas immediately adjacent to the sutures.[2] Remodelling is not limited to the ecto- and endocranial surfaces but also occurs on the internal surfaces, e.g. those facing the marrow spaces, where the reverse depository and resorptive activities occur.

Overall calvarial morphological developmental changes may be summarized as follows:

(1) By 26–28 weeks of gestation the calvarium has significant ossification of the frontal and parietal bones, although the anterior fontanelle, metopic, coronal and sagittal sutures remain open.
(2) Compared with the second trimester, a 60% increase in calvarial length and 70% increase in width has occurred by birth, with the rate of increase in biparietal width exceeding that of the anterior cranial fossa. Again, the anterior fontanelle remains open, along with the metopic, coronal and sagittal sutures.
(3) By 15–18 months of age the calvarium is 10% longer than that of the neonate, although biparietal width is approximately the same: this reflects delayed growth of the frontal relative to the temporal lobes of the brain. The posterior fontanelle has become closed at this phase and the anterior fontanelle has also begun to ossify. The metopic suture is fused, whereas the coronal and sagittal sutures remain patent.
(4) At 30–36 months of age the parietal eminences are rounding, the anterior fontanelle is completely ossified, the metopic suture obliterated, and the coronal and sagittal sutures are not only narrowing but are becoming more interdigitated.
(5) Subsequently, the calvarium develops a more rectangular configuration, with the adult form being only slightly larger than that of the adolescent.

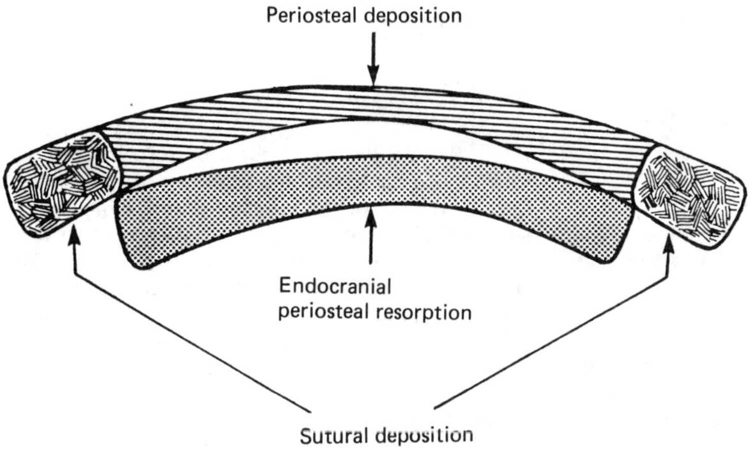

Figure 17.2 Cranial vault remodelling

Thus, although the proportion of the total body mass represented by the head decreases from the fourth month of gestation onwards, at birth the head is still nearly half the total mass. This presents an impediment to the passage through the birth canal. At birth, therefore, there is literal distortion of the head, facilitated by the relatively large unossified fontanelles between the flat calvarial bones. With compression during delivery, the calvarium can increase in length and decrease in width to ease its passage through the birth canal. The relative lack of mandibular prenatal growth also makes delivery easier, since a prominent chin would impede passage through the birth canal.

Birth is, however, still a major physiological problem, associated with a temporary interruption of physical growth for the following 1–2 weeks, as epitomized by the incremental lines in the skeleton and teeth.

Growth and development of component cranial regions

Cranial base

The cranial base consists (in the median plane) of a segment, termed the basicranial axis, stretching from the pituitary region to the anterior border of the foramen magnum; an anterior extension from the pituitary region to the junction of the frontal and nasal bones and a posterior extension from the anterior to posterior border of the foramen magnum. The cranial base interconnects the neuro- and viscerocranium, so that its maldevelopment may be reflected by anomalous viscerocranial development and location and/or disturbed neurocranial growth. The cranial base develops partly by intramembranous ossification and partly by endochondral ossification. The bones of the cranial base are preceded by discrete chondrification centres, which coalesce into a single basal cartilaginous plate, perforated by vascular and neural structures that subsequently become the cranial foramina after the completion of endochondral ossification. Enlargement of the cranial base thus results from proliferative cartilaginous growth between ossified areas (synchondroses) and sutural displacement secondary to increased intracranial volume.

The principal zone of cranial base growth is the spheno-occipital synchondrosis which persists until adulthood. Growth changes at this region are primarily related to nasopharyngeal and maxillary expansion throughout childhood and puberty. Indeed, growth changes in this region are partly responsible for the forwards and downwards displacement of the viscerocranium during development. The ossified basicranial areas increase by surface apposition and resorption, with significant resorption on the endocranial aspect to allow cranial fossa deepening associated with neural development.

Progressive cranial base flexion begins in the embryonic period and continues until adulthood. Such flexion is associated with neurocranial expansion, caudal redirection of the foramen magnum and movement of the face from beneath the anterior cranium. At birth, the cranial base is grossly flattened, whereas by six years of age, both occipital and sphenoid bones are angled with respect to their synchondrosis. Such cranial base flexion may be associated with laryngeal descent and the capacity for speech,[2] upright posture and/or enlarged brain.[7,8]

As growth changes in the cranial base are important to understanding the development of the skull as a whole, it will now be considered from two vantage points.

Extracranial aspect

At birth, the basilar bones are still separated by synchondroses. While the majority of these ossify during childhood, the spheno-occipital synchondrosis remains patent throughout adolescence to form the sole medial cartilaginous growth site. The sphenoethmoidal joint, despite the replacement of cartilage by fibrous tissue, probably remains another growth site until about 6–8 years.

The typical synchondrosis comprises a central reserve zone flanked on either side by zones in which hyaline cartilage proliferate interstitially, undergoes cellular hypertrophy and then degenerates to be replaced by bone. In the two hyaline cartilage regions, the following sequence of events may be identified:

(1) Mitosis of chondrocytes.
(2) Daughter chondrocytes form into regular columns.
(3) Chondrocytic hypertrophy and mineralization, followed by necrosis.
(4) Invasion by osteogenic tissue with true bone formation.
(5) Replacement of this primitive bone by mature organized bone.

Growth at the spheno-occipital synchondrosis is the principal contributor to cranial base enlargement, although substantial contributions may also be made at the midsphenoidal synchrondrosis. The spheno-ethmoidal synchondrosis, when present, is the main site at which the anterior extension increases in length.[9] Further increments are received from bone deposition at the anterior border of the foramen magnum[10] and local remodelling in the region of the pituitary fossa. Growth in length of the posterior extension of the cranial base results from bone resorption on the posterior border of the foramen magnum being greater than bone deposition on its anterior margin.

A further mechanism involved in producing overall cranial enlargement is surface remodelling.[10] At its simplest, the cranial floor consists of two cortical plates separated from each other by cancellous bone, although in some regions other structures intervene (e.g. the paranasal air sinuses in the body of the sphenoid bone). The predominant remodelling pattern consists of bone deposition on the periosteal surface of the ectocranial cortical plate and resorption from the corresponding surface of the endocranial plate. The endosteal surfaces of the plates undergo remodelling activities the converse of those taking place periosteally. In this way, the whole cranial floor is moved relatively downwards. This type of growth, cortical drift, helps to produce the requisite amount of braincase enlargement with less disruption of the spatial relationships of the structures associated with the cranial base than could be achieved by growth solely at the joints. Thus, encircling the endocranial surface of the braincase is a complete circumcranial reversal line of bone growth, below the line the endocranial surface is resorptive and above the line the surface is depository. Extending medially from the reversal line to the midline of the cranial base are reciprocal gradients between the amount of growth taking place due to cortical drift and that due to deposition at the joints. In general, the remodelling processes producing the cortical drift progressively increase as the midline is approached, while growth at the joints diminishes.

A number of regional variations are superimposed upon the overall pattern of cortical drift. For example, the endocranial surfaces of the petrous temporal bone form isolated regions of deposition in the generally resorptive cranial floor so that their relative degree of prominence is maintained. Similarly, the endocranial walls of the sella turcica are areas of bone deposition, although the floor is generally resorptive. Since the endocranial surface of the remainder of the sphenoidal body and wings are resorptive, the sella turcica increases its relative prominence within the cranial cavity. The maxilla moves progressively closer to the foramen magnum as a result of the increasingly acute cranial base angulation at the spheno-occipital synchondrosis. Growth of the cranial base therefore undergoes rapid development in the first three years of life and subsequently slows down.

Intracranial aspect

From late second trimester to adulthood, the intracranial cranial base shows progressive elongation and anterior fossa expansion. By the 26–28th week of gestation, the intracranial base is dominated by the posterior cranial fossa, although occipital ossification is incomplete and the posterolateral fontanelles patent. During the first 18 months of life, the intracranial base increases 25% in anteroposterior length, 20% on maximum width and 15% in interpterion width. Between 15 and 30 months of age, there is a 25% increase in anterior clinoid to frontal bone length, whereas no significant change occurs in the anterior clinoid to posterior skull length. By four years of age, the intracranial base assumes adult characteristics, with marked anterior and middle cranial fossa development. Compared with the morphology at birth, there has been a 50% increase in total skull length, 40% resulting from anterior fossa elongation. By contrast, there has been a 35% increase in skull width and 30% increase in interpterion width. The dimensions of the intracranial base increase slightly throughout childhood and adolescence, without significant shape change. Compared with the neonate, however, the adult intracranial base lengthens 40%, with a 25% increase in maximum width, primarily reflecting significant postnatal expansion of the anterior cranial fossa.

Mid-face

Growth of the mid-face embraces orbital, nasal, paranasal and maxillary development. Whereas orbital expansion occurs predominantly before birth, following the neural growth pattern, growth of the maxilla,, nasal and paranasal cavities follows the somatic growth pattern. Most of the bones of the mid-face are of dermal origin with intervening sutures.

Sutural growth

The facial sutures provide a group of principal growth sites within the upper facial skeleton in the three planes of space.[11]

(1) *The circummaxillary group:* between the maxilla and the frontal, nasal, lacrimal, ethmoid, palatine, vomer and zygomatic bones in addition to the pterygoid processes of the sphenoid.
(2) *The craniofacial group:* separating the nasal, lacrimal, facial part of the ethmoid, palatine, vomer and zygomatic bones from the frontal, perpendicular plate of the ethmoid, temporal and sphenoid bones.
(3) *The sagittal group:* comprising the medial palatal, internasal and intermaxillary sutures and the mandibular symphysis.

Growth at the first two groups contribute to anteroposterior and vertical craniofacial enlargement, with increase in facial width occurring at the sagittal group.

Nasal region

In the nasal region, there is an extensive area of cartilage, representing the original nasal capsule, which plays an important role in facial growth.[12,13] The vomer ossifies in the mucoperichondrium from two centres that develop about the eighth week of gestation. The centres extend and unite beneath the lower margin of the cartilage to form the vomerine groove into which the inferior margin of the cartilage is received. The ossification centre for the mesoethmoid appears about the time of birth in the midline of the cartilage of the prechordal part of the cranial base and extends into the septal cartilage to form the perpendicular ethmoid plate. The mesoethmoid remains separated from the vomer by the sphenoidal tail of the septal cartilage for the first two years of life. During the third year, ossification extends into the sphenoidal tail with the formation of the definitive septovomerine joint. As a result, the piriform aperture relocates from between the orbits to below them, primarily as a result of the increased size of the nasal cavity. Lateral nasal cavity expansion has little effect on the superior portion of the osseous nose, whereas the nasal bridge widens, resulting in the more vertical configuration of the orbital rim.

The anterior walls of the nasal cavity are formed by the frontal processes of the maxillae. The external (cutaneous) periosteal surfaces of these processes are depository, whereas the internal mucosal surfaces are resorptive. The nasal bones undergo similar remodelling changes. The result is a widening of the anterior nasal aperture and an increasing protrusion of the nasal bridge. Within the nasal cavity, the mucosal surfaces of the lateral walls are generally resorptive, with bone deposition occurring on the opposing periosteal surfaces of the medial orbital walls and medial walls of the maxillary sinuses. The height of the nasal cavity is increased by resorption from the upper surface of the palate.

Facial development

By 26–28 weeks gestation, the anterolateral and posterolateral fontanelles are patent, together with the coronal, squamosal, lambdoid, occipitomastoid, temporosphenoidal, frontosphenoidal, zygomatico-frontal, zygomaticosphenoidal and zygomatico-temporal sutures. At this stage, the mid-face lies beneath the cranial base.

By birth, cranial length has increased by 50%, and 30% in height, although the mid-face still lies beneath the cranial base. With advancing age, the facial skeleton gradually moves forwards and downwards, possibly reflecting continued cartilaginous nasal septal growth.[14]

The growth increments at the sutures and nasal septum are associated with extensive remodelling of the external and internal surfaces of the bones of the facial skeleton.[10] A large area over the anterior external surface of the facial skeleton is resorptive in nature. The buccal surface of the root of the maxillary zygomatic processes is resorptive. Whereas the lingual periosteal surface of the maxillary arch is entirely depository, the posterior region of the maxillary tuberosity is a site of rapid bone deposition. If the maxillary arch is viewed from below, then there is bone deposition on the inner aspect and bone resorption on the outer aspect. These changes are associated with complementary remodelling changes on the internal endosteal surfaces and the surfaces lining the tooth sockets. In coronal section, the palate and upper arch may be described by another V-shape, except the V is inverted and truncated. The outer aspect of this V, formed by the floor of the nasal cavity and paranasal sinuses and the buccal periosteal surfaces of the dental arch, is resorptive, while the inner aspect (the downward-facing periosteal surface of the palate) is depository. Thus, there are two overlapping V-shaped systems in the midface: the dental arch, where the V is horizontal, and the palate, where the V is coronal. Together, these contribute to growth in dental arch length, width and height, and nasal cavity height. Growth of the vertically orientated V reduces the downward facial growth contributed by increments at the sutures and nasal septum, while growth in the horizontally orientated V reduces the forward growth component produced at these sites. As a result, the downward growth of the facial skeleton is accentuated but its forward growth is reduced.

Within the body of the maxilla, the paranasal sinuses are enlarged by resorption from the internal surfaces of their floors and walls, except medially where deposition takes place, complementing the resorption on the opposing inner-facing surfaces of the lateral walls of the nasal cavity.

The maxillary zygomatic process has a cutaneous, anterolaterally facing surface which is an area of bone resorption, as opposed to the temporal surface which undergoes deposition. The net result is that the zygomatic process is moved posteriorly relative to the body of the maxilla.

Detailed growth changes in the mid-face have been studied by the use of implants and serial cephalographs.[15,16] These have shown that the maxilla undergoes a small and variable degree of rotation during growth. At the same time, there are varying degrees of bone resorption on the nasal aspect of the maxilla and apposition on the palatal aspect (*Figures 17.3, 17.4*). In most patients, the net effect is little change in upper jaw orientation during growth, i.e. the palatal plane remains stable.[17] In individuals with a short face (short anterior face

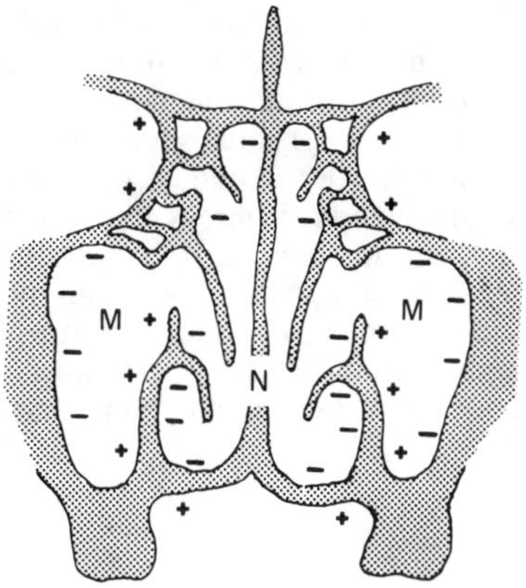

Figure 17.3 Growth changes in the nasal cavity (N) and maxillary sinus (M). In this coronal section through the facial skeleton, (+) indicates net bone deposition and (−) net bone resorption.

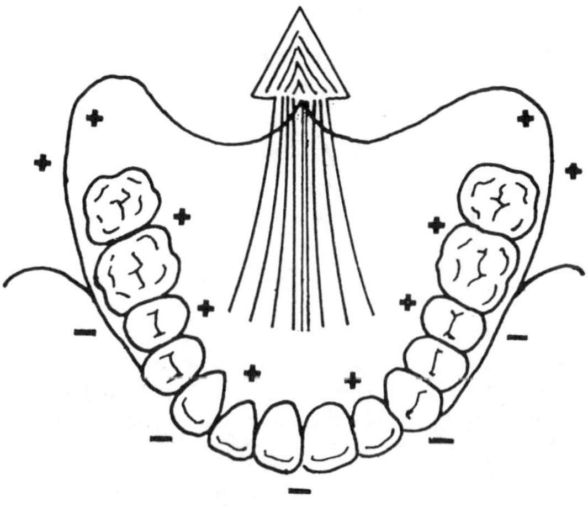

Figure 17.4 Remodelling in the maxillary arch viewed from the mouth; (+) indicates net bone deposition and (−) net bone resorption.

height), however, there is excessive forward rotation of the mandible during growth, resulting in a square mandibular outline, deep bite occlusion and crowded lower incisors. In long face individuals (excessive anterior face height), on the otherhand, the palatal plane rotates downwards and posteriorly, the net result often being an anterior open bite occlusion associated with mandibular deficiency.

This rotational maxillary movement influences the tooth eruption paths. The path of maxillary tooth eruption is downwards and somewhat forwards. In normal growth, the maxilla may rotate a few degrees forward but frequently rotates slightly backward. The forward rotation would tend to tip the incisors forwards, increasing their prominence, while backward rotation directs the anterior teeth more posteriorly than would have been the case without the rotation, relatively uprighting them and decreasing their prominence. Thus craniofacial growth changes are intimately associated with those of the dentition.

The face is generally vertically orientated, with three processes being involved:

(1) Retention of a small anterior basicranial angle into adult life.
(2) Resorption from the anterior surface of the facial skeleton.
(3) Limited forward growth component at the sutures and nasal septum.

It is assumed that the limited anterior facial growth is related to the general hominid evolutionary trend towards head balance on the vertebral column, a component adaptation to the upright posture and bipedal locomotion.[18]

Mandible

In order to achieve the correct occlusal relationships between the upper and lower teeth, the growth rates of the maxilla and mandible must be highly correlated (*Figure 17.5*). Both adhere to the somatic growth pattern with an adolescent growth spurt. The mandible, however, lacks the complex sutural and endochondral systems which are so important to mid-face growth. The mandible articulates with the glenoid fossa of the temporal bone via the

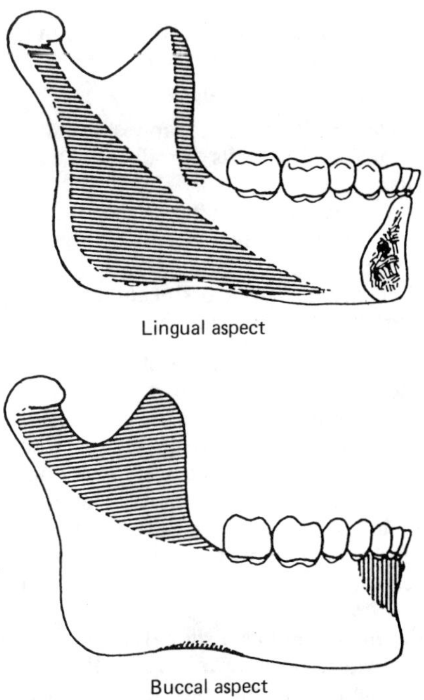

Figure 17.5 Mandibular growth changes with bone resorption predominating in the shaded areas.

temporomandibular joint. Thus, the location of the mandible relative to the skull is partly dependent upon mid-face and cranial base growth changes. Mandibular arch widening therefore cannot significantly exceed the bicondylar width, which in turn is dependent on the width of the glenoid fossae and lateral expansion of the cranial base. Whereas the mandibular condyle was considered the primary feature of mandibular growth, more recent evidence has identified a number of other variables, including depository–resorptive activity on the mandibular body and ramus, with endochondral ossification in the condylar region allowing for multidirectional growth and remodelling capacity in response to compressive forces.

During mandibular development, several secondary cartilages appear. The principal mandibular secondary cartilages are found in the coronoid, angular and condylar processes. The coronoid and angular cartilages are active growth centres during the early stages of development but have disappeared at or shortly after birth.[19] By contrast, the condylar cartilage persists throughout the growth period and even beyond. The fact that other secondary cartilages develop in close proximity to dermal bones suggests that chondrogenic and osteogenic cells arise from the same undifferentiated cell pool.[20]

Damage to the condyle during childhood leads to a severe reduction in mandibular growth, while condylar hyperplasia is associated with an enlarged mandible.[21,22] There are, however, differences between growth changes at the condylar head of the mandible and primary cartilaginous sites, e.g. epiphyseal cartilages of long bones.

(1) The condylar head grows by apposition to its superior surface of cells produced in the intermediate layer.
(2) The chondrocytes in the condylar head do not divide or form into columns and emerge still viable at the ossification face.
(3) Removal of cartilage at the ossification face may result from chondroclastic activities.

In general, the condyle projects posterosuperiorly from the mandible, so that bone increments at the cartilage increase both the vertical height of the ramus and the anteroposterior depth of the whole bone: the actual proportion of each depends upon the condylar orientation on the mandible. In fact, as the condylar head projects laterally as well as posterosuperiorly, increments at the condylar cartilages also increase the bilateral mandibular width (*Figures 17.6–17.9*).

Initially, the mandible has a short ramus relative to a long body whereas, by term, the height of the body has increased, reflecting the development of the primary tooth buds. At this stage, the mandibular symphysis is still patent but both sides fuse within the first two years of life. Subsequently, the mandibular body increases in size to accommodate the eruption of both deciduous and permanent dentitions. A number of studies have shown that the posterior ramal border is one of the sites of most rapid bone deposition, whereas the anterior ramal border (coronoid process) is predominantly resorptive.[15] As a result, a powerful posteriorly directed component is added to the intrinsic growth of the mandible, yet the anteroposterior dimensions of the body and ramus maintain their relative

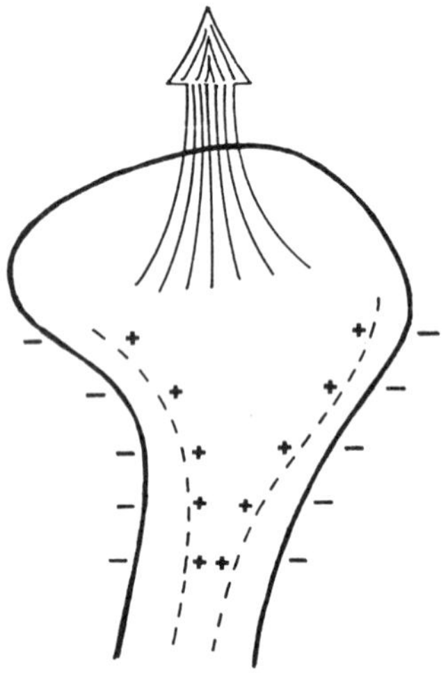

Figure 17.6 Growth changes in the mandibular condylar region. Arrow indicates direction of condylar cartilaginous growth changes, with net bone deposition (+) and net bone resorption (−) on the buccal and lingual cortical plates.

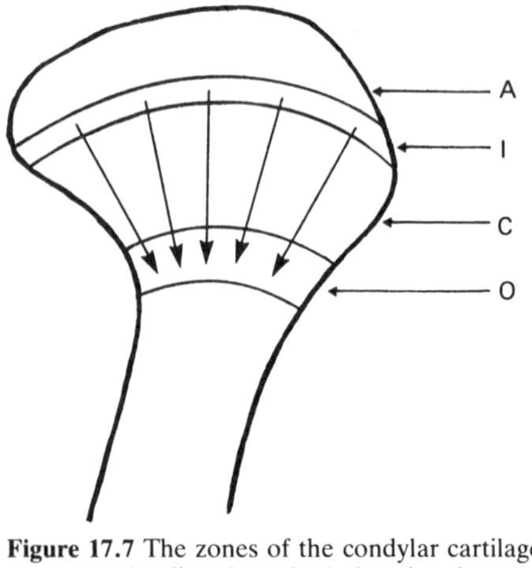

Figure 17.7 The zones of the condylar cartilage. Arrows represent the direction of relative chondrocyte movement in the intermediate zone. A, articular fibrocartilage; I, intermediate zone; C, condylar cartilage; O, zone of ossification

proportions. In fact, the mandibular ramus undergoes complex remodelling changes in addition to those occurring on the anterior and posterior borders.[23] The buccal periosteal surface of the coronoid process and the adjacent area extending below the sigmoid notch on to the lateral surface of the condylar process is resorptive, while the lingual periosteal surface of the process, posterior to the temporal crest, is depository. Since the lingual surface faces upwards and inwards, and the buccal surfaces downwards and outwards, these remodelling changes result in the two coronoid processes growing upwards, with their apices moving apart.

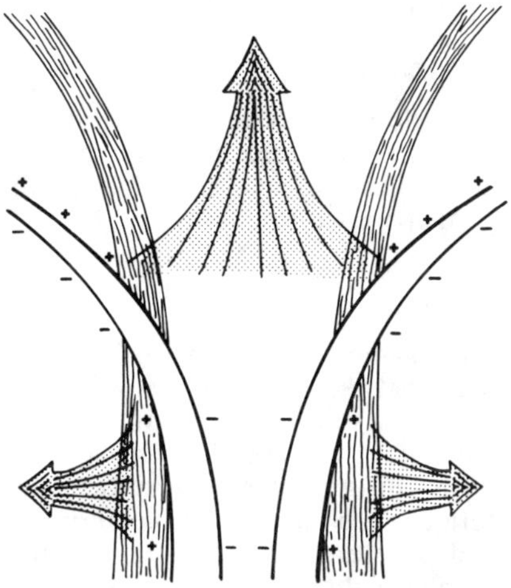

Figure 17.8 Bone growth. Differential patterns of net bone appositon (+) and resorption (−) lead to changes in overall form.

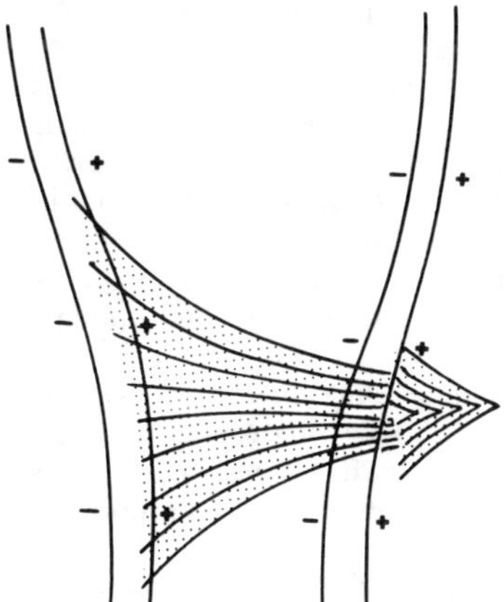

Figure 17.9 Bone growth. Differential patterns of net bone appositon (+) and resorption (−) lead to shifts in local bone contours.

The lingual surface of the coronoid process faces upwards, inwards and posteriorly, so that additions on this surface, coupled with resorption on the buccal and anterior surfaces, result in the coronoid process moving posteriorly with concomitant elongation of the mandibular corpus. As the ramus grows by bone deposition along the posterior border, the regions that previously lay at its border become progressively incorporated into the ramus. In other words, growth of the mandible, like that of the mid-face, is a complex process, requiring detailed mechanisms for control.

During postnatal development, growth in mandibular width is completed first, followed by growth in length and then growth in height. In fact, growth in width of both jaws, including the width of the dental arches, tends to be completed before the adolescent growth spurt. As the jaws (both maxilla and mandible) grow in length posteriorly with permanent tooth eruption, both molar and bicondylar widths show small increases, with the anterior width dimensions stabilizing earlier. Growth in mandibular length, however, continues through puberty, being completed by 14–15 years in girls (2–3 years after first menstruation) and 18 years in boys (4 years after sexual maturity). Growth changes in mandibular height and concomitant tooth eruption continues to 17–18 years in girls and 20–25 years in males.

With the use of metallic implants,[16] serial radiographic analyses have indicated that rather complex growth changes occur in the mandible. Rather than comprising a single bone, the mandible may in fact be considered to comprise:

(1) The alveolar processes, whose growth and development are dependent upon tooth function.
(2) The coronoid processes and mandibular angle, whose growth and development are dependent on the activity of the muscles of mastication.
(3) The condylar process, whose growth and development is associated with the glenoid fossa.
(4) The mandibular core, whose growth and development may be associated with the inferior alveolar nerve.

In the core area (body) of the mandible, growth changes include rotation, which comprises upward movement anteriorly and downward movement posteriorly. In fact, this rotation may involve two mechanisms: rotation around the condyle and rotation around the mandibular body.[16]

Between four years of age and adulthood, the mandible may rotate up to 15°, 25% of which occurs at the condyle and 75% within the mandibular body. During the time the mandibular body rotates forwards an average 15°, the mandibular plane angle (representing the orientation of the jaw viewed from the outside) decreases approximately 2–4°. In other words, mandibular rotation is masked to a certain extent by surface deposition and resorption. Thus, the posterior part of the lower border of the mandible must be an area of resorption, while the anterior aspect of the lower border is either unchanged or undergoes slight apposition. The postnatal mandibular growth changes are therefore far more complex than traditionally envisaged, although much more data are required for a complete definition of mandibular variability.

Factors influencing craniofacial development

Craniofacial development is characterized by the occlusal relationships between the maxillary and mandibular teeth. Epidemiological studies, however, indicate that the prevalence of malocclusion is much greater in modern times compared with 1000 years ago.[24] For instance, tooth crowding and malalignment was unusual until recently, although mild jaw discrepancies may have been common in some primitive populations. Skeletal studies have also suggested that in some isolated populations there may have been prevalence for prognathic mandibles (e.g. in South Pacific Islanders)[25] or mild buccal (molar) cross-bites (e.g. in Australian aborigines).[26] There is also evidence for a reduction in tooth size, tooth number and jaw size during evolution, although changes occurring over the past 1000 years cannot be considered evolutionary in nature. Certainly, a progressive reduction in jaw size, if not well matched with a decrease in tooth size and number, could contribute to tooth crowding and malalignment. Such gradual changes could not have accounted for the sudden increase in dental malocclusions and overcrowding within the past 1000 years.

Conceivably, the present marked prevalence in tooth malalignment may reflect a more marked reduction in jaw size in modern times as a result of a reduction in dietary consistency,[27] although other factors may also be involved.

As previously stated, the jaws can be considered to comprise a core of bone to which the functional processes are attached. The functional processes will be altered if the function is lost or changes. For instance:

(1) Alveolar bone exists only to support the teeth. If a tooth fails to erupt, then the alveolar bone will not form in that area, whereas if a tooth is extracted, there will be alveolar bone resorption in the area.
(2) The muscular processes, e.g. the coronoid process, primarily function for muscle attachment. Increased masticatory activity with a coarse diet will therefore be associated with increased mass of such muscular processes and vice versa.

Craniofacial development and growth is also influenced by a number of functional patterns and habits.

Sucking habits

As a general rule, sucking habits during the primary dentition years have little, if any, long-term effects. If these habits persist beyond the time that the permanent teeth begin to erupt, however, malocclusion is likely, characterized by the following:

(1) Flared and spaced maxillary incisors.
(2) Lingually positioned lower incisors.
(3) Anterior open bite.
(4) Narrow upper arch.

This characteristic malocclusion associated with sucking arises from direct pressure on the teeth by persistent thumb pressure and alteration in the resting cheek and lip pressure patterns.

Tongue thrusting

Individuals with an anterior open bite malocclusion place their tongue between their incisors when they swallow, while those who have a normal incisor relationship do not. The general consensus now holds that tongue thrusting does not in fact cause such an anterior open bite[28] but comprises a physiological adaptive mechanism to seal the front of the mouth during deglutition.

Mouth breathing

Because respiratory needs are the primary determinant of jaw and tongue posture, and to a lesser extent that of the head, it is reasonable to suppose that mouth breathing could result in different head, jaw and tongue postures. Such postural changes might affect the equilibrium that governs jaw growth and tooth position. To breathe through the mouth, as opposed to through the nose, three postural changes are required: lowering the mandible; positioning of the tongue downwards and forwards, and extending the head.

Such postural changes may indeed be associated with the so-called long face syndrome, comprising downwards and backwards mandibular growth rotation, excessive posterior tooth eruption, a tendency for maxillary constriction, excessive overjet and anterior open bite.[29,30,31] More recent studies suggest that other factors may also be involved, although mouth breathing may be a contributory factor.

Such complex functional changes that may affect craniofacial development complicate evaluation of the genetic and environmental contributions.

Genetic versus environmental factors

Craniofacial maldevelopment could be produced by inherited (genetic) characteristics. For instance: there may be an inherited disproportion between tooth size and jaw size resulting in crowding or spacing; there may be an inherited disproportion between the size and shape of the upper and lower jaws resulting in improper occlusal relationships.

Primitive populations, in which malocclusion is less frequent than in modern groups, are characterized by genetic isolation and uniformity. If everyone in a group carried the same genetic information for tooth and jaw size, there would be no possibility of an offspring developing a malocclusion. Genetic factors that introduced disturbances into the masticatory system would tend to be eliminated, since malocclusions associated with a primitive diet might result in death due to malnutrition.

One of the characteristics of modern Western civilization is large population migrations into urban centres, with associated increased opportunities for intermarriage. More recent research based on Hawaiian populations[32] and twins,[33] however, suggests that only a proportion of malocclusion traits can be attributed to hereditary factors. Also, although tooth crowding is undoubtedly related in part to the continued reduction in jaw size during human evolution, it seems unlikely that there are specific genes for dental occlusion. Thus, although genetic influences are obviously important for masticatory development, environmental factors must also play a role. There is, however, no theoretical explanation of how a coarser diet and more powerful masticatory function could significantly alter dental arch size.

Cross-bites and individual tooth malalignments appear to arise from the interaction between the initial position of the tooth buds and the pressure environment that guides their eruptive path. Certainly, forces from the lips, cheeks, tongue and fingers can influence the vertical and horizontal tooth positions. Minor malalignments may therefore be primarily of functional origin, whereas major problems may have additional genetic or developmental components.

Jaw malpositions or malformations may therefore reflect a variety of factors, including: inherited patterns; defects in embryonic development; trauma and functional influences. The fact that ideal occlusion does not occur in all primitive populations suggests that variations are compatible with normal function. Conceivably, with a modern diet, greater variations in jaw morphology and location can be tolerated, whereas they were previously incompatible with long-term survival and reproductive success in more primitive societies. Recent research therefore indicates that genetic factors may be more important than traditionally envisaged, although the role of both genetic and environmental interactions on craniofacial growth and development have yet to be apportioned.

Control of skull growth

This brings us to consider the various mechanisms that control skull growth.

Role of growth sites

Because of their structural similarity to the postcranial epiphyseal cartilages, the view is frequently expressed that the primary cartilaginous growth sites of the skull play a major role in determining the enlargement of the cranial base and mid-face.[34,35] There is, however, clinical evidence that the septal cartilage of the nasal cavity is not indispensable for facial growth.[36,37]

Sutures

There is general agreement that sutures respond to growth changes in the calvarium, rather than providing the motive force for calvarial growth.[38]

Condylar cartilage

Although growth changes have been noted at the condylar cartilage, the general consensus holds that this is a responsive rather than motive change.[39]

Functional matrix theory

The head may be composed of a number of distinct regions, termed functional components, each responsible for a particular function or set of functions. Each component may itself be composed of a functional matrix, made up of the structures performing the function, and a skeletal unit which supports and protects the functional matrix. In fact, two types of functional matrix may exist.

(1) Capsular matrices in the form of the soft tissues surrounding the brain and around functional spaces, e.g. the mouth, pharynx.
(2) Periosteal matrices, e.g. skeletal muscle, which is attached to its skeletal unit through the periosteum.

The essential part of this functional matrix theory[40] is the notion that the growth and function of the functional matrix play a major determining role in the differentiation, development and growth of the associated skeletal unit. Certainly soft tissues, especially skeletal muscles, affect craniofacial growth and morphology. There is, however, no general agreement that the response to soft tissues is as dominating as proponents of functional cranial analysis believe. The mechanisms by which mechanical stresses in the soft tissues might affect bone remain obscure.

Conclusions

Rather than comprising a single bone, the craniofacial skeleton comprises a number of component regions, not only exhibiting different growth rates, but also influencing the growth of other regions. There cannot therefore be one mechanism for the control of skull growth and development: this indicates the need for further research in attempting to define the obvious multifactorial controlling factor(s).

Review questions

1. What is the role for sutures in craniofacial growth?
2. What factors favour the functional matrix theory for the control of skull growth?
3. Describe the changes that occur during the development of the cranial base.
4. Contrast the growth patterns of the neurocranium and mandible.
5. Briefly list the growth changes that occur in the mid-facial region.

References

1. MOORE, W.J. and LAVELLE, C.L.B. (1975) *Growth of the Facial Skeleton in the Hominoidea*. New York: Academic Press
2. ENLOW, D.H. (1982) *Handbook of Facial Growth*. Philadephia: W.B. Saunders
3. BERGSMA, D. (1975) *Morphogenesis and Malformation of Face and Brain*. New York: Alan R Liss
4. BOSMA, J.F. (1976) *Symposium on Development of the Basicranium*. Bethesda, Md.: US Department of Health, Education and Welfare
5. JOHNSTON, M.C. and LISTGARTEN, M.A. (1972) The migration, interaction and early differentiation of orofacial tissues. In *Development Aspects of Oral Biology*, edited by H.S. Slavkin and L.A. Bavetta. New York: Academic Press
6. PRITCHARD, J.J., SCOTT, J.H. and GIRGIS, F.G. (1956) The structure and development of cranial and facial sutures. *J. Anat.*, **90**, 73–86
7. ZUCKERMAN, S. (1955) Age changes in the basicranial axis of the human skull. *Am. J. Phys. Anthropol.*, **13**, 521–539
8. FORD, E.H.R. (1958) Growth of the human cranial base. *J. Anat.*, **90**, 63–72
9. BAER, M.J. (1954) Patterns of growth of the skull as revealed by vital staining. *Hum. Biol.*, **26**, 80–126
10. ENLOW, D.H. (1968) *The Human Face*. New York: Harper & Row
11. SCOTT, J.H. (1956) Growth at the facial sutures. *Am. J. Orthodont.*, **42**, 381–387
12. SCOTT, J.H. (1953) The cartilage of the nasal septum (a contribution to the study of facial growth). *Br. Dent. J.*, **95**, 37–43
13. LATHAM, R.A. (1970) Maxillary development and growth: the septo-premaxillary ligament. *J. Anat.*, **107**, 471–478
14. MCNAMARA, J.A., RIOLO, M.L. and ENLOW, D.H. (1976) Growth of the maxillary complex in the rhesus monkey. *Am. J. Phys. Anthropol.*, **42**, 15–24
15. BJORK, A. (1968) The use of metallic implants in the study of facial growth in children: method and application. *Am. J. Phys. Anthropol.*, **29**, 243–254
16. BJORK, A. (1955) Cranial base development. *Am. J. Orthod.*, **41**, 298–325
17. BJORK, A. and SKIELLER, V. (1983) Normal and abnormal growth of the mandible: a synthesis of longitudinal cephalometric implant studies over a period of 25 years. *Eur. J. Orthod.*, **5**, 1–46
18. BJORK, A. and SKIELLER, V. (1976) Postnatal growth and development of the maxillary complex. In *Factors Affecting Growth of the Midface*, edited by J. McNamara. Ann Arbor: Centre for Human Growth and Development
19. SYMONS, N.B.B. (1952) The development of the human mandibular joint. *J. Anat.*, **86**, 326–332
20. HALL, B.K. (1970) Cellular differentiation in skeletal tissues. *Biol. Rev.*, **45**, 455–484
21. SARNAT, B.G. and ENGLE, M.B. (1951) A serial study of mandibular growth after removal of the condyle in the macaca rhesus monkey. *Plast. Reconstr. Surg.*, **7**, 364–380
22. RUSHTON, M.A. (1944) Growth at the mandibular condyle in relation to some deformities. *Br. Dent. J.*, **76**, 57–68
23. JOHNSTON, P.A., ATKINSON, P.J. and MOORE, W.J. (1976) The development and structure of the chimpanzee mandible. *J. Anat.*, **122**, 467–477
24. WOLPOFF, W.H. (1980) *Paleoanthropology*. New York: Alfred A. Knopf
25. BAUME, L.J. (1974) Uniform methods for the epidemiologic assessment of malocclusion. *Am. J. Orthod.*, **66**, 251–272
26. CAMPBELL, T.D. and BARRETT, M.J. (1953) Dental observations on Australian aborigines. *Aust. Dent. J.*, **57**, 1–6
27. CORRUCINI, R.S. (1983) Epidemiological survey of occlusion in North India. *Br. J. Orthod.*, **10**, 44–47
28. PROFFIT, W.R. and MASON, R.M. (1975) Myofunctional therapy for tongue-thrusting: background and recommendations. *J. Am. Dent. Assoc.*, **90**, 403–411
29. VIG, P.S., SHOWFETY, K.J. and PHILLIPS, C. (1980)

Experimental manipulation of head posture. *Am. J. Orthod.*, **77**, 258–268
30. HARVOLD, E.P. (1981) Primate experiments on oral respiration. *Am. J. Orthod.*, **79**, 359–372
31. WARREN, D.W. (1984) A quantitative technique for assessing nasal airway impairment. *Am. J. Orthodont.*, **86**, 306–314
32. CHUNG, C.S. (1971) Genetic and epidemiologic studies of oral characteristics in Hawaii's school children. *Am. J. Hum. Genet.*, **23**, 471–495
33. LUNDSTROM, A. (1984) Nature vs nurture in dentofacial variation. *Eur. J. Orthod.*, **6**, 77–91
34. BAUME, L.J. (1968) Patterns of cephalofacial growth and development. A comparative study of the basicranial growth centres in rat and man. *Int. Dent. J. (Lond.)*, **18**, 489–513
35. SCOTT, J.H. (1958) The cranial base. *Am. J. Phys. Anthropol.*, **16**, 319–348
36. LATHAM, R.A. (1968) A new concept of the early maxillary growth mechanism. *Eur. Orthod. Soc.*, **44**, 53–63
37. MOSS, M.L. and RANKOW, R.M. (1968) The role of the functional matrix in mandibular growth. *Angle Orthod.*, **38**, 95–103
38. ZOLLER, R.M. and LASKIN, D.M. (1969) Growth of the zygomaticomaxillary suture in pigs after sectioning the zygomatic arch. *J. Dent. Res.*, **48**, 573–578
39. GIANELLY, A.A. and MOORREES, C.F.A. (1965) Condylectomy in the rat. *Arch. Oral Biol.*, **10**, 101–106
40. MOSS, M.L. and SALENTIJN, L. (1969) The primary role of functional matrices in facial growth. *Am. J. Orthod.*, **55**, 566–577

18

Craniofacial morphogenesis

Introduction

A quarter of a million babies (approximately 7% of all live births in the United States) have some mental or physical defect. These are usually either present at birth or become apparent sometime after birth. Craniofacial malformations are common among these defects, which may include structural, functional or biochemical abnormalities. Cleft lip and/or cleft palate is the most prevalent of such defects, affecting approximately 1:600 white infants. The incidence of cleft palate and/or cleft lip is higher among orientals, native Americans and Eskimos, but lower among blacks. Other craniofacial malformations include the following:

(1) Jaw deformities.
(2) Dental anomalies.
(3) Defects in cranial or facial ossification.
(4) Excessive spacing or narrowing between the eyes.
(5) Facial asymmetries, e.g. disproportionate facies.
(6) Craniofacial defects comprising parts of certain syndromes, e.g. fetal alcohol syndrome.

Causes of craniofacial deformity

Congenital malformations now loom large as significant causes of infant mortality and morbidity. This reflects, in part, the better control of infections and other conditions that have traditionally taken their toll among the newborn. A high percentage of malformations is also observed among embryos or fetuses lost in the first trimester, or in later miscarriages and stillbirths. In the case of malformations restricted to the craniofacial area, a small proportion can be traced to specific genetic or chromosomal disorders. A slightly larger proportion may result from potent environmental factors, e.g. malnutrition, maternal disease, radiation exposure, alcohol or other drugs, and problems in pregnancy and delivery. The majority are multifactorial in origin, however, centring on interactive processes in which particular genes alter the ability of the developing fetus to adapt to environmental factors.

The effects of craniofacial abnormalities may be profound for the patient, for the family and for society. The disability or disfigurement often entails immediate and long-term exposure to surgical, medical and auxiliary support services. The complications of craniofacial malformations may be severe, since vision, eating, hearing, breathing and speaking depend, in part, on an intact craniofacial skeleton.

Dentofacial malrelations (i.e. discrepancies between tooth and dental arch form) occur more frequently, are often not so severe, and are often responsive to orthodontic treatment and/or orthognathic surgery. Sometimes dentofacial malrelations cause no major eating or breathing disturbances and may go uncorrected. Dentofacial malrelations, however, may affect chewing, swallowing, breathing and speech. They may also impair oral hygiene practices or predispose to oral habits that lead to muscle fatigue, pain and other symptoms. Dentofacial malrelations may also diminish self-image and discourage social integration.' Genetic factors obviously contribute to the shaping of the face and oral structures. Environmental factors are also known to be significant and operate *in utero* and after birth. Deficient nutrition, teratogens and other prenatal exogenous factors may also lead to dentofacial anomalies. Postnatal diet may influence dentofacial development through functional and nutritional means. Other factors include facial trauma, abnormal breathing patterns and postural or oral habits, e.g. thumb-sucking.

Recently, increasing evidence suggests that such abnormalities may, in fact, be primarily determined in the initial stages of craniofacial development.

Craniofacial mesenchyme

In addition to providing sensory and autonomic ganglia, the neural crest contributes connective tissue elements to craniofacial development. Specifically, the connective tissue of the following regions are known to be derived from the neural crest:

(1) Dermis of the face.
(2) Lower jaw.
(3) Tongue.
(4) Thymus.
(5) Thyroid gland.
(6) Parathyroid glands.[1]

Thus, failure of sufficient quantities of cephalic neural crest cells to translocate and interact with developing organs may lead to abnormal development of the heart, thymus, parathyroids, palate, ears and other structures originating in the cephalic part of the embryo. These defects may occur singly or may be multiple (the latter often being denoted as specific syndromes). Many craniofacial malformations found in association with heart defects may reflect a common neural crest cell deficiency.

Timing of craniofacial deformity

The developmental mechanisms leading to craniofacial skeletogenesis begin prior to the early stages at which these structures are morphologically visible. At such early stages, the tissues from which all skeletal elements will emerge are entirely mesenchymal.[2] They comprise the following:

(1) A population of stellate-shaped cells which contact one another via their cytoplasmic processes.
(2) An extracellular matrix comprising collagens, glycosaminoglycans and glycoproteins.[3,4]

Most of this mesenchyme is formed from the epiblast at the primitive streak during the gastrulation phase of embryonic development. Following a period of dispersion and proliferation, this mesodermal mesenchyme becomes epithelial, forming segmental somites, the mesomere and lateral plate tissues. Subsequently, most of these epithelial compartments become transformed again on to mesenchymal populations, some of which will form the axial and appendicular musculoskeletal tissues. In the head region, the metameric pattern of paraxial mesoderm condensation is less well defined. Definitive somites can be seen as far rostrally as the otic region, the most cranial component contributing to the unsegmented occipital complex and hypoglossal musculature. Rostral to the first somite, the paraxial mesoderm forms seven completely segregated clusters (somitomeres), which contribute to the sphenoid and otic skeletal complexes and the extrinsic ocular musculature.[5,6]

There is also a second, and most important, source of mesenchyme, the neural crest. The neural crest tissue (*Figure 18.1*) is derived from the neural fold ectoderm during the process of neurulation.

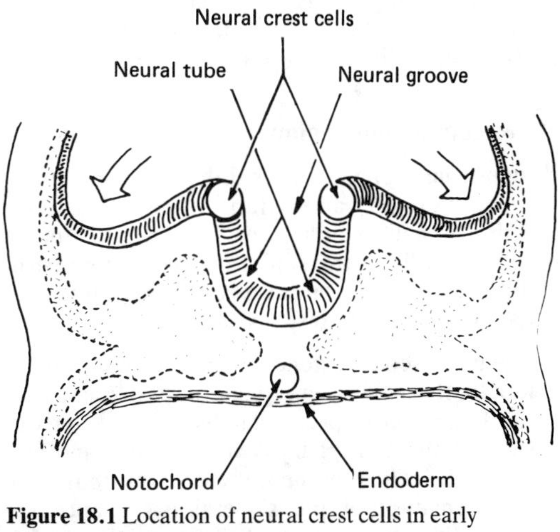

Figure 18.1 Location of neural crest cells in early neurogenesis.

The neural crest is the thickened ectoderm around the edge of the embryonic neural plate. As the neural plate closes to form the neural tube, the neural crest cells are released from their position in the neural fold.[7] Although the neural fold comprises three different cell types, only the cells which emigrate are termed neural crest cells. The mechanism for the release of the neural crest cells from the neural fold is obscure. However, the basement membrane underlying the neural crest cells breaks down and the neural crest cells extend their cytoplasmic processes and actively migrate away from the neural fold.[7] Once the neural crest cells are free from the neural fold, they actively migrate away, or are passively translocated, to their final destination.[1]

The neural crest

The neural crest may be divided into two regions: the cranial neural crest and the trunk neural crest.[8]

The *trunk neural crest* cells primarily contribute to the following:

(1) Dorsal root ganglia.
(2) Sympathetic ganglia.
(3) Schwann and satellite cells.
(4) Adrenal medulla.
(5) Melanocytes.

The *cranial neural crest* forms many mesenchymal derivatives, in addition to nervous elements and melanocytes.[9] In contrast to the trunk neural crest cells, the majority of the cephalic neural crest cells remain superficial, dispersing between the surface ectoderm and either paraxial mesoderm or the prosencephalon, depending on their level of origin. Subsequently, most of these cells become located beside and beneath the pharynx and forebrain.[10] Such cellular migrations are facilitated by, and dependent upon, the appearance of hyaluronate-rich, fibronectin-lined extracellular pathways.[11]

Fate of component regions

All superficial cephalic tissues shift from dorsolateral to ventrolateral locations during the same period. Thus the cephalic neural crest cells do not move alone through the extracellular matrix. Rather such cellular migrations comprise an integrated co-ordinated set of tissue displacements.

(1) The neural crest, extending from the diencephalon to the midmetencephalon, participates in the formation of periocular tissues and derivatives of the first pharyngeal (maxillomandibular) arch.[8] Thus the neural crest contributes to the formation of the skeletal tissue and the connective tissues for the musculature and organs derived from the pharyngeal arches and accompanying pharyngeal pouches. (The muscles of the region are derived from the somitomeres, i.e. cranial somite-like mesoderm).
(2) The neural crest, extending from the cranial myelencephalon to the middle of the optic placode, contributes to the hyoid (second) arch.
(3) The neural crest, from the midplacode level to the third somite, seeds the third and fourth arches and the sixth arch area, in addition to the thymus and parathyroid gland connective tissue and calcitonin (C) cells of the thyroid gland.[12]
(4) The neural crest cells in the third and fourth arches and sixth arch area migrate to the outflow tract of the heart – the conotruncal region.[13]
(5) The neural crest cells of all the arches form the walls of the large arteries deriving from the pharyngeal arches, except the lining endothelium.[12]

There is therefore a continuum of cranial structures which are dependent on the neural crest cell contributions. These extend from the orbital region throughout the face and neck to the heart. Most of the cephalic neural crest forms a continuous mesenchymal population from the prosencephalon to the level immediately in front of the larynx. This ectomesenchyme is the source of all connective tissues in the regions that will form the face and mouth, including odontoblasts.[14] In other words, most gross craniofacial anomalies may be traced back to some disturbance in neural crest cells *per se*, or their migration.

Mechanisms of craniofacial development

During the initial stages of craniofacial development, two overlapping processes occur, morphogenesis and cytodifferentiation.

The *morphogenetic phase* involves movement of appropriate numbers of mesenchymal cells from their sites of origin to their sites of terminal differentiation. This involves neural crest cell movement from the neural fold region to, and around the pharynx, optic vesicles and prosencephalon.

The *cytodifferentiation phase* comprises cellular differentiation at a given area, in addition to specific extracellular matrix formation.

These two interactive processes are linked to the generation of craniofacial pattern and form.

The cephalic paraxial mesoderm forms before the neural crest cells emerge. The first members of this mesenchyme to appear are those that will form the most rostral somitomeres and prechordal mesoderm. These appear at the time of maximal primitive streak elongation.[15] As the streak regresses, additional paraxial mesoderm is formed and subsequently becomes organized into a series of seven loosely condensed somitomeres.

The neural crest cells migrate on to this mesodermal fabric. Except for those members of the crest population which contribute to peripheral nervous system formation,[16] the neural crest cell populations move laterally and ventrally over the outer surface of the somitomeres, beneath the superficial ectoderm. Prior to their advance, the surface ectoderm separates from the somitomeres, forming a transient cell-free space.[11] This separation reflects the action of a variety of enzymes, including hyaluronidase, produced from both the surface epithelium and neural crest cells.[11,17] Caudal to the optic vesicle, the neural crest populations migrate ventrally to the level of the pharynx, invading the regions between the pharyngeal pouches, to form the branchial arches. The more rostral members move over the prosencephalon, around the surface of the optic vesicles, to contribute to maxillary and frontonasal process formation.[31] For normal craniofacial development, these neural crest cell populations must become dispersed according to region-specific patterns of cellular migration.[16] Just as neural crest cells are unique in their ability to respond to migration-supporting environments, these particular environments are unique in their ability to support patterned migrations. As a result of these initial dispersions, neural crest and mesenchymal cell populations subsequently occupy separate regions of the head, with a well-defined interface between the two. This neural crest–mesoderm interface is not impenetrable, as it may be crossed by:

(1) Angiogenic cords, which subsequently develop into blood vessels.
(2) Nerve fibres.
(3) Prospective Schwann cells.
(4) Voluntary skeletal muscle primordia.

Neural crest contributions to the craniofacial region

Neural crest-derived populations provide a most significant contribution to cranial morphogenesis. In addition to the primary osseous components, many connective tissues are neural crest in origin.[12,18] Skeletogenesis by neural crest cells is normally dependent upon products released by the adjacent epithelial tissues. This applies both to cranial bones formed by intramembranous and endochondral ossification. Such cytodifferentiation of these neural crest cell populations requires the interaction between the mesenchymal cells and the products of nearby tissues. In this manner, the subsequent cytodifferentiation of neural crest-derived tissues is similar to the initial stages of neural crest cell migration.

The neural crest tissues therefore contribute by themselves, or in conjunction with mesoderm, to three types of cranial tissue.

Tissues primarily of neural crest cell origin

(1) Peripheral neurones:
  (a) sympathetic nervous system;
  (b) parasympathetic nervous system;
  (c) afferent peripheral nerves;
  (d) efferent peripheral nerves.
(2) Schwann sheath cells:
  melanocytes.

Tissues of mesodermal–neural crest origin

(1) Dermis.
(2) Cartilage.
(3) Endochondral bone.
(4) Intramembranous bone.
(5) Connective tissues.
(6) Perivascular muscle.
(7) Involuntary muscle.

Tissues of mesodermal origin

(1) Cardiac muscle.
(2) Voluntary muscle.
(3) Haemopoietic cells.
(4) Angiogenic cells.
(5) Nephrogenic cells.

Each neural crest cell, or cell line, must therefore become committed or restricted in order to express a particular phenotype. The results of research based on transplanting and explanting neural crest tissues in embryos have shown that specific neural crest populations are programmed at a very early developmental stage, possibly during the initial period of neural crest cell formation.[8] For instance, the spatial pattern of skeletogenesis within the branchial arch appears to be programmed in the neural crest population before it actually leaves the neuroepithelium, with differences in skeletal morphology between branchial arches being based on the original location of the crest primordium along the neuroaxis. Such early establishment of regional differences in neural crest populations should not be surprising, since these cells are derived from the neural plate, which is the first tissue in the body to acquire polarity and some regional autonomy.

Craniofacial anomalies

In view of this influence of neural crest cells on subsequent cranial morphogenesis, an increasing number of specific craniofacial anomalies can be traced to very early developmental stages. By the completion of neural crest cell migration in the fourth week of intra-uterine life, neural crest cells have contributed to virtually all of the loose mesenchymal tissue in the facial region lying between the surface ectoderm and the underlying forebrain and eye. Most of the neural crest cells in the facial area later differentiate into skeletal and connective tissues, including the jaws and teeth.

A few examples are listed to emphasize the importance of neural crest cells in craniofacial anomalies:

(1) Extirpation of the chick forebrain neural crest tissue results in cleft lip and palate formation.[19]
(2) Severe facial asymmetry in some patients may be related to unequal amounts of neural crest cell migration on the two sides of the face.
(3) In the congenital Treacher Collins syndrome, there is underdevelopment of both maxilla and mandible resulting from a generalized lack of mesenchymal tissue. Experimentally, this syndrome may be produced by the administration of drugs which decrease cell mobility.[20] Such experiments suggest that the neural crest cells with the longest migration path (i.e. those taking a circuitous route to the lateral and lower areas of the face) are most affected, whereas those going to the central area tend to complete their migratory movement. This explains why midline defects, including clefts, are rarely part of the syndrome. Some degree of asymmetry may be present but both sides are affected.
(4) Many teratogenic agents, e.g. fetal alcohol syndrome, mimic neural crest extirpation, leading to craniofacial and heart defects.

Mandibular morphogenesis

Although the neural crest provides an important contribution to craniofacial development, the subsequent morphogenetic mechanisms are still largely unknown. This is illustrated by consideration of mandibular morphogenesis. The mandible is, in fact, a complex structure, comprising various units at different levels of organization.

(1) The complete bony mandible.
(2) The component mandibular elements: Meckel's cartilage; bone; muscle; condylar secondary cartilage; nerves; etc.
(3) The component mandibular tissue cells: osteocytes; chondrocytes; myoblasts; neurones; etc.
(4) The mandibular extracellular tissue compartments: cartilage; bone.
(5) The mandibular intra- and extracellular substances: collagen; glycosaminoglycans; fibronectin; glycoproteins; mineral complexes, e.g. calcium apatite.

All these elements may contribute to mandibular morphogenesis.[21,22]

In general terms, mandibular morphogenesis is guided by growth and morphogenesis of Meckel's cartilage. For instance, genes or drugs which specifically act on chondrocytes disrupt the shape and form of Meckel's cartilage, leading to overall mandibular shape disruption.[23] The shape of such primordial cartilages is, in turn, a function of their individual chondrocytes.[24] Morphogenesis of chondrocytes and their extracellular matrices is dependent upon correct assembly and organization of molecules within those matrices.[21] As Meckel's cartilage undergoes ossification, it is acted upon by muscles, innervated by nerves, vascularized by blood vessels and covered by connective tissues.

These represent extrinsic control mechanisms of mandibular morphogenesis. Such extrinsic controls function in addition to the intrinsic controls already occurring in the cells.[22] In other words, both intrinsic and extrinsic factors influence the initial phases of craniofacial morphogenesis.

As with any other craniofacial region, mandibular growth comprises both size and shape changes. If such growth results in altered shape, then that growth must be polarized: if equal growth occurred in all directions, there would be an increase in size but not shape; if growth predominates along one axis (i.e. disproportionate growth) morphological shape will be altered. Such shape changes are again influenced by both intrinsic and extrinsic factors.[22]

As previously stated, cells which ultimately form cartilage, bone, connective tissue and tooth dentine arise from neural crest cells.[24] Delayed migration may result in neural crest cells failing to reach and/or populate a specific craniofacial region.[25] Neural crest cell migration may also be impaired when extracellular spaces fail to form, as in some genetic disorders.[26] Interruption of neural crest cell mitosis can lead to excessive cell death and abnormal morphogenesis.[27] Once the neural crest cells reach the facial processes, their mitotic rate is increased,[28] perhaps partly through increased interaction of neural crest derived cells with one another[29] and partly through epithelial–mesenchymal interactions which stimulate mitosis.[30]

At this early developmental stage the mandible is no more than a process filled with a homogeneous mass of mesenchyme and covered by epithelium (27 days of age for man). Nerves and blood vessels soon penetrate the mandibular processes. The mesodermal core begins to differentiate into myotubes which arise from cranial mesoderm rather than the neural crest. As a result of inductive interactions with the mandibular epithelium, neural crest-derived mesenchyme begins to condense and differentiate as cartilage – the primordium of Meckel's cartilage. Such condensations involve the aggregation of like cells to a centre, either by increased local cell division or by cellular aggregation towards a centre. This phase allows like cells to interact. This is critical for initiation of cytodifferentiation. Such cytodifferentiation may not be initiated if condensations are too small (as in some genetic defects). Subsequent condensations herald bone and tooth formation. Once this phase of cytodifferentiation has been initiated, morphogenesis and growth begin, with Meckel's cartilage playing a key role in the case of the mandible.[31]

The basic form of a skeletal element is set very early in development, before the onset of cytodifferentiation. The basic morphogenetic properties, which determine the shape of a particular morphogenetic unit, depend either on intrinsic neural crest cell properties or the mesenchyme which forms from them. Thus processes that act later during craniofacial development are all important, but affect: subsequent differentiation; the rate of growth and minor architectural features, e.g. grooves and canals for the passage of blood vessels and nerves.

Given the basic craniofacial form at the early stages of development, subsequent morphological changes will be affected by a number of processes. These processes, however, have little role in the initiation of craniofacial malformations, but become increasingly important in subsequent craniofacial development. They include the following:

(1) Mitotic rate of chondroblasts, osteoblasts, myoblasts.
(2) Innervation.
(3) Vascularity.
(4) Rate of secretion and deposition of extracellular matrix.
(5) Epigenetic interaction with adjacent tissues.
(6) Epithelial–mesenchymal interactions.

In general, therefore, craniofacial anomalies may be regarded as reflecting one or more of the following:

(1) Absence of the neural crest because of defective initial inductive interactions.
(2) Abnormal neural crest cell migrations, either because the cells themselves are defective or because of abnormalities in the extracellular matrix encountered by migrating neural crest cells.
(3) Defective differentiation of neural crest cells caused by either intrinsic defects, e.g. increased adhesiveness, or as a result of defective inductive tissue interactions.
(4) Abnormalities in tissues such as nerves, muscles or blood vessels, with which the neural crest cells must interact.

As with all developmental abnormalities, the earlier the embryonic stage of development in which the defect occurs, the more major and life-threatening will be the malformation.

Conclusions

It is obvious that craniofacial growth is far more complex than traditionally envisaged. In view of the powerful influences emanating from the neural crest, genetic factors would appear to have a predominant influence over craniofacial morphogenesis, although their migrations and subsequent cytodifferentiation may be affected by both local and general environmental factors. Craniofacial form is, however, an integrated complex, with growth and development of the various component units variably influencing those of others. Obviously a great deal more research is required to elucidate the functional activity of these factors. Such research will however require elucidation of the factors influencing craniofacial form at the cellular rather than the macroscopic level.

Review questions

1. List the various tissues of the skull derived from neural crest cells.
2. With two examples, identify the causes of craniofacial malformation.
3. Give an account of the embryonic development of the mandible.
4. How could environmental and genetic factors affect craniofacial morphogenesis?
5. Describe the embryological origin of the neural crest.

References

1. NODEN, D.M. (1984) Craniofacial development: new views on old problem. *Anat. Rec.*, **208**, 1–13
2. HAY, E.D. (1968) Organization and fine structure of epithelium and mesenchyme in the developing chick embryo. In *Epithelial–Mesenchymal Interactions*, edited by R. Fleischmajer and R.E. Billingham. Baltimore: Williams & Wilkins
3. MANASEK, F.J. (1975) The extracellular matrix: a dynamic component of the developing embryo. *Curr. Top. Devel. Biol.*, **10**, 35–102
4. SLAVKIN, H.C. and GREULICH, R.C. (1975) *Extracellular Matrix Influences on Gene Expression.* New York: Academic Press

5. MEIER, S. (1979) Development of the chick embryo mesoblast. *Devel. Biol.*, **73**, 25–45
6. ANDERSON, C.B. and MEIER, S. (1981) The influence of the metameric pattern in the mesoderm on migration of cranial neural crest cells in the chick embryo. *Devel. Biol.*, **85**, 385–402
7. TOSNEY, K.W. (1982) The segregation and early migration of cranial neural crest cells in the avian embryo. *Dev. Biol.*, **89**, 13–24
8. NODEN, D.M. (1983) The role of the neural crest in patterning of avian cranial skeletal, connective and muscle tissues. *Dev. Biol.*, **96**, 144–165
9. NODEN, D.M. (1980) The migration and cytodifferentiation of cranial neural crest cells. In *Current Research Trends in Prenatal Craniofacial Development*, edited by R.M. Pratt and R.L. Christiansen. New York: Elsevier/North Holland
10. JOHNSTON, M.C. (1966) A radioautographic study of the migration and fate of cranial neural crest cells in the chick embryo. *Ant. Rec.*, **156**, 143–156
11. PRATT, R.M., LARSEN, M.A. and JOHNSTON, M.C. (1975) Migration of cranial neural crest cells in a cell-free hyaluronate-rich matrix. *Dev. Biol.*, **44**, 298–305
12. LELIEVRE, C.S. and LEDOUARIN, N.M. (1975) Mesenchymal derivatives of the neural crest: analysis of chimaeric quail and chick embryos. *J. Embryol. Exp. Morphol.*, **34**, 125–154
13. KIRBY, M.L. and STEWART, D.E. (1983) Neural crest origin of cardiac ganglion cells in the chick embryo: identification and extirpation. *Dev. Biol.*, **97**, 433–443
14. LELIEVRE, C.S. (1978) Participation of neural crest-derived cells in the genesis of the skull in birds. *J. Embryol. Exp. Morphol.*, **47**, 17–37
15. MEIER, S. (1981) Development of the chick embryo mesoblast: morphogenesis of the prechordal plate and cranial segments. *Devel. Biol.*, **83**, 49–61
16. NODEN, D.M. (1978) The control of avian cephalic neural crest cytodifferentiation. *Dev. Biol.*, **67**, 313–329
17. GREENBERG, J.H. and PRATT, R.M. (1977) Glycosaminoglycan and glycoprotein synthesis by cranial neural crest cells *in vitro*. *Cell Diff.*, **6**, 119–132
18. NODEN, D.M. (1978) The control of avian cephalic neural crest cytodifferentiation. *Dev. Biol.*, **67**, 296–312
19. JOHNSTON, M.C. (1964) Facial malformation in chick embryo resulting from removal of neural crest. *J. Dent. Res.*, **43**, 822
20. POSWILLO, D. (1975) The pathogenesis of the Treacher Collins syndrome (mandibulofacial dysostosis). *Br. J. Oral Surg.*, **13**, 1–26
21. HALL, B.K. (1978) *Developmental and Cellular Skeletal Biology*. New York: Academic Press
22. THOROGOOD, P.V. (1983) Morphogenesis of cartilage. In *Cartilage*, edited by B.K. Hall. New York: Academic Press
23. BERGSMA, D. (1979) *Birth Defects Compendium*. New York: Alan Liss
24. HALL, B.K. (1980) Chondrogenesis and osteogenesis in cranial neural crest cells. In *Current Research Trends in Prenatal Craniofacial Development*, edited by R.M. Pratt and R.L. Christiansen. New York: Elsevier/North Holland
25. MORRISS, G.M. and THOROGOOD, P.V. (1978) An approach to cranial neural crest cell migration and differentiation in mammalian embryos. In *Development of Mammals*, edited by M.H. Johnson. Amsterdam: North Holland
26. WESTON, J.A. (1980) Role of the embryonic environment in neural crest morphogenesis. In *Current Research Trends in Prenatal Craniofacial Development*, edited by R.M. Pratt and R.L. Christiansen. New York: Elsevier/North Holland
27. JOHNSTON, M.C. and SULIK, K.K. (1979) Some abnormal patterns of development in the craniofacial region. *Birth Defects*, **15**, 23–42
28. MINKOFF, R. and KUNTZ, A.J. (1977) Cell proliferation during morphogenetic change. *J. Embryol. Exp. Morphol.*, **40**, 101–113
29. SOLURSH, M. (1983) Cell–cell interactions and chondrogenesis. In *Cartilage*, edited by B.K. Hall. New York: Academic Press
30. HALL, B.K. (1983) Epithelial–mesenchymal interactions in cartilage and bone development. In *Epithelial–Mesenchymal Interactions*, edited by R.H. Sawyer and F. Fallon. New York: Praeger Press
31. DIEWERT, V.M. (1980) Correlation between mandibular retrognathia and induction of cleft palate with 6-aminonicotinamide in the rat. *Teratology*, **19**, 213–228

19

Mechanisms of tooth eruption

Introduction

The complex process of tooth eruption results in the movement of a tooth from its developmental to its functional position. Since the functional position of a tooth is liable to undergo changes throughout life, e.g. due to orthodontic therapy or to compensate for the loss of occlusal substance due to attrition, human tooth eruption is a continuous rather than a limited process. Conventionally, the process of tooth eruption is divided into three phases:

(1) *Pre-eruptive phase*, during which the enamel organ, lying within the developing jaw, reaches full size, along with completion of tooth crown calcification.
(2) *Prefunctional phase*, which commences with root formation and is completed when the tooth reaches the occlusal plane (the crown penetrates the oral mucosa to appear in the oral cavity during this phase).
(3) *Functional phase*, which includes the generally small tooth movements that occur after the tooth has reached the occlusal plane.

Tooth eruption – the problem

Rather than comprising a single process, tooth eruption may in fact involve a number of processes. The existence of a single mechanism to account for the complex movements of a tooth during eruption is therefore a naive assumption. For instance, the high rate of collagen turnover during tooth eruption may suggest that this tissue provides the major eruptive force. Alternatively, it may also be a reflection of the marked functional readjustments that occur within this tissue to accommodate the tooth movements during the process of eruption. Also, there is a general assumption that teeth erupt with a certain force. However, such an eruption force must be balanced by some restraining influence to prevent continued eruptive tooth movements after the attainment of the correct occlusal location (*Figure 19.1*).

Not all mammalian teeth erupt by the same mechanism. Although gomphosis (a ligamentous attachment to bone) is the only form of tooth attachment in mammals,[1] mammalian teeth can be

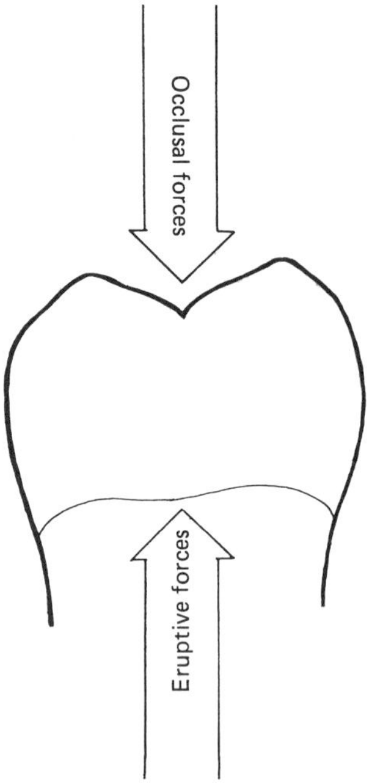

Figure 19.1 Diagram to illustrate the opposing occlusal and eruptive forces on a tooth

subdivided into three broad categories on the basis of their eruptive characteristics.

In the *continuously growing tooth*, there is no gross separation between the anatomical crown and the anatomical root. Continuous growth of the tooth at the apex and continuous eruption occur throughout the life of the animal. The clinical crown is constantly replaced by a root covered with enamel in progressive stages of development.[2] With the loss of tooth substance due to occlusal attrition, more tooth substance is extruded from the socket to maintain the clinical crown. This form of tooth is characteristic of animals with rapid occlusal wear and eruption (e.g. rodent incisor teeth).

The *continuously extruding tooth* has a defined crown and anatomical root. The tooth begins by partially emerging from the investing tissues, revealing only a fraction of the large enamel surface. The enamel beneath the gingiva is covered with cementum, enabling supra-alveolar fibres to be attached to the tooth. As the tooth is worn, more of the anatomical crown extrudes and the epithelial attachment migrates apically, but, since no new tooth structure is being formed, the continuous tooth eruption results in a gradual loosening and final exfoliation of the tooth. This form of tooth is characteristic of the lower incisors of sheep and cattle.

Human teeth may be characterized as *continuously erupting teeth* with investing tissues. In the absence of periodontal disease, the teeth do not extrude if further eruption occurs. Also, eruption does not occur by enlargement of the clinical crown but rather by additions to the alveolar process.[3]

Whether the basic mechanisms of tooth eruption in these three categories are analogous remains obscure.

There are marked physiological and morphological contrasts between human teeth and rodent incisors, yet these latter form the predominant experimental model for the investigation of tooth eruption. Care must therefore be taken in extrapolating the results from laboratory rodents to the human situation. Using callipers,[4] enlarged radiographs,[5] calibrated microscopes[2] or variable capacitance displacement transducers,[6] eruption rates of 200–1100 μm/day have been recorded in the mouse, guinea pig and rabbit. In human teeth, eruption rates of the order of 140 μm/day during the most rapid period[7] have been recorded, dropping to 5 μm/day as the teeth reach the occlusal plane.[8] The greater eruption rates of rodent incisors facilitate their accurate measurement: a major reason for the use of these teeth in experimental models.

Investigation of human tooth eruption

There are three major categories of techniques that have been used to investigate human tooth eruption.[9]

Clinical studies have been based on the mucogingival junction,[10] a datum line joining the incisal edges of the deciduous lateral incisors,[7] average occlusal plane[11] or ankylosed teeth,[8] as fixed reference points from which to measure tooth eruption rates. Measurement of enlarged orientated photographs[7] and direct measurements on dental casts[11] have provided information on the postemergent rate of erupting teeth. Once a tooth reaches the occlusal plane, further data on eruption rates are difficult to obtain. The eruption rates determined by use of the occlusal plane for reference are lower than the true eruptive rates, due to the vertical movement of the entire occlusal plane during facial growth.[12] The points provided by the stable mucogingival junction and cementogingival junction provide the best clinical reference points from which to measure eruption.[10]

Histological studies provide detailed pictures of tooth movement during eruption. Such studies have shown the slow drift of the tooth follicle before apparent eruptive movements begin, and the slow mesio-occlusal drift of adult teeth.[13] In addition, vital staining techniques have been used experimentally to identify the specific tissue activities during tooth eruptive movement.

Although the *evaluation of radiographs* has facilitated the analysis of human tooth eruption, the validity of such studies is compromised by the dearth of fixed reference points. Indeed, conventional cephalometric datum points, e.g. lower border of the mandible, inferior alveolar canal, developing tooth follicles, ankylosed teeth, deciduous lateral incisors, radiographic markers placed at the mucogingival junction, tooth follicles prior to root formation, bone trabeculations in the anterior portion of the mandibular symphysis or palate, in addition to metallic implants, comprise just some of the reference points that have been used to measure tooth eruption from radiographs. It is anticipated that the use of image analysis and subtraction radiography may soon provide more detailed data in this regard, especially when associated with the application of more accurate techniques of geometric analysis.[14]

Human tooth eruption

Based on orthopantomographic studies of children and adolescents,[7,8,9,11] six stages of tooth eruption have been defined (*Table 19.1*).

Follicular growth

Permanent tooth germs that bud from the deciduous teeth generally assume a lingual position relative to their precursors.[13] As the deciduous teeth develop and erupt, the permanent tooth follicles undergo somewhat complex migrations from their initial to their pre-eruptive positions.[15] Once crown formation has begun, however, the follicles of the posterior teeth move buccally with little, or any, radiographic evidence of occlusal or mesiodistal movement. In fact, the tooth crypt is analogous to a cyst at this stage, symmetrically expanding vertically and mesiodistally. The centre of the tooth crypt, however, remains at the same distance from the inferior (alveolar) dental canal: this apparent immobility persists until the entire crown has calcified and approximately 2–4 mm of the root have developed. Eruptive movement of the tooth *per se* begins soon after the root begins to form. This supports the notion that metabolic activity within the periodontal ligament provides a major component of tooth eruption.

Pre-emergent eruptive spurt

During the second phase, root formation continues as the tooth begins a period of rapid eruption in the occlusal direction.' All points on the developing tooth move occlusally, including the lengthening tooth root. This phase of eruption describes a

Table 19.1 Classifications of tooth eruption

Tooth events	*Brodie*[40]	*Noyes and Schour*[39]	*Weinmann*[13]	*Carlson*[9]	*Darling and Levers*[8]	*Steedle and Proffit*[28]
Initiation of calcification	Movement of the crypt	Stage I–preparatory stage	Second period. First phase pre-emergence	Crown formation	Concentric growth of the tooth follicle	Follicular growth
Initiation of root development		Stage II–migration toward the oral epithelium		Period of eruption	Bodily movement of the tooth toward the occlusal plane	Pre-emergent eruptive spurt
Gingival emergence	Rupture of the crypt and gingival emergence	Stage III–emergence of crown tip into the oral cavity	Second phase–emergence to contact			Post-emergent eruptive spurt
First occlusal contact		Stage IV–first occlusal contact	Third phase–post-occlusal contact			
Occlusal plane stages						
Period of quiescence		Stage V–full occlusal contact		Movement of the occlusal plane	Establishment of a state of equilibrium	Juvenile occlusal equilibrium
Pubertal growth					Bodily movement associated with the adolescent growth spurt	Circumpubertal occlusion eruptive
Period of adulthood		Stage VI–continuous eruption			Equilibrium which persists into adult life	Adult occlusal equilibrium

smooth course, although the rate increases as gingival emergence is approached.[16] Two processes are therefore necessary for this eruptive phase.

(1) There must be resorption of the overlying bone (and of the overlying deciduous roots in the case of permanent teeth).
(2) The eruption mechanism itself must move the tooth in the direction where the path has been cleared.

These two processes usually operate in concert, although this is not always the case. For instance, bone resorption does not occur in patients with the cleidocranial dysplasia syndrome, and this contributes to the abnormal patterns of tooth eruption.

Postemergent eruptive spurt

At the time of gingival emergence, the rate of human tooth eruption is at its greatest.[7] From this point, the eruption rate appears to slow as the tooth approaches the occlusal plane and comes under the influence of both masticatory and other intra-oral forces.

Juvenile occlusal equilibrium

Once the permanent teeth reach occlusion, occlusal movement stops or is incredibly slow for several years, while the occlusal plane remains at the same distance from the inferior alveolar canal. Whether the vertical drift is non-existent or minimal, this period of relative quiescence ends at the beginning of puberty, when the second active phase of eruption begins.

Circumpubertal occlusal eruptive spurt

Between 11 and 16 years of age, the teeth in occlusion begin a second active eruption phase lasting 2–3 years. This period is characterized by an increase in lower facial height through additions to the alveolar height, a feature that may not occur simultaneously in the maxilla and mandible. At this period, the facial tissues undergo a period of accelerated growth, with lengthening of the facial and masticatory muscles and lowering of the mandible and associated soft tissues, although compensatory alveolar growth maintains the freeway space (*Figure 19.2*). This eruptive spurt slows as the face reaches maturity and a state of relative equilibriumis re-established by 18 years of age.

Adult occlusal equilibrium

Once physical maturity is reached, vertical tooth movement does not stop abruptly. Throughout life, small increases in lower facial height and continued eruption occur. Lower facial height increases 0.3 mm per year in the second decade, 0.1 mm per year in the third decade and 0.07 mm per year in the seventh decade. During this period, a gradually decreasing eruption rate continues to compensate for facial growth. Indeed, the general consensus holds that mesio-occlusal eruption continues in adult life, with interproximal and occlusal attrition providing the predominant aetiologic factor. In the latter years, however, continued tooth eruption may be greatly overshadowed by tooth loss, marked occlusal abrasion and periodontal breakdown, leading to a reduction in facial height. Thus during adult life, teeth continue to erupt at an extremely slow rate. If its antagonist is lost at any age, however, a tooth can erupt more rapidly, demonstrating that the eruption mechanism remains active and capable of producing significant tooth movement even late in life.

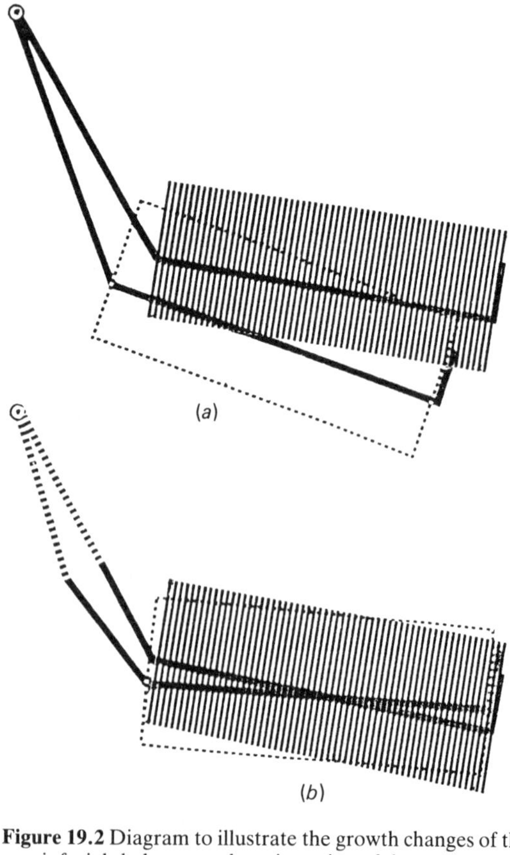

Figure 19.2 Diagram to illustrate the growth changes of the craniofacial skeleton on the orientation of the upper (hatched) and lower dental arches. *a*, young patient; *b*, mature patient.

Control of tooth eruption

Almost every structure in the vicinity of the tooth has, at one time, been assigned to provide the motive force of tooth eruption. Generally, theories that attribute the eruption mechanism to the basal area (root elongation, pulp and dentinal proliferation) have been repudiated, while those that assign the motive force to elements of the periodontal ligament are gaining adherents.

Gubernacular cord

It has been suggested that the gubernacular cords, which comprise fibrous connective tissue strands connecting the follicles of the permanent teeth to the oral mucosa, have an important role in controlling the movement of developing teeth through the growing jaws.[17] During tooth eruption, the gubernacular cords decrease in length but increase in thickness and become less dense. Whether the gubernaculum provides a duct, a path of least resistance or is actively engaged in pulling the tooth out from the underlying tissues, has, however, yet to be established. This tissue certainly cannot be implicated once the tooth has breached the oral mucosa. Nevertheless, surgical removal of the connective tissue overlying human unerupted teeth may lead to their eruption.

Alveolar bone growth

Alternatively it has been suggested that continued alveolar bone deposition results in the eruption of teeth to their occlusal location.[18] However, tooth eruption is frequently associated with root formation down into the underlying alveolar bone, i.e. associated with bone resorption rather than deposition.

Root growth

As the prefunctional phase of eruption occurs at a time coincident with root formation, root growth has been implicated as a motive force of tooth eruption.[19] Conceivably, pressure generated from the growing root-end may result in the resorption at the base of the alveolar socket, rather than overlying tooth eruption. Accordingly, a connective tissue band at the base of the socket has been postulated to prevent the translation of stresses from root growth resulting in alveolar bone resorption rather than tooth eruption. Unfortunately, this tissue, the hammock ligament, has not been detected in all teeth. Also, human teeth may erupt to their final occlusal position prior to root formation, i.e. root development may proceed after the attainment of the occlusal location. Alternatively, impacted or unerupted human permanent incisors or canines, in which the roots have fully formed, may erupt into a functional position within the dental arch following surgical exposure. Unerupted teeth with completed roots sometimes drift considerable distances within the jaws, although the motive force for such movements remains obscure.

Intrapulpal pressure

Once a tooth has penetrated into the oral cavity, there must be some form of pressure gradient favouring eruption. Conceivably, such a pressure gradient may be derived from vascular pressure within the pulp cavity, although whether a pulpal pressure of 9 mmHg is sufficient to result in tooth eruption has yet to be determined.

Periodontal ligament

In contrast to a tooth being pushed out of the socket, another group of theories contends that it may be pulled out by the periodontal ligament. In fact, the three most likely theories ascribe the driving force of tooth eruption to the cross-linking and shrinkage of collagen, the contractility and mobility of fibroblasts and the thixotropic gel-like nature of the periodontal membrane. There is no doubt that the predominant force of tooth eruption appears to reside in the periodontal ligament, although without isolated systems for investigation, causal relationships will be difficult to establish. One view maintains that tractional forces are generated within the oblique fibre system of the periodontal ligament due to the cross-linking and aggregation that occurs during collagen maturation.[20] During collagen fibril formation, tension could develop due to:

(1) Decrease in entropy during electrostatic attraction of disordered tropocollagen macromolecules and alignment along lines of stress.
(2) Linear polymerization, producing a decrease in length of macromolecules.
(3) Shrinkage associated with dehydration.

Alternatively, the fibroblasts within the periodontal ligament may generate an eruptive force either by their contractility or locomotor activity.[21] Certainly the similarity of eruption rates in continuously erupting teeth of different-sized animals favours the theory of a periodontally induced process of tooth eruption. The collagen contraction theory, however, necessitates a continuous turnover cycle for collagen within the periodontal ligament to maintain eruption, since contraction would occur only during the maturation phase. Such high turnover rates within the periodontal ligament may, however, indicate that the rate of tooth movement is not the sole factor which governs turnover time of components within the periodontal ligament. One method of assessing the role of collagen in producing an eruptive force centres on the administration of drugs that interfere with its maturation process. The lathyritic agent aminoacetonitrile (AAN) inhibits cross-linkage within collagen, and when administered to laboratory rodents, marked reductions in tooth eruption rates have been noted in one study[22] but not in others.[23]

Many investigations have been concerned with the mechanism whereby the periodontium succeeds in anchoring the tooth adequately yet allows the tooth to move. For continuously erupting rodent incisors, periodontal fibres coming from the alveolar bone and those coming from the cementum may meet in an intermediate plexus. This intermediate plexus supposedly comprises precollagenous fibres which allow continuous rebuilding and rearrangement of the periodontal ligament without changes in bone or cementum.[24] However, the verification of the intermediate plexus as a finite periodontal component rather than an artefact, awaits further investigation.

Periodontal ligament fibres are generally considered to be laid down at the commencement of the prefunctional phase of eruption, when they exhibit an oblique orientation suitable for the collagen contraction hypothesis of tooth eruption. There are, however, studies that indicate that a considerable proportion of a tooth root may be formed prior to oblique periodontal fibre formation.[25] Furthermore, the finding that the teeth in irradiated laboratory rodents erupt into the oral cavity without tooth root formation suggests that periodontal ligament-generated forces may not be solely responsible for tooth eruption. Similarly, teeth appear to erupt into the oral cavity normally in patients with hypophosphatasia (an autosomal recessive disorder associated with a gross deficiency of both cementum and periodontal ligament).[26] Conceivably, tooth eruption comprises a complex series of processes, with various facets being more important than others at different phases.

Physiology of tooth eruption

Tooth eruption can be considered as a static equilibrium problem. At any given time, eruptive tooth forces are opposed by forces that inhibit occlusal movement. A force of 8.4 g has been shown to prevent human tooth eruption under controlled conditions,[27] whereas forces less than 1 g may prevent rodent incisal tooth eruption.[28] The data from such studies are difficult to interpret, however, until the exact contribution of the periodontal ligament to tooth eruption has been defined.

In the early stages of tooth eruption, permanent tooth germs move relative to the deciduous teeth. Although the buds of the permanent premolars are at first located occlusal to the deciduous teeth, their migration to a cervical, and later an apical, position can be explained by the eruptive movements of the deciduous molars. Tooth follicles expand buccally, occlusally and apically, and at no time from the beginning of cusp calcification to the onset of root development is there evidence that significant bone deposition occurs apical to the follicle. With several millimetres of root development, occlusal movement begins to occur. As the volume of the periodontal ligament increases with root lengthening, the rate of tooth eruption increases. When more than one half of root development has occurred, gingival emergence is accelerated by removal of overlying tooth and bone. If the deciduous teeth are extracted prior to one half of root formation, emergence is delayed, presumably because additional bone must be resorbed.

Bone resorption appears to occur independently of eruption. If dead crown shells or metal replicas are substituted into dental follicles just prior to eruption, resorption of overlying bone continues and eruption occurs on schedule.[29] Failure of the tooth to keep pace with bone resorption, as in primary failure of eruption, may therefore be an important clinical sign of a problem with the eruption mechanism.

Once the tooth has penetrated the bone, fibroblasts responsible for collagen turnover must keep pace with the erupting tooth or eruption may be slowed, even in the presence of an intact and active mechanism. In the pre-emergent eruptive spurt, the rate of movement is determined by the generative and adaptive capacity of elements of the dental follicle and by resorption, first of the overlying bone and then of the deciduous teeth or gingival tissues. Conceivably, the rate of bone resorption or gingival remodelling is the predominant rate-limiting factor of pre-emergent eruption, rather than the activity of the eruption mechanism.

Post-eruptive tooth movements

At gingival emergence, the tooth is erupting at its most rapid rate, still protected from the masticatory and soft-tissue forces by the adjacent teeth, with the bone and gingiva no longer limiting factors. In the majority of cases, the rate of eruption slows as the tooth approaches the occlusal plane. In fact, the forces of occlusion are considered to be a primary factor in the inhibition of tooth eruption, although there is no direct evidence on this point. Nevertheless, although human teeth achieve equilibrium when in occlusion, their eruption rates are renewed following loss of their antagonists in the opposing jaw, i.e. over-eruption occurs following tooth loss in the opposing jaw.

Since the intermittent forces of occlusion are known to vary in size, duration, frequency and direction, their investigation is complicated. Upon application of an intermittent force, initial displacement in the apical direction is related exponentially to the magnitude of the force. Light forces displace the tooth easily, but as the force approaches 100 g, the amount of movement per increment of force becomes substantially less.[30] This phenomenon has been attributed to a gradual displacement of periodontal tissue fluid until the collagen fibres begin to resist root displacement. At approximately 50 g, distortion of the alveolar plates begins to occur as the stressed collagen fibres transfer the force to the alveolus, resulting in bone bending.[31] With heavy continuous loading, the tooth moves apically at a constant rate after the initial intrusion until the limit is reached.

Tooth recovery from axial loading occurs in two phases. The initial rapid linear phase is followed by a slower declining phase, requiring a total of 60–90 s to return to the preloading postion.[32] Such a biphasic response is consistent with the recoiling of the bone of the socket in an elastic manner and the gradual reversion of the collagen fibres to the wavy condition as the fluid is replenished in the periodontal ligament. Repeated force application every 2–5 s inhibits complete recovery, with a postrecovery extrusive effect being attributed to dilatation of the stressed periodontal blood vessels (inflammation of the periapical tissues). Periods of sleep or occlusal rest result in a relatively more extruded position of the tooth within its socket, while eating and daily activities produce a relatively more intruded position.[33]

The long-term effects of intermittent axial loading of a tooth have not been recorded, due to difficulties in monitoring tooth location over long periods. However, patients with loss of occlusal antagonists or generalized muscular weakness display excessive eruption of the posterior teeth. By contrast, patients with scoliosis who have therapy involving a body cast with a neck brace to support the head, demonstrate a reduction in posterior tooth eruption and proclination of the anterior teeth from increased pressure on the inferior border of the mandible.

Conceivably, after an erupting tooth emerges into the oral cavity, the mechanical forces of intermittent occlusal loading are capable of disturbing the generative or adaptive mechanisms of the periodontal ligament. Although the teeth quickly return to their preloading position, eruption is slowed by intermittent occlusal forces. Return of the tooth to its preloading position, therefore, does not indicate a return to the preloading eruption rate, i.e. occlusal forces either mechanically set back the remodelling process or significantly modify the activity of the cells responsible for movement. In both instances, eruption slows and the pattern of movement changes as the initial occlusal equilibrium is achieved.

Table 19.2 Magnitude and duration of force against the teeth during function

Factor	*Force magnitude*	*Force duration*
Tooth contacts		
Mastication	Very heavy	Very short
Swallowing	Light	Very short
Tissue pressures of lip, cheek and tongue		
Swallowing	Moderate	Short
Speaking	Light	Very short
Resting	Very light	Long
External pressures		
Habits	Moderate	Variable
Orthodontic treatment	Moderate	Variable
Intrinsic pressures		
Periodontal fibres	Light	Long
Gingival fibres	Variable	Long

The tongue, lips and cheeks are also primary factors which impede tooth eruption (*Table 19.2*). For instance, there is evidence that changes in resting tongue pressure result from changes in head posture,[34] although such changes may be secondary to changes in craniofacial skeletal development. Although the tongue may be between the teeth at times during sleep, or when the mandible is in the rest position, it need not be interposed in order for tongue pressures to affect tooth eruption. Friction from contact of the tongue or cheek with the side of the tooth could potentially provide a force of a few grams which may be sufficient to equal the force of eruption, i.e. resting tongue and lip pressures are in the 5–15 g range.[35] Jaw growth and eruptive tooth movements are known to interact during normal craniofacial development. For instance, the rotation of the face necessitates compensatory adaptations of the paths of tooth eruption during the circumpubertal eruptive spurt.[36] By grouping these rotations according to the direction of condylar growth, it has been shown that four-fifths of the mandibular rotation is masked by compensatory remodelling at the gonial angle. Such complex skeletal changes reinforce the notion that facial growth in this phase does not follow a specific unalterable growth pattern. Interactive skeletal and dental compensations maintain the pattern, but these same adaptations can be affected by environmental influences to alter normal facial growth. Light continuous forces from the tongue at rest are therefore probably important modulators of eruptive movements, especially during the circumpubertal eruptive spurt.

These forces may be responsible for the maintenance of the freeway space in the presence of rapid facial growth or moderate attrition, and may act as rate-limiting factors during these periods in combination with occlusal forces.

Once tooth eruption slows in early childhood, the activity of certain specific groups of periodontal fibres may be important for the control of tooth eruption. For instance, the supracrestal fibres of the periodontal ligament attached between tooth and alveolar bone have been shown to exert a force to return a displaced tooth to its original location.[37] The trans-septal group of periodontal fibres have also been shown to approximate the teeth when the interproximal contacts are broken, which suggests that these fibres may exist under tension in the natural state.[38] The ability of the supracrestal fibres to resist remodelling under tension suggests how the erupting tooth can cause incremental addition to alveolar bone height. Movement of the tooth as a result of eruptive forces may generate tension in the supracrestal fibre groups of the mature periodontium, which is transmitted to the periosteum, stimulating the osteoblasts of the alveolar crest to deposit bone. The overall metabolic activity of the gingiva and periosteum, as influenced by both systemic factors and the degree of tension, may then determine the rate by which the alveolar height increases: this mechanism is similar to the periosteal tension hypothesis postulated for other areas of the body.

Such a concept of tooth-eruption control in the adult provides evidence for the relationship between severe occlusal attrition and facial height. There is a general consensus that tooth eruption compensates for only 60% of the loss of occlusal tooth substance. In other words, continued tooth eruption may only partially compensate for the loss of tooth substance due to attrition, so that further attrition may result in a loss of tooth height and consequent reduction in facial height.

The inhibitory effect of the supracrestal complex, modified in the presence of periodontal disease, may also account for the variation in eruption which occurs with a loss of antagonist in adults. Thus unopposed teeth maintained in a state of periodontal health may not significantly overerupt in the adult. Conceivably, therefore, the systemic and local factors that control eruptive movements in this adult phase differ both quantitatively and qualitatively from earlier stages, and are characterized by the addition of gingival and alveolar growth limitations to the rate-limiting factors. Such concepts reaffirm the importance of timing in tooth eruption problems. The rapid compensatory adaptations during several phases of tooth eruption provide excellent opportunities for influencing the development of vertical problems. It is, however, unfortunate that rate-limiting factors can also have a more dramatic effect when rapid eruption is occurring than during the stages of relative quiescence.

Assessment of developmental age

Dental development correlates reasonably well with chronological age[39] but occurs as a relatively independent process (*Table 19.3*). Of all the indicators of developmental age, dental age correlates least well with the other developmental indices.[40] By contrast, skeletal age correlates well with physical growth status: thus, the latter is primarily used as a maturity index of skeletal maturation of the patient as a whole.

Table 19.3 Average chronology of tooth development

Tooth	*Calcification begins*		*Cown completed*		*Eruption*		*Root completed*	
	Maxilla	*Mandible*	*Maxilla*	*Mandible*	*Maxilla*	*Mandible*	*Maxilla*	*Mandible*
Primary								
Central incisor	14 w	14 w	1½ m	2½ m	10 m	8 m	1½ y	1½ y
Lateral incisor	16 w	16 w	2½ m	3 m	11 m	13 m	2 y	1½ y
Canine (cuspid)	17 w	17 w	9 m	9 m	19 m	20 m	3¼ y	3¼ y
1st molar	15 w	15 w	6 m	5½ m	16 m	2½ y	2¼ y	2¼ y
2nd molar	19 w	18 w	11 m	10 m	29 m	27 m	3 y	3 y
Permanent								
Central incisor	3 m	3 m	4½ y	3½ y	7¼ y	6¼ y	10½ y	9½ y
Lateral incisor	11 m	3 m	5½ y	4 y	8¼ y	7½ y	11 y	10 y
Canine (cuspid)	4 m	4 m	6 y	5¾ y	11½ y	10½ y	13½ y	12¾ y
1st premolar (bicuspid)	20 m	22 m	7 y	6¾ y	10¼ y	10½ y	13½ y	13½ y
2nd premolar (bicuspid)	27 m	28 m	7¾ y	7½ y	11 y	11¼ y	14½ y	15 y
1st molar	32 w	32 w	4¼ y	3¾ y	6¼ y	6 y	10½ y	10¾ y
2nd molar	27 m	27 m	7¾ y	7½ y	12½ y	12 y	15¾ y	16 y
3rd molar	8 y	9 y	14 y	14 y	20 y	20 y	22 y	22 y

w = weeks *in utero*; m = months; y = years.

Assessment of chronological age by the status of tooth eruption is a subject bounded more by subjective intuition than scientific data.

Tooth movement

If a tooth is moved by an extrinsic force, e.g. an orthodontic applicance, it will eventually be located in a new position in the jaw and, if stabilized there, will be supported in its new position by a remodelled periodontium with a periodontal space of normal width. If the tooth is considered to be moved bodily within the jaw, as opposed to tipping, such tooth movements will be accompanied by alveolar bone resorption on one side of the tooth socket and deposition on the other. Such gross changes in alveolar bone morphology will be accompanied by remodelling changes at the microscopic level, until the normal morphology of the tissues in the region are established. Such tooth movements are not only associated with changes in the alveolar bone but also with compensatory changes at the level of the periodontal ligament and its associated ground substance.

The basic mechanics of such tooth movements remain obscure. For instance:

(1) Movement of the position of a tooth within the alveolus may result in circulatory changes associated with changes in tissue oxygen tension.
(2) Circulatory changes may be accompanied by changes in the pH of the local environment.
(3) Changes in pressure or blood supply to the periodontal tissues may be associated with mast cell or macrophagic degranulation.
(4) Whereas large pressure changes may be associated with tissue necrosis, more physiological forces are used for the movement of teeth in orthodontic therapy.

The movement of teeth during orthodontic therapy may cause damage to the dental pulp. This may become apparent in dentinogenesis, formation of pulp stones, death of the pulp, internal or external root resorption. Interference to the blood supply to a tooth is the most likely pathogenesis of these phenomena.

Conclusions

Tooth eruption seems to be compensatory and is controlled by rate-limiting factors which vary in the various phases of tooth eruption. Although the force of eruption influences the rate of bone resorption, such resorptive processes occur independently of eruption and are rate-limiting factors in the pre-emergent stages of tooth eruption. After emergence, intermittent occlusal loading may disrupt the generative or adaptive mechanisms of the periodontal ligament so that eruption slows. Light continuous forces from the resting tongue and other soft tissues can also significantly limit the eruption of teeth during periods of rapid growth. Growth limitations of the alveolar bone and gingiva may play an important role in the control of tooth eruption in the adult. These factors, combined with a reduction of metabolic activity of elements of the periodontal ligament, may account for the relative stability of non-periodontally involved teeth. Much more research is, however, required before the processes involved in tooth eruption are fully explained. For instance, there is virtually no data as to why premature tooth eruption occurs in patients with hemifacial atrophy or adrenogenital syndrome or, conversely, why there is delayed tooth eruption in such conditions as patients with large crowns, hypercementosis, supernumerary teeth, hypopituitarism or cleidocranial dysostosis. Even impacted third molars, the most common tooth eruption disturbance, cannot always simply be explained on the basis of lack of space in the dental arch.

Review questions

1. What mechanism of tooth eruption can you strongly support?
2. List the component phases of movement from the follicular stage to the time the tooth attains its occlusal location.
3. What factors influence tooth eruption?
4. How can tooth movements occur in the adult?
5. What factors determine the final position of a tooth in the adult dental arch?

References

1. NOBLE, H.W. (1969) The evolution of the mammalian periodontium. In *Biology of the Periodontium*, edited by A.H. Melcher and W.H. Bowen. New York: Academic Press
2. ADDISON, W.H.F. and APPLETON, J.L. (1915) The structure and growth of the incisor teeth of the albino rat. *J. Morphol.*, **26**, 43–96
3. ANNEROTH, J. and TALARI, A. (1976) Eruptive movements of teeth in human adults. In *The Eruption and Occlusion of Teeth*, edited by D.F.G. Poole and M.V. Stack. Boston: Butterworth
4. SCHOUR, I. and VAN DYKE, H.B. (1931) Effect of replacement therapy on eruption of the incisor of the hypophysectomized rat. *Proc. Soc. Exp. Med. Biol.*, **29**, 378–382

5. MAIN, J.H.P. and ADAMS, D. (1965) Measurement of the rate of eruption of the rat incisor. *Arch. Oral Biol.*, **10**, 999–1008
6. MOXHAM, B.J. (1979) Recording the eruption of the rabbit mandibular incisor using a device for continuously monitoring tooth movements. *Arch. Oral Biol.*, **24**, 889–899
7. BURKE, P.H. and NEWELL, D.J. (1958) A photographic method of measuring eruption of certain human teeth. *Am. J. Orthod.*, **44**, 590–602
8. DARLING, A.I. and LEVERS, B.G. (1976) The pattern of eruption of some human teeth. *Arch. Oral Biol.*, **20**, 89–96
9. CARLSON, H. (1944) Studies on the rate and amount of eruption of certain human teeth. *Am. J. Orthod.*, **30**, 575–588
10. TALARI, A. and AINAMO, J. (1974) An orthopantomographic study of the width of attached gingiva. *J. Dent. Res.*, **53**, 1110
11. SMITH, R.G. (1980) A clinical study into the rate of eruption of some human permanent teeth. *Arch. Oral Biol.*, **25**, 675–681
12. BJORK, A. and SKIELLER, V. (1972) Facial development and tooth eruption: an implant study at the age of puberty. *Am. J. Orthod.*, **62**, 339–383
13. WEINMANN, J.P. (1941) Bone changes related to eruption of the teeth. *Angle Orthod.*, **11**, 83–99
14. BOOKSTEIN, F.L. (1983) Geometry of craniofacial growth invariants. *Am. J. Orthod.*, **83**, 221–234
15. OOE, T. (1968) Changes of position and development of human anterior tooth germs after birth. *Okajimas Folia Anat. Jap.*, **44**, 83–97
16. BURKE, P.H. (1954) Eruption analysis of maxillary first incisors in a patient with unilateral absence of the second incisor. *Trans. Eur. Orthod. Soc.*, 343–349
17. SCOTT, J.H. (1948) The development and function of the dental follicle. *Br. Dent. J.*, **85**, 193–199
18. BRASH, J.C. (1928) The growth of the alveolar bone and its relation to the movements of the teeth including eruption. *Dent. Rec.*, **73**, 460–476
19. HUNTER, J. (1778) *Natural History of Human Teeth.* London: Johnson
20. WEINREB, M.M., MICHAELI, Y. and SILBERMAN, G. (1969) Role of attrition and occlusal contact in the physiology of the rat incisor. IV. Prevention of attrition in the articulating incisor. *J. Dent. Res.*, **48**, 120–130
21. NESS, A.R. (1967) Eruption – a review. In *The Mechanisms of Tooth Support.* Bristol: Wright & Sons
22. THOMAS, N.R. (1965) The process and mechanism of tooth eruption. *PhD Thesis*, University of Bristol
23. BERKOVITZ, B.K.B. (1972) The effect of demecolcine and of triethanomelamine on the unimpeded eruption rate of normal and root resected incisor teeth in rats. *Arch. Oral Biol.*, **17**, 937–947
24. SICHER, H. and BHASKAR, S.N. (1972) *Orban's Oral Histology and Embryology*, 7th edn. St. Louis: C.V. Mosby
25. MAGNUSSON, B. (1968) Tissue changes during molar tooth eruption. *Trans. R. Schs. Dent. Stockh. Umea*, **13**, 1–122
26. GORLIN, R.J. and GOLDMAN, H.M. (1970) *Thoma's Oral Pathology*, 6th edn. St. Louis: C.V. Mosby
27. SMEDLEY, L.C. (1975) A technique for measuring the eruptive force of the human second bicuspid. *Thesis for Certificate in Orthodontics.* Temple University, Philadelphia
28. STEEDLE, J.R. and PROFFIT, W.R. (1985) The pattern and control of eruptive tooth movements. *Am. J. Orthod.*, **87**, 56–66
29. MARKS, S.C. and CAHILL, D.R. (1984) Experimental study in the dog of the nonactive role of the tooth in the eruptive process. *Arch. Oral Biol.*, **29**, 311–322
30. PICTON, D.C.A. (1969) The effect of external forces on the periodontium. In *Biology of the Periodontium*, edited by A.H. Melcher and W.H. Bowen. London: Academic Press
31. PARFITT, G.J. (1960) Measurement of the physiological mobility of individual teeth in an axial direction. *J. Dent. Res.*, **39**, 608–618
32. PICTON, D.C.A. (1964) The effect of repeated thrusts on normal axial tooth mobility. *Arch. Oral Biol.*, **9**, 55–63
33. PARFITT, G.J. (1976) The dynamics of a tooth in function. *J. Periodontol.*, **47**, 102–107
34. VIG, P.S., WOOD, L.W. and PROFFIT, W.R. (1982) The influence of cranial posture on tongue and lip pressure. *J. Dent. Res.*, **61**, 327
35. PROFFIT, W.R. (1978) The facial musculature in its relation to the dental occlusion. In *Muscle Adaptation in the Craniofacial Region*, edited by D.S. Carlson and J.A. McNamara. Ann Arbor: The Center for Human Growth and Development, University of Michigan
36. BJORK, A. (1969) Prediction of mandibular growth rotation. *Am. J. Orthod.*, **55**, 585–599
37. EDWARDS, J.G. (1970) A surgical procedure to eliminate rotational relapse. *Am. J. Orthod.*, **57**, 35–46
38. MOSS, J.P. and PICTON, D.C.A. (1974) The effect on approximal drift of cheek teeth of dividing mandibular molars of adult monkeys (*Macaca irus*). *Arch. Oral Biol.*, **19**, 1211–1214
39. NOYES, H.J. and SCHOUR, I. (1938) *Dental Histology and Embryology*, 5th edn. Philadelphia: Lea & Febiger
40. BRODIE, A.G. (1934) Present status of knowledge concerning movement of the tooth germ through the jaw. *J. Am. Dent. Assoc.*, **24**, 1830–1838

20

Orthodontic tooth movement

Introduction

The effect of orthodontic therapy on the supporting structures provides an insight into the dynamics of the alveolar bone and the periodontal ligament. In this regard, there are two basic rules:

1. Whenever the tooth root causes compression of the periodontal ligament, there is alveolar bone resorption.
2. Whenever the periodontal ligament is stretched, new alveolar bone is deposited.

Thus, orthodontic tooth movement primarily involves changes in the alveolar bone as a result of compression or tension in the periodontal ligament. In the usual course of events, cementolysis on the root surface or root resorption rarely occur. In some cases, however, root resorption does occur, with disastrous consequences of tooth instability. The fact that this may occur, even with the correct use of orthodontic therapy, serves to emphasize the dearth of knowledge concerning the factors controlling root form.

Tooth supporting tissues

Periodontal ligament

The oblique fibres of the periodontal ligament primarily function to transfer masticatory-generated pressure on the tooth to the supporting alveolar bone. Such pressures may result in temporary alveolar bone buckling, although the physiological significance of this has yet to be investigated. Superior to this the main fibre group, the supra-alveolar fibres, may be subdivided into the following categories:

(1) Dentogingival.
(2) Dentoperiosteal.
(3) Transseptal.
(4) Alveologingival.
(5) Circular group.

In addition to being variously grouped, the periodontal fibres comprise several different types. For instance, fairly thin connective tissue fibres occur in the interstitial and marrow spaces, whereas dense fibres and fibre bundles traverse between the tooth root cementum, alveolar bone and gingivae.

Such fibre bundles generally comprise closely packed fibrils of indefinite length.[1] These collagen fibrils are primarily of fibroblastic origin, comprising aggregated peptide chains of amino acids arranged in the form of a helix.[2] The fibrils are organized in an amorphous ground substance consisting of a variety of substances, including glycosaminoglycans, water and salts, in addition to capillary blood and lymph vessels, nerves and a variety of different cell types.

Compression of the periodontal ligament in orthodontic tooth movement may be reflected by:

(1) Compression of blood vessels predisposing the adjacent tissue to anoxic (hypoxic) necrosis.
(2) Direct trauma to the component cells, initiating an inflammatory response.
(3) Resorption of the adjacent alveolar bone, permitting tooth movement.

The primary objective of orthodontic tooth movement is to obtain the optimum degree of alveolar bone resorption to facilitate the precise movement of the tooth (or teeth) to a new, but stable, location within the dental arch. There is a general consensus that ideal orthodontic treatment primarily results in a diminution of the component periodontal ligament tissue fluid without altering the component ground substance. In fact, this periodontal ground substance may play a crucial role in binding the periodontal fibrils together and facilitating the adhesion of the component periodontal fibres on to the resorbed alveolar bone surfaces.[3]

In fact, the events are far more complicated than this brief scenario, since the component periodontal tissue undergoes constant renewal, although whether this rate of renewal is changed following compression has yet to be determined.

On the opposite side of the tooth root, orthodontic tooth movement will result in periodontal fibre tension. There is even less data concerning this aspect of tooth movement, since such tension may result in: stretching of existing periodontal fibres; rapid fibrogenesis by periodontal fibroblasts and periodontal ligamentous trauma associated with inflammatory changes in both the membrane itself and in the adjacent alveolar bone.

Alveolar bone

The alveolar bone is not uniform in thickness around a tooth. Rather, there are often morphological contrasts:

(1) The alveolar bone walls of the middle and marginal regions of the tooth socket are often quite dense, with few marrow spaces.
(2) The alveolar bone in the apical region on the lingual (or palatal) aspect of the tooth may incorporate large marrow spaces.[4]
(3) The thin alveolar bone walls on the labial and lingual sides of the teeth are frequently dense compared with those on the mesial and distal aspects. (This facilitates tooth movement to occur preferentially in either a mesial or distal direction.)

If the teeth are orthodontically displaced mesially or distally as soon as the lamina dura has been eliminated by resorption, the tooth roots may be rapidly displaced through the spongiosa of the alveolar bone.[5] In addition, compared with the alveolar bone in the adult, there are larger marrow spaces in the child and adolescent, often presenting as a spongiosa extending into the alveolar crest. This morphological difference in alveolar bone form contributes to the relative ease of orthodontic tooth movement in the adolescent and/or child compared with the adult. In addition, since osteoclasts are predominantly derived from bone marrow precursor cells, more extensive marrow spaces may facilitate their rapid appearance. The method by which forces applied to a tooth during orthodontic treatment are translated to component cells of the alveolar bone remains, unfortunately, enigmatic.

Orthodontic tooth movement

Where there is compression of the periodontal ligament, this is always associated with increased alveolar bone resorption (although alveolar bone is not different from bone in other locations, with bone resorption and osteogenesis occurring simultaneously to varying degrees). Since the periodontal ligament is frequently as narrow as 0.25 mm or less, the component fibres will be compressed between the root and alveolar bone surfaces. Initially, therefore, further tooth movement cannot occur until the alveolar bone surface has undergone some resorption. Thus little or no tooth movement may occur after an initial period of 5–6 days, predominantly involving periodontal compression, although this duration may be significantly shortened if stronger orthodontic forces are used. Although osteoclasts appear to be the principal cells involved in such alveolar bone resorption, both macrophages and fibroblasts are capable of phagocytosis, together with polymorphonuclear leucocytes. In addition, the zone of compressed alveolar bone may be associated with a mild inflammatory tissue response including component capillary blood vessel dilatation and occasional disruption. Such changes are, however, highly variable, depending upon a variety of factors including magnitude and duration of the orthodontic force. In the case of heavy orthodontic forces, there may be marked changes in the compressed region of the periodontal membrane, including degeneration, degradation and necrosis of the component collagen fibres and cells, primarily being phagocytosed by macrophages assisted by polymorphonuclear leucocytes and fibroblasts.[6,7]

The location of such changes will, in part, be determined by the dynamics of the orthodontic tooth forces. For instance, these changes primarily occur in the region of the alveolar crest when there is a tipping tooth movement, whereas the changes predominate in the mid-root region if a tooth is moved bodily within the arch.[3]

Thus the changes on the compression side of the tooth may be summarized as follows:

(1) Gradual compression of the periodontal ligament, associated with degenerative changes.
(2) Migration of osteoclasts to the region from the marrow spaces.
(3) Gradual increase in the number of young fibroblasts and macrophages at the site of alveolar bone resorption.
(4) Once started, osteoclastic bone resorption tends to occur for the next 10–12 days, unless there is a change in the forces.
(5) Subsequently, there is widening of the periodontal ligament associated with further osteoclastic recruitment and further bone resorption occurring over a large alveolar bone surface.

Whether or not these changes on the compression side of the periodontal membrane are precisely synchronized with those on the tension side has yet to be determined.

Alveolar bone changes

Bone formation

Recruitment, differentiation, mitosis and functional activity of osteoblasts and fibroblasts within the periodontal ligament and associated alveolar bone predominate in the tension side of the tooth socket.[8] This is followed by the initial deposition of osteoid bone as bridges between the stretched periodontal fibres. When sufficient thickness of osteoid bone has formed, further mineralization occurs, along with subsequent replacement by organized trabecular and cortical alveolar bone. This also occurs, to a limited extent, on the alveolar bone surface where the resorptive changes predominate.

Bone induction

One of the main problems impeding our understanding of the mechanics of orthodontic tooth movement centres on the dearth of knowledge concerning the factors influencing local bone growth and development.

Orthodontic tooth movement through alveolar bone depends on the precise spatial and temporal regulation of bone growth and differentiation. In this regard, bone formation may be considered to comprise a developmental cascade that includes the following:

(1) Chemotaxis and proliferation of progenitor cells.
(2) Differentiation; matrix calcification.
(3) Vascular invasion.
(4) Bone formation and mineralization.

This very complex process may be influenced by a variety of factors at a number of different levels.

Sources of osteoblasts and osteoclasts

There are two main cellular systems associated with alveolar bone and bone marrow – the haemopoietic and stromal cell systems. These two systems furnish the cells required for the control of orthodontic tooth movement.

Haemopoietic system

The osteoclast appears to be a product of one of the cell lines of the haemopoietic system stem cells.[9–11] There is, however, no rigorous definition of such a stem cell. Undoubtedly they have a high capacity for cell renewal throughout life, in addition to the ability to differentiate into a variety of functional cell populations. Stem cells account for only a very small proportion of the haemopoietic cells and are not morphologically distinct. In fact the total population of haemopoietic cells may be divided into a number of compartments (colony-forming units). It is generally assumed that transitions between compartments are unidirectional from high self-renewal towards increasing specialization of differentiated functions and associated loss of proliferative potential.[12,13] The three main colony-forming units of the haemopoietic system ultimately give rise to erythroid cells, megakaryocytic cells and granulocytic and monocytic cells.

Osteoclast formation is a multistep process, including cellular proliferation, differentiation and fusion. In fact, four separate classes of osteoclast have been described, each class representing a stage in their developmental process.

Osteoclast progenitors

Osteoclast progenitors are proliferating cells without recognizable characteristics. It is not known whether these progenitors are identical to macrophage progenitors.

Osteoclast precursors

Osteoclast precursors are postmitotic cells and generally have but one nucleus.

Osteoclasts

Osteoclasts comprise fused precursor cells. Precursor cells may fuse with one another or with existing osteoclasts. In addition, existing osteoclasts may fuse with each other to form even larger cells. Osteoclasts should not therefore be regarded as individual multinucleated cells but rather as the active stage in the lifetime of cells that participate in the polykaryon.

Postosteoclasts

Theoretically, the existence of a fourth class of cells, postosteoclasts, is possible, i.e. mononuclear cells derived from osteoclasts by fission. It is therefore possible that mononuclear postosteoclasts may start a new cycle of activity by fusion after appropriate stimulation, or they may simply die after fission.

Stromal system

The stromal system is a fibroblastic network which acts as a support for haemopoietic cells and is an important part of the environment which influences their proliferation and differentiation.[14–16] Stromal cells are commonly assumed to include:

(1) The soft connective tissue layer of pre-osteoblasts and osteoblasts associated with bone surfaces.
(2) The reticular and endothelial cells of the sinusoidal vessels present throughout the marrow cavity and spaces within bones.[17,18]
(3) The adipocytes of marrow, which are a subline of fibroblastic cells.[19]

Four differentiation stages of the osteoblastic cell line have been defined.

(1) Cuboidal osteoblastic cells with cell surface receptors for parathyroid hormone. These cells are capable of secreting a number of phenotype-specific macromolecules, such as osteocalcin and Type I collagen.
(2) In the adult, bone-lining cells occupy the majority of bone surfaces considered inactive or resting, because they are not being remodelled. Such lining cells are probably inactive osteoblasts in terms of matrix production and probably are mainly associated with the functional separation of the bone fluid compartment and the extracellular fluid compartment. These cells may also serve as nutritional support cells for osteocytes via gap junctions between cell processes of osteocytes and bone-lining cells.
(3) The osteocyte is the most mature differentiation stage of the osteoblastic line. A certain proportion of osteoblasts become incorporated into newly forming matrix which is first uncalcified osteoid and, at a later stage, calcified bone.
(4) Pre-osteoblasts are the immediate precursors of osteoblasts. They are situated beyond the line of osteoblasts and may still be capable of mitosis. The osteoprogenitor cells are therefore undifferentiated mesenchymal cells, which interconnect the osteogenic (osteoblastic stem) cells with the more differentiated osteoblasts, bone-lining cells, osteocytes and pre-osteoblasts.

Thus the precursors of the osteogenic (osteoblastic and chondroblastic) cells are cellular components of the stromal system of bone and marrow and appear to be derived from a stromal stem cell.[20] It is supposed that there are stromal stem cells within the bone and marrow which yield committed progenitors, each giving rise to a different stromal cell line. Stromal tissue is a heterogeneous collection of loose and dense connective tissue which is distributed throughout the organs of the body. Such stromal cells include the mesenchymal cells, which are components of the connective tissue mesh, and the endothelial and reticular cells of the microvasculature. There is, however, scant information concerning the cellular dynamics of these stromal cells in non-skeletal tissues.

Types I and II collagen are the main collagenous components of bone, whereas non-collagenous molecules include osteocalcin, osteonectin, sialoprotein and bone proteoglycan. These substances may all be products of osteogenic cells,[21] although there may be different subpopulations of osteoblastic cells with varying degrees of functional activity. Other stromal cell lines include fibroblastic cells which are capable of synthesizing Type I collagen, which may also be precursors of some osteogenic cells. There are also reticular cells, capable of synthesizing Type III collagen.[22]

Thus, stromal cell systems associated with bone and marrow differentiate into osteogenic, adipose, fibroblastic and reticular lines, but the actual stromal stem cell responsible has yet to be adequately defined. Stromal stem cells in tissues outside the skeleton may be induced to differentiate into osteogenic cells under certain environmental conditions. Similarly, macrophages and osteoclasts are essentially of haemopoietic cell origin. The question remains as to which factors affect the physiological activity of these two cell lines and the degree of interaction between them.

Local environment

The local environment of bone formation is probably a composite of interacting cells and the adjoining extracellular matrix, in which matrix-cell interactions are of major regulatory significance. Such matrix components as collagens, proteoglycans, fibronectin, osteonectin and other non-collagenous proteins undoubtedly influence the activities of bone cells and their precursors. Bone specific local growth factors of cellular and matrix origin may combine to modulate the differentiation process, along with systemic factors, e.g. growth hormone, insulin, parathyroid hormone, calcitonin and steroids. The nutritional status, physical activities and age-related tissue vitality may also play an important role.

Extracellular matrix components

The extracellular matrix of bone may have an important influence on bone growth and resorption. The principal component of extracellular bone matrix is collagen[23–25] which functions as a substratum for osteoprogenitor and/or osteolytic cell function. Most normal cells attach to surfaces such as collagen via the cell surface glycoprotein fibronectin.[26,27] Fibronectin has an affinity for collagen, fibrin and heparin.[26,27] A related form of fibronectin is also present in blood plasma, where it cross-reacts with cell surface fibronectin. In addition, the geometric arrangement of the extracellular bone matrix collagen may have a profound influence on the rate and extent of bone formation and/or resorption by providing osteogenic or osteolytic cell anchorage.

As extracellular bone matrix is predominantly in the solid state, it provides an ideal medium for the local control of bone cell activities. Bone matrix may aid osteogenesis or osteolysis by regulating the release of chemotactic, mitogenic and differentiation factors into the local milieu as needed during bone formation and regeneration or lysis.

Bone cells may also elaborate factors that regulate their own growth and functional activity (autocrine factors).[27] It is also known that electrical,[28] mechanical[29] and gravitational[30] forces influence the bone matrix. Although the cellular mechanisms underlying these effects are unclear, prostaglandins and/or other locally elaborated factors may function as the transducing agents.

Systemic factors

It is possible that systemically elaborated hormones and locally secreted factors act together to regulate bone cell differentiation and function.[31–33] For instance, the pituitary growth hormone is the dominant systemic influence on three-dimensional skeletal growth and development.[34] In addition, insulin appears to modulate several systemic factors influencing bone, including Vitamin D metabolites.[35] Whereas glucocorticoids have a profound effect, either at the level of collagen synthesis, alkaline phosphatase activity[36] or mineralization,[37] calcitonin[38] and thyroid hormone[39] also affect osteoblastic activity.

The influence of dietary minerals and vitamins on bone mineralization is well known, although their detailed metabolic functioning remains obscure. For instance, magnesium depletion appears to retard bone formation and mineralization, whereas Vitamin A appears to affect bone cell differentiation.[40] Vitamin D metabolites, on the other hand, appear to have a biphasic effect, with an increase in alkaline phosphatase activity at high local vitamin levels but a reduction in alkaline phosphatase activity at low levels.[41]

Conclusions

Orthodontic movement of teeth in the dental arch is obviously a complex and very imperfectly understood process. Certainly osteoclasts, derived from marrow stem cells, are responsible for calcified bone resorption, although the phagocytic role of macrophages, polymorphonuclear leucocytes and fibroblasts has received scant investigation. It is also unclear whether odontoclasts are unique cells responsible for cemental resorption of the tooth root, or merely osteoclasts lying adjacent to the tooth root. The early steps of osteoclastic differentiation appear to be initiated by colony-stimulating factors, although the origin of such factors has yet to be defined. Possible mechanisms involved in bone resorption include the local production of lactate or of acid (hydrogen ions), possibly as a result of carbonic anhydrase activity and/or specific transport mechanisms, e.g. sodium and hydrogen ion exchange. Osteoclasts may also secrete calcium-chelating organic anions, e.g. citrate, to assist in the solubilization of the mineral phase. Transcellular calcium transport may also be a necessary part of the process. Bone matrix components are probably degraded by the action of extracellular proteinases, e.g. collagenase, proteoglycanase and other metalloproteinases whose optimal activities are at physiological pH. Lysosomal acid hydrolases, including the proteolytic cathepsins, may also contribute, and osteoclasts may be one of the only cell types in which lysosomal hydrolases are involved in extracellular digestion in a locally acid environment.

On the other hand, osteoblasts are known to be responsible for the synthesis of extracellular bone matrix components and for the priming of the matrix for its subsequent mineralization. Osteoblasts differentiate from periosteal lining cells on the bone cortex in addition to the stromal cells of the bone marrow. They are therefore from a different lineage from osteoclasts, although this does not rule out the fact that factors derived from osteoblastic cells may regulate osteoclastic cells, and vice versa. Type I collagen is the major protein synthesized by osteoblasts and undergoes its final stage of maturation to produce fibrils in the extracellular compartment with release of procollagen peptides into the circulation. Osteoblasts also produce glycosaminoglycans, especially chondroitin 4-sulphate and specific proteoglycans. Osteoblasts shed small vesicles from their plasma membranes which appear in the extracellular matrix as sites of initial calcium phosphate crystal nucleation and growth. Other osteoblastic products that may regulate mineralization include the glycosaminoglycans and proteoglycans as well as osteocalcin, osteonectin and sialoproteins. Proteins may also enter bone from plasma and influence subsequent pysiological activity.

Osteocytes, derived from osteoblasts and embedded in bone, may not only control mineral exchange between bone and plasma but, in view of their widespread canaliculi interconnections, may also have an overall modifying bone cell influence.

Although bone cells are responsive to orthodontic forces, in addition to many hormones and drugs, the physiological processes actually involved have yet to be delineated. For instance, osteoclasts may be activated by many factors including:

(1) Parathyroid hormone.
(2) Vitamin D_3.
(3) Thyroxine.
(4) Prostaglandins, e.g. PGE_2.
(5) Interleukin 1.
(6) Transforming growth factors.
(7) Colony-stimulating factors.
(8) Lymphotoxin.
(9) Epidermal growth factor.
(10) Tumour necrosis factor.

By contrast, only calcitonin, oestrogens and gamma-interferon appear to inhibit osteoclastic activity. Which one, or which combination, of these factors occurs following the orthodontic movement of teeth in the dental arch remains, for the present, obscure.

Similarly, a variety of factors activate osteoblastic activity, including:

(1) Vitamin D metabolites.
(2) Insulin.
(3) Insulin-like growth factors (e.g. somatomedin).
(4) Anabolic steroids.
(5) Thyroxine.
(6) Prostaglandins.
(7) Various ill-defined factors, e.g. bone-derived growth factors, skeletal growth factor, bone morphogenic protein.

In addition, osteoblastic activity appears to be inhibited by glucocorticoids and possibly β transforming growth factors.

Whether alveolar bone, in view of its close affiliation with neural crest cells, is unique, compared with the skeleton as a whole, has yet to be discerned. Although many skeletal features are genetically determined, those upon which structural competence depends, e.g. cortical thickness and organization of the trabeculae, are influenced by functional forces. It seems most likely that the osteoblasts are more responsive to orthodontically-induced stresses than osteoclasts, primarily reflected by increased prostaglandin (PGE_2) induced cAMP and DNA synthesis.[42] The alternative hypothesis, that mechanical forces stimulate osteoblastic activity through piezoelectric signals, is difficult to prove;[43] the process is probably mediated by a different intracellular mechanism.[44] Finally, the alveolar bone will be modelled after tooth movement (the retentive stage of orthodontic treatment). This regulatory mechanism is even more complex, involving multiple interactions between cells and their chemical messengers.[45] Thus, the orthodontic movement of teeth within the dental arch may involve interaction between the following mechanisms:

(1) Cell–cell interaction.
(2) Cell–matrix interaction.
(3) Systemic hormonal and mechanical factors.
(4) Immune processes.

The physiological basis of orthodontic tooth movement has yet to fully elucidated.

Review questions

1. Contrast the changes in the alveolar bone on the compression and tension sides of the tooth socket.
2. How does the origin of osteoblasts differ from osteoclasts?
3. What local environmental factors influence orthodontic tooth movement?
4. What systemic factors influence orthodontic tooth movement?
5. What are the effects of excessive orthodontic forces on the tooth?

References

1. SELVIG, K.A. (1964) An ultrastructural study of cementum formation. *Acta Odontol.*, **22**, 105
2. OLSEN, B.R. (1963) Electron microscope studies on collagen. *Z. Zellforsch.*, **59**, 199
3. REITAN, K. (1959) Tissue arrangement during retention of orthdontically rotated teeth. *Angle Orthod.*, **29**, 105
4. REITAN, K. (1964) Effects of force magnitude and direction of tooth movement on different alveolar bone types. *Angle Orthod.*, **34**, 244
5. REITAN, K. (1960) Tissue behaviour during orthodontic tooth movement. *Am. J. Orthod.*, **46**, 881

6. KVAM, E. (1970) A study of the cell-free zone following experimental tooth movement in the rat. *Eur. Orthod. Soc. Rep. Congr.*, **45**, 419
7. RYGH, P. (1974) Elimination of hyalinized periodontal tissues associated with orthodontic tooth movement. *Scand. J. Dent. Res.*, **82**, 57
8. REITAN, K. (1951) The initial tissue reaction incident to orthodontic tooth movement as related to the influence of function. *Acta Odontol. Scand. Suppl.*, 6
9. JOTEREAU, F.V. and LE DOUARIN, N.M. (1978) The developmental relationship between osteocytes and osteoclasts, a study using quail-chick nuclear marker in endochondral ossification. *Dev. Biol.*, **63**, 253–265
10. GOTHLIN, G. and ERICSSON, J.L.E. (1976) The osteoclast. *Clin. Orthop.*, **120**, 201–238
11. LOUTIT, J.F. and NISBET, N.W. (1982) The origin of osteoclasts. *Immunobiology*, **161**, 193–203
12. TILL, J.E. and MCCULLOCH, E.A. (1980) Hemopoietic stem cell differentiation. *Biochim. Biophys. Acta*, **605**, 431–459
13. KELLER, G.M. and PHILLIPS, R.A. (1982) Detection *in vitro* of a unique multipotent hemopoietic progenitor. *J. Cell Physiol. (Suppl.)*, **1**, 31–36
14. WEISS, L. (1981) Haemopoiesis in mammalian bone marrow. *Ciba Found. Symp.*, **84**, 5–21
15. SORRELL, J.M. and WEISS, L. (1980) Cell interactions between hematopoietic and stromal cells in the embryonic chick bone marrow. *Anat. Rec.*, **197**, 1–19
16. DEXTER, T.M. (1982) Stromal cell associated haemopoiesis. *J. Cell Physiol. (Suppl.)*, **1**, 87–94
17. WEISS, L. (1980) The hemopoietic microenvironment of bone marrow. *Ciba Found. Symp.*, **71**, 3–19
18. OWEN, M. (1980) The origin of bone cells in the postnatal organism. *Arthritis Rheum.*, **23**, 1073–1080
19. LANOTTE, M., SCOTT, D., DEXTER, T.M. and ALLEN, T.D. (1982) Clonal preadipocyte cell lines with different phenotypes derived from murine marrow stroma. *J. Cell Physiol.*, **111**, 177–186
20. FRIEDENSTEIN, A.J. (1976) Precursor cells of mechanocytes. *Int. Rev. Cytol.*, **47**, 327–355
21. TRIFFITT, J.T. (1980) The organic matrix of bone tissue. In *Fundamental and Clinical Bone Physiology*, edited by M.R. Urist. Philadelphia: J.B. Lippincott
22. REDDI, A.H. (1981) Cell biology and biochemistry of endochondral bone development. *Collagen Res.*, **1**, 209–226
23. REDDI, A.H. (1976) Collagen and cell differentiation. In *Biochemistry of Collagen*, edited by G.N. Ramachandran and A.H. Reddi. New York: Plenum
24. REDDI, A.H. (1982) Regulation of local differentiation of cartilage and bone by extracellular matrix: a cascade type mechanism. In *Limb Development and Regeneration*, edited by P.F. Kelly, R.O. Goetinck and J.A. MacCabe. New York: A.R. Liss
25. KLEINMAN, H.K., KLEBE, R.J. and MARTIN, G.R. (1981) Role of collagenous matrices in adhesion and growth of cells. *J. Cell Biol.*, **88**, 473–485
26. YAMADA, K.M. and OLDEN, K. (1978) Fibronectins – adhesive glycoproteins of cell surface and blood. *Nature*, **275**, 179–184
27. PECK, W.A. and BURKS, J.K. (1977) Proliferation and specialization of bone cells cultured in serum-free medium. In *Mechanisms of Localized Bone Loss*, edited by J. Horton, T. Tarpley and W. Davis. Washington: Information Retrieval Inc.
28. BECKER, R.O. (1978) Electrical osteogenesis – pro and con. *Calc. Tissue Res.*, **26**, 93–97
29. RODAN, G.A. (1981) Mechanical and electrical effects on bone and cartilage cells. In *Orthodontics*, edited by H.G. Barres. Philadelphia: University of Pennsylvania Press
30. HATTNER, R.S. and MCMILLAN, M.D. (1968) Influence of weightlessness upon the skeleton: a review. *Aerosp. Med.*, **39**, 849–855
31. REDDI, A.H. (1982) Local and systemic mechanisms regulating bone formation and remodelling: an overview. In *Current Advances in Skeletogenesis*, edited by M. Silbermann and H.C. Dlavkin. Amsterdam: Excerpta Medica
32. RAISZ, L.G. and KREAM, B.E. (1981) Hormonal control of skeletal growth. *Ann. Rev. Physiol.*, **43**, 225–238
33. SILBERMANN, M. (1982) Hormones and cartilage. In *Cartilage*, edited by B.K. Hall. New York: Academic Press
34. REDDI, A.H. and SULLIVAN, N.E. (1980) Matrix-induced endochondral bone differentiation. *Endocrinology*, **10**, 1291–1299
35. SCHNEIDER, L.E., SCHEDL, H.P., MCGAIN, T. and HASSLER, M.R. (1977) Experimental diabetes reduces 1,25-dihydroxy vitamin D in the rat. *Science*, **196**, 1452–1454
36. CANALIS, E.M. (1983) Effect of glucocorticoids on Type I collagen synthesis, alkaline phosphatase activity and deoxyribonucleic acid content in cultured rat calvaria. *Endocrinology*, **112**, 93–939
37. RATH, N.C. and ANBAR, M. (1982) Effect of adrenalectomy and aldosterone on mineralization of ectopically-induced bone. In *Current Advances in Skeletogenesis*, edited by M. Silbermann and H. Slavkin. Amsterdam: Excerpta Medica
38. WEISS, R.E., SINGER, F.R., GORN, A.H., HOFER, D.P. and NIMMI, M.E. (1981) Calcitonin stimulates bone formation when administered prior to initiation of osteogenesis. *J. Clin. Invest.*, **68**, 815–818
39. BURCH, W.M. and LEBOVITZ, H.E. (1982) Triiodothyronine stimulates maturation of porcine growth plate cartilage *in vitro*. *J. Clin. Invest.*, **70**, 496–504
40. MAJESKA, R.J. and RODAN, G.A. (1982) The effect of $1,25(OH)_2D_3$ on alkaline phosphatase in osteoblastic osteosarcoma cells. *J. Biol. Chem.*, **257**, 3362–3365
41. SCHWARTZ, R. and REDDI, A.H. (1979) Influence of magnesium depletion on matrix-induced endochondral bone formation. *Calcif. Tissue Int.*, **29**, 15–20
42. YEH, C-K. and RODAN, G.A. (1984) Tensile forces enhance prostaglandin E synthesis in osteoblastic cells grown on collagen ribbons. *Calcif. Tissue Int.*, **36**, S67–S71
43. EDITORIAL (1981) Electromagnetism and bone. *Lancet*, **i**, 815–816

44. BINDERMAN, I., SHIMSHONI, Z. and SOMJEN, D. (1984) Biochemical pathways involved in the translation of physical stimulus into biological message. *Calcif. Tissue Int.*, **36**, S82–S85

45. BARON, R., VIGNERY, A. and HOROWITZ, M. (1984) Lymphocytes, macrophages and the regulation of bone remodelling. *Bone Mineral Res.*, **2**, 175–243

21

The healing of bone fractures

Introduction

A fracture occurs whenever the upper limit of bone strain is exceeded. In the case of the jaws, fracture may result from excessive force during tooth extraction or, more commonly, from physical violence resulting from an argument. The process of bone healing is considered here primarily to emphasize that bone growth and repair may occur as a local process, in addition to overall maturation of the skeleton as a whole (*Table 21.1*).

The speed of healing and perfection of repair of a fracture depend on whether the break has occurred in a previously normal bone or at some site of pre-existent disease (pathological fracture). They also depend on the nature and extent of the fracture. Fractures may be complete or incomplete (green-stick), closed (simple) with intact overlying tissue, comminuted, when the bone has been splintered, and compound, when the fracture site communicates with the skin or mucosal surface. Incomplete closed fractures heal most rapidly, with almost complete reconstruction of the pre-existing architecture. Comminuted and compound fractures, by contrast, heal much less rapidly, often associated with permanent post-fracture distortion or deformity. In compound fractures bone splinters comprise impediments to repair, whereas there is always a danger of infection in a comminuted fracture, leading to bone destruction, impairment of the blood supply and fibrosis: all of which interfere with normal bone repair. As this work is primarily devoted to physiology, the healing of simple bone fractures is the primary concern.

Mechanics of bone repair

The healing of a fracture represents a continuous process, although it is traditionally divided into three phases for ease of description.

Haematoma

Immediately after a fracture there is considerable haemorrhage into the fracture site from ruptured blood vessels within the bone, periosteum and adjacent soft tissues. Coagulation of this blood gives rise to a loose fibrin mesh that not only seals off the

Table 21.1 Factors affecting bone fracture healing

Factor	*Effect*
Haematoma	
Plasma fibronectin	Anchors cells in the ground substance Required for collagen formation
Endothelial cell-derived growth factor	Mitogenic
Callus formation	
Platelet derived growth factor	Mitogenic: fibroblasts; bone cells Activates monocytes and promotes bone resorption
Epidermal cell growth factor	Mitogenic: cartilage, bone Inhibits Type I bone collagen synthesis
Fibroblast growth factor	Mitogenic: cartilage, fibroblasts
Insulin-like growth factor	(Somatomedin C) Chondrocyte proliferation Chondrocyte proteoglycan synthesis
Nerve growth factor	Mitogenic
Bone formation/remodelling phase	
Epidermal growth factor	Promotes bone resorption
Fibroblast growth factor	Promotes bone resorption
Insulin	Synergistic effect with BGP
Interleukins (monocyte products)	
(IL 1)	Fibroblast proliferation Collagenase production Prostaglandin production
(IL 2)	T cell growth factor (lymphokine): resorption via OAF production

fracture site but also provides a framework for the subsequent ingrowth of fibroblasts and new capillary blood vessels. The blood clot then undergoes organization, eventually producing a soft tissue callus that provides some anchorage for the bone fragments but no structural rigidity.

Callus formation

After a few days, newly formed cartilage and bone matrix are evident in the fibrovascular response. Some of the component fibroblasts, osteoblasts and chondroblasts are undoubtedly derived from the adjacent periosteum and endosteum, although osteoblasts and chondroblasts may also be derived from primitive mesenchymal cells at the site, as may some of the fibroblasts. By the end of the first week, well-developed new bone and cartilage are dispersed throughout the soft tissue callus. Subsequently this new calcified tissue units the two bone fracture surfaces, resulting in the formation of provisional/temporary callus. In the course of the ensuing weeks, this callus becomes increasingly well developed, although the component bone trabeculae tend to be randomly arranged and unequal in size.

Organization phase

Over the ensuing weeks and months, the provisional callus is replaced by mature bone, with the component trabeculae arranged according to the prevailing functional demands. Provided there are no complications, it may be difficult to identify the true location of a fracture site some years after the event.

The fracture cascade

A fracture results in a well-defined cascade of tissue responses that include removal of tissue debris, re-establishment of the vascular supply and the production of new bone tissue.

A fracture initially involves disruption of the local blood supply to the region, resulting in:

(1) Haemorrhage.
(2) Anoxia.
(3) Cell death.
(4) An aseptic inflammatory response.

This is then followed by:

(1) Revascularization.
(2) Resorption of necrotic tissue.
(3) Proliferation–differentiation of pluripotential osteoprogenitor cells in the periosteum, endosteum and narrow stroma, to functional fibroblastic, chondrogenic and/or osteogenic cells.

Inflammatory stage

This cascade of processes is believed to be initiated by the inflammatory reaction but can be delayed or halted at any stage by infection, instability of the two fragments, or the interposition of soft tissues with no osteogenic potential between the fragments.

The initial inflammatory response results in the release of vasoactive angiogenic pyrogens from the necrotic bone and vascular tissue. In addition, vasodilatation occurs in the vessels surrounding the fracture within hours of the injury.[1] The blood clot (haematoma) that develops as a consequence of these changes is subsequently invaded by a variety of blood-formed elements, including: macrophages (for fibrin resorption); fibroblasts (for the formation of a fibrous tissue scar); osteoblasts and inflammatory cells.

Cellular proliferation

Fracture healing initially requires the proliferation of cells with a chondrogenic potential, subsequently being replaced by a cellular population with osteogenic and osteoclastic potential. Chondrogenic and osteogenic cells appear to be derived from cells resident around the fracture site, whereas the primary source of osteoclastic cells appears to be from circulating cells of the monocytic–macrophagic lineage.[2,3] The osteogenic cells appear to be derived from the cambium layer of the periosteum and the endosteum (including the marrow and haversian spaces). This phase begins 8–12 h after injury and temporarily overlaps the hyperaemic phase. Interestingly, this proliferative phase not only affects the regions adjacent to the fracture but also the bone as a whole, and even the periosteum of uninvolved bones. Within the affected bone, the periosteal proliferative activity is more marked at the fracture site, although if there is a degree of motion between the fracture surfaces, other periosteal and endosteal cells all differentiate to form some hyaline cartilage and/or fibrocartilage to brace the fracture site.[4] By three weeks post-fracture, the callus chondrification is complete. It subsequently calcifies and is replaced endochondrally by fibre/lamellar bone in a manner analogous to the conversion of normal epiphyseal growth cartilage tissue to metaphyseal bone trabeculae.

In some instances, metal plates, particularly in long bone or jaw fractures, are used to approximate the two bone ends and limit their movement. In such cases, healing occurs without forming an intermediate cartilage–fibrocartilage tissue; osteoclastic cutting zones traverse the fracture line, and the defect is bridged by newly deposited osteonal lamellar bone. Thus, when a narrow gap persists between the fragments, the space may be filled by simple lamellar bone orientated perpendicularly to the long axis. This tissue is subsequently remodelled.[5] In the healing of linear fractures of the plate-like bones of the skull, new bone is generated directly by the modulation of periosteal osteoprogenitor cells to the osteoblast class.[6]

Bone repair represents a response to injury that is classified as a regionally accelerated phenomenon (RAP).[7] Certainly, the local changes involve increased acidity, including changes in tissue Po_2 and Pco_2 due to anoxia and vascular stasis (haematoma). Such changes may initiate periosteal and endosteal proliferative activity, although increased parathyroid activity may also be involved.

Skeletal repair

It is known that mitogenic peptides are produced by many of the cells that populate the fracture site. These regulatory chemical messengers may be classified into the following types:

(1) *Autocrine:* when the elaborating and target cell is the same.
(2) *Paracrine:* when the peptide produced travels to the target cell by diffusion.
(3) *Endocrine:* when the bloodstream is required to transport the peptide to a distant target cell.

These peptides can then stimulate the proliferation of mesenchymal cells to form chondroblasts and osteoblasts, depending upon the prevailing environmental conditions.

Chronological sequence of fracture site healing

This section is included here primarily to emphasize the interaction between reparative and defence reactions of the host.

Inflammatory reaction

This is the initial response of the host to bone fracture. The inflammatory reaction involves polymorphonuclear leucocytes, lymphocytes and monocytes, some of the last fusing to form macrophages. Macrophages are also present in the haematoma, and these cells may produce a macrophage-derived growth factor that is mitogenic for osteoblasts and chondrocytes.[8] The haematoma also contains blood platelets which release platelet-derived growth factor that stimulates fibroblastic proliferation.[1] The release of this peptide is stimulated by the arachidonic acid precursor of prostaglandins.[9]

Callus stage

When periosteal and endosteal mesenchymal cells begin to differentiate and form the fibrocartilaginous callus, the chondroblasts produce peptides which are not only mitogenic for chondroblasts but also morphogenic for the formation of type II collagen.[10,11] The hyaluronic acid synthesized by these differentiating cells may also inhibit their continued proliferation, i.e. there is a feedback mechanism.[12] The osteoprogenitor cells which differentiate to form osteoblasts (endosteum and marrow) may also produce mitogenic growth factors.[13] Such growth factors are obviously important in the initiation of new bone formation; other factors released from the degradation of bone fragments may also be involved. Macrophages and osteoclasts release collagenases that facilitate the degradation and removal of devitalized bone, whereas monocytes may interact with T lymphocytes, resulting in the release of a lymphokine–osteoclast activating factor.[14] Interestingly, other lymphokines may be released that activate macrophages.

Remodelling phase

Many of the cellular mechanisms which operate to remove devitalized bone continue until the fracture is healed. Resorption liberates a collagenase-resistant glycoprotein (BMP) that is not only mitogenic but also stimulates chondroblastic activity.[15] Also, resorption of collagen may result in the release of factors chemotactic for fibroblasts and macrophages.[16] Interestingly, collagen, fibrin and other molecules may also be chemotactic for fibroblasts, so that bone repair demonstrates not only the involvement of numerous interacting processes but also a degree of redundancy in the process as a whole. The attraction of osteoclast-precursor cells to sites of resorption, and their ability to fuse and/or attach to the matrix, appears to depend upon cell surface and matrix surface oligosaccharides.[17] Matrix components such as collagens, fibronectin, laminin, hyaluronic acid and proteoglycans may not only influence cellular biosynthetic activities, but may also be chemokinetic and chemotactic influences that speed cellular translocations.[18] The activities of cells within a fracture therefore involve:

(1) The production of, and responses to, mitogenic autocrine and paracrine growth factors.
(2) The synthesis of matrix-bound differentiation factors.
(3) The responses to the specific bone morphogenetic glycoprotein (mitogenic-cartilage induction) during early callus remodelling.

The endocrines, vitamins and interactions between growth factor *per se* may also exert moderating effects.

Abnormalities of fracture healing

Fibrous union

If the component units of a bone fracture cannot be sufficiently immobilized, then either cartilaginous or fibrous union may occur. Ultimately, this fibrous scar tissue at the fracture site may be replaced by bone, but this will be a very slow process.

Non-union

A complete lack of bony union at a fracture site usually reflects the fact that soft tissues are interposed between the two bony surfaces.

Delayed union

This usually reflects the following:

(1) There is some movement between the two fracture surfaces or the two fracture surfaces are too firmly compressed one to another.
(2) Infection, by causing persistent inflammatory reactions, may delay or impair the healing process.
(3) Poor blood supply: a feature that probably accounts, in part, for the delayed healing of fractures in the elderly patient.
(4) Pathological fractures: any fracture that occurs as a result of a pathological process, e.g. osteogenesis imperfecta, tumours.

Extraction wound healing

The healing of a socket following a tooth extraction is essentially the same process as the healing of a bone fracture.

(1) Immediately following tooth extraction, there is local haemorrhage followed by blood clotting.
(2) Tissue damage associated with the extraction is followed by a short-lived mild inflammatory reaction at the edges of the socket.
(3) There is an ingrowth of capillary buds and fibroblasts from the connective tissues of the socket walls.
(4) The blood clot is ultimately replaced by this granulation tissue.
(5) Epithelium begins to migrate over the top of the socket to form an epithelial seal.
(6) Coarse woven bone is then formed within the granulation tissue, subsequently filling the socket.
(7) Some months later this tissue is replaced by mature bone whose component trabeculae are organized to accommodate the changed functional demands. This is associated with resorption and remodelling of the existing socket so

that ultimately it may be difficult to determine radiographically the location of the original socket.

Conclusions

The question yet to be answered is whether bone fractures heal by creeping substitution or by osteo-induction.

The term *creeping substitution* refers to the histologically observed ingrowth of new vessels, to the subsequent appearance of first resorptive osteoclasts and to the generation of osteoblasts from perivascular connective tissue cells. Such a system embraces the angiogenic role of tissue degradation products, the mitotic effect of endothelial growth factor and a variety of serum-borne growth factors, in addition to serum and autocrine mitogenic factors.

Osteo-induction is accomplished by the diffusion of bone morphogenetic glycoprotein from resorbing bone matrix, resulting in the initial proliferation and differentiation of mesenchymal cells to chondroblasts. In fact, both processes probably occur. The main point is that the healing of bone fractures, as in the growth of bone, can no longer be considered in simple morphological terms.

Review questions

1. What is the role of inflammation in bone healing?
2. What factors might be expected to influence bone healing?
3. What is the role of the remodelling phase in bone healing?
4. List the various phases involved in bone healing in chronological order.

References

1. RHINELANDER, F.W., PHILLIPS, R.S., STEER, W.M. and BEER, J.C. (1968) Microangiography in bone healing. II. Displaced closed fractures. *J. Bone Joint Surg.*, **50A**, 643
2. ZAMBONIN-ZALLONE, A., TETI, A., PRIMAVERA, M.V., NALDINI, L. and MARCHISIO, P.C. (1983) Osteoclasts and monocytes have similar cytosketal structures and adhesion property *in vitro*. *J. Anat.*, **137**, 57
3. KAHN, A.J. and SIMMONS, D.J. (1975) Investigation of cell lineage in bone using a chimera of chick and quail embryonic tissue. *Nature*, **258**, 325
4. COHEN, J. (1956) Cartilage production in human fracture callus. *Lab. Invest.*, **5**, 53
5. HART, M.B., WU, J-J., CHAO, E.Y.S. and KELLY, P.J. (1985) External skeletal fixation of canine tibial osteotomies. *J. Bone Joint Surg.*, **67A**, 598
6. SIMMOMS, D.J. (1979) In *Fundamental and Clinical Bone Physiology*, edited by M.R. Urist. Philadelphia: J.B. Lippincott
7. JAWORSKI, Z.F.G. (1983) Histomorphometric characteristics of metabolic bone disease. In *Bone Histomorphometry*, edited by R.R. Recker. Boca Raton, Fla.: CRC Press
8. RIFAS, L., SHEN, V., MITCHELL, K. and PECK, W.A. (1984) Macrophage-derived growth factor for osteoblast-like cells and chondrocytes. *Proc. Natl. Acad. Sci. USA*, **81**, 4558
9. LINDER, B.L., CHERNOFF, A., KAPLAN, K.L. and GOODMAN, D.G. (1979) Release of platelet-derived growth factor from human platelets by arachidonic acid. *Proc. Natl. Acad. Sci. USA*, **76**, 4107
10. AZIZKHAN, J.C. and KLAGSBRUN, M. (1980) Chondrocytes contain a growth factor that is localized in the nucleus and is associated with chromatin. *Proc. Natl. Acad. Sci. USA*, **77**, 2762
11. SHEN, V., RIFAS, L., KOHLER, G. and PECK, W.A. (1985) Fetal rat chondrocytes sequentially elaborate separate growth- and differentiation-promoting peptides during their development *in vitro*. *Endocrinology*, **116**, 920
12. LASH, J.W. and VASAN, N.S. (1983) Glycosaminoglycans in cartilage. In *Cartilage: Structure, Function and Biochemistry*, edited by B.K. Hall. New York: Academic Press
13. WERGEDAL, J.E. and BAYLINK, D.J. (1984) Characterization of cells isolated and cultured from human bone. *Proc. Soc. Exp. Biol. Med.*, **176**, 27
14. RAISZ, L.G., LUBEN, R.A., MUNDY, G.R., DIETRRICK, J.W., HORTON, J.E. and TRUMMEL, C.L. (1975) Effect of osteoclast activating factor from human leukocytes on bone metabolism. *J. Clin. Invest.*, **56**, 408
15. URIST, M.R. and STRATES, B.S. (1970) Bone formation in implants of partially and wholly demineralized bone matrix. *Clin. Orthop.*, **71**, 271
16. SOMERMAN, M., HEWITT, A.T., VARNER, H.H., SCHIFFMAN, E., TERMINE, J. and REDDI, A.H. (1983) Identification of bone matrix derived chemotactic factor. *Calcif. Tissue Int.*, **35**, 481
17. BANG, G. and URIST, M.R. (1967) Bone induction in excavation chambers in matrix of decalcified dentin. *Arch. Surg.*, **94**, 781
18. NEWMAN, S.A., FRENZ, D.A., TOMASEK, J.J. and RABUZZI, D.D. (1985) Matrix-driven translocation of cells and non-living particles. *Science*, **228**, 885

22

Teeth

Introduction

Tissue calcification involves the deposition of a mineral phase in an extracellular matrix. Such calcification does not merely comprise mineral precipitation, provided adequate ions are present in sufficient concentration. Rather, mineralization is a highly cellular process, with the outcome of the mineralization process being determined to a large extent by the organic matrix. Mineralization of bones and teeth is a tightly controlled, highly regulated process dependent upon the interplay between a number of intra- and extracellular factors. Bone, dentine and cementum are of mesodermal origin, whereas enamel is primarily of ectodermal origin. The mesodermally derived tissues (dentine and cementum) are similar in composition, comprising hydroxyapatite crystals deposited in a matrix of Type I collagen and non-collagenous components, including: phosphoproteins; proteoglycans; osteonectin; proteolipids and various glycoproteins.

The respective tissues are formed by contiguous cell layers, with mineral formation occurring in the preformed matrix some time after its formation. The matrix is chemically modified and additional matrix components appear extracellularly at mineralization. Simultaneously, new matrix secretion occurs some distance away.

Amelogenesis is somewhat different, in that the enamel is initially formed in its full thickness. This primary enamel then becomes fully mineralized in a consecutive process, with selective amelogenin removal. Thus, within a single tooth structure, mineralization occurs by two distinct processes. Moreover, the fact that so many defects may occur in odontogenesis (*Table 22.1*) gives testimony to the fact that odontogenesis is a very complex process.

Table 22.1 Defects of tooth form and number

Environmental

- Developmental
  - Odontomes
  - Hypodontia
    - Microdontia
    - Missing teeth
    - Ankyloglossum superior syndrome
    - Cyanotic heart disease
    - Holoprosencephaly (cyclopia)
    - Aglossia–adactyly syndrome
    - Oculoauriculovertebral dysplasia (Goldenhar)
    - Hemifacial microsomia
  - Hyperdontia
    - One large maxillary central incisor and growth hormone responsive dwarfism
    - Molarization of pre-molars
    - Supernumerary teeth
    - Accessory cusps and ridges
    - Accessory roots
    - Enamel pearls
    - Macrodontia
    - Gemination
- Traumatic
  - Hypodontia
    - Tumours
    - Radiation
  - Dilaceration
- Inflammatory
  - Resorption
- Chemical and metabolic
  - Supravalvular aortic stenosis – infantile hypercalcaemic syndrome
  - Maternal thalidomide

Hereditary

- Defect primary in tooth germ
  - Axial core defects
  - Dens invaginatus and dens indente
    - Dens evaginatus (occlusal tubercle)
  - Taurodontism
    - Isolated taurodontism
    - With amelogenesis imperfecta
    - Tricho–dento–osseous syndrome
    - X-polyploidy
    - Scanty hair, oligodontia and taurodontia, SOT syndrome
    - Oral–facial–digital syndrome II (Mohr)
    - Microcephalic dwarfism
    - Trisomy 21 (Down)
  - Cynodont teeth with large pulp chambers
    - Thistle-shaped pulp chambers
    - Lobdontia (Keen)
  - Hypodontia
    - Peg or missing maxillary lateral incisors
    - Missing bicuspids
    - Missing third molars
    - Missing mandibular lateral incisors
    - Missing maxillary central incisors
    - Missing 81 incisors
    - Missing mandibular incisors and maxillary lateral incisors
    - Multiple teeth
  - Supernumerary teeth
    - Mesodens
    - Maxillary lateral incisors
    - Premolars
    - Cuspids
    - Gemination
- Defect in teeth accompanied by generalized disorder
  - Gardner's syndrome (odontomas)
  - Otodental syndrome – globodontia and high frequency hearing loss
  - Short thin dilacerated roots and short stature
  - Hypodontia
    - Hypodontia and nail dysgenesis
    - Hypodontia, nail dysgenesis and hypotrichosis
    - Hypodontia and hypotrichosis
    - Hypohidrotic ectodermal dysplasia
    - Chondroectodermal dysplasia (Ellis–van Creveld)
    - Deafness, ectodermal dysplasia, polydactylism, syndactylism
    - Ectodermal dysplasia, deafness and ocular anomalies
    - Charlie M. syndrome (Gorlin)
    - Mesoectodermal dysgenesis
    - Incontinentia pigmenti
    - Oculomandibulodyscephaly
    - Focal dermal hypoplasia
    - Lipoid proteinosis
    - Hurler's syndrome (MPS I)
    - Hunter's syndrome (MPS II)
    - Trisomy 21 (Down)
    - Cranio–oculodental syndrome
    - Craniofacial dysostosis
    - Cleft palate, stapes fixation, oligodontia
    - Pyknodysostosis
    - Orodigitofacial syndrome
    - Mandibulofacial dysostosis
    - Progressive hemifacial atrophy
    - Poikiloderma congenita
    - Otopalatodigital syndrome
    - Progeria
    - Cherubism
    - Cleft lip/palate and cleft lip/palate syndromes
    - Ehlers–Danlos syndrome
    - Encephalofacial angiomatosis (Sturge–Weber)
    - Osteopetrosis
    - Dyskeratosis congenita, infrequent malformed teeth
    - Odontotrichemolic hypohidrotic dysplasia
    - Hypohidrotic ectoderma dysplasia with cleft lip/palate, ocular, genital and digital anomalies
    - Coffin–Siris syndrome
    - Palmo–plantar keratosis, hypodontia, hypotrichosis, cysts of eyelids
    - Premolar aplasia, hyperhidrosis and canities prematura (Book), missing premolars
    - Ectodactyly, ectodermal dysplasia and cleft lip/palate, the EEC syndrome (Rudiger–Haase–Passarage syndrome), small and conical teeth
    - Gorlin–Chaudry–Moss syndrome (hypertrichosis – missing or bell-shaped roots, craniofacial dysostosis, heart, genital and eye abnormalities)
    - Hypertrichosis lanuginosa
    - Melanoleucoderma
    - Otodental syndrome, missing premolars
  - Hyperdontia
    - Natal teeth
      - Oculomandibulodyscephaly
      - Pachyonychia congenita, Type II
      - Chondroectodermal dysplasia
      - Cyclopia
      - Osteogenesis imperfecta
    - Permanent dentition
      - Cleidocranial dysostosis
      - Gardner's syndrome
      - Achondroplasia
      - Cleft lip/palate syndromes
      - Tricho–rhino–phalangeal syndrome (Giedion)
    - Macrodontia
      - Congenital hemihypertrophy (Curtius)
      - Angiosteohypertrophy
      - Taurodontism
      - Otodental syndrome (Levin & Jorgenson)
      - Rothmund–Thompson syndrome (anomalous cusps)

Odontogenesis

The tooth germ consists of three parts:

(1) *The enamel organ:* the formative group of tissues responsible for enamel formation (amelogenesis).
(2) *The dental papilla:* the formative organ of the pulpo-dentine complex.
(3) *The dental follicle:* the formative organ that differentiates into the tooth supporting tissues.

As with so many craniofacial tissues, neural crest cells contribute to the tooth germ, particularly to preodontoblasts,[1] i.e. the odontoblasts comprise ectomesenchymal tissue. The epithelium of the primitive oral cavity (stomodeum) consists of a layer of low columnar/cuboidal cells of ectodermal origin, separated by a basement membrane from the subjacent mesenchymal tissue. Although this latter comprises ectomesenchyme of neural crest cell origin, whether the cephalic crest cells are specified as dental papilla cells prior to or during their migration is unclear. These cells interact with the oral epithelium to give rise to the dental lamina.

At six weeks of age, the first signs of odontogenesis occur in the form of the primary epithelial band. This band is the result of oral epithelial proliferation resulting in projections into the underlying ectomesenchyme. Between 6 and 8 weeks, this primary epithelial band gives rise to two processes:

(1) *The vestibular band:* this lies buccal to the dental lamina and forms a trough-like vestibule between the cheeks and lips and the gingiva.
(2) *The dental lamina:* a shelf-like structure that projects lingually into the underlying ectomesenchyme.

In the region of future deciduous tooth formation, this dental lamina maintains temporary contact with the overlying epithelium. In the posterior region, where the future permanent molars develop, the lamina projects distally into the future ascending ramus and maxillary tuberosity regions. In these two latter locations, contact between the dental lamina and overlying epithelium is lost.

Tooth development occurs in a series of stages. These stages merely provide convenient descriptors, since tooth development is in fact a continuous process. In addition, each tooth within the dental arch develops at different times, i.e. within the arch the tooth germs will be at different stages in their development.

Stages of tooth germ development

Bud stage

From about the seventh week of intra-uterine life, a series of buds begins to develop on the dental lamina. These buds are in fact tooth germ primordia. They comprise mainly an ectodermal component, albeit with a central ectomesenchyme condensation, which subsequently gives rise to the dental papilla. The dental papilla subsequently undergoes differentiation, resulting in superficial odontoblast formation. The remainder of the dental papilla differentiates into dental pulp tissue. This whole primitive tooth germ is surrounded by a dental sac, which not only provides nutrition and protection to the developing tooth, but also subsequently gives rise to cementum and the periodontal ligament.

Cap stage

The cap stage of tooth formation is characterized by invagination of the enamel organ, reflected by partial enclosure of the dental papilla. At this cap stage, three distinct cell layers may be denoted.

The *external enamel epithelium* comprises a monolayer of cuboidal cells that is contiguous on the outer surface with the ectomesenchyme of the dental sac. On the inner aspect it is bounded by the stellate reticulum. Structurally, the cells of the external enamel epithelium are unremarkable, suggestive of a relatively inert biological function at this stage.

The *internal enamel epithelium* comprises a layer of columnar cells bounded by the dental papilla on its deep surface and the stellate reticulum superiorly. The cells of the internal enamel epithelium are supported by a prominent basement membrane that separates them from the ectomesenchyme of the dental papilla. This layer forms the concave papillary surface of the enamel organ and condenses to a knot. This latter projects into the papilla at or near the centre of the concavity. It is a transient structure of no apparent significance.

At the cervical edges of the enamel organ, the two layers of internal and external enamel epithelia are continuous and comprise a zone of active cellular proliferation, ultimately leading to tooth root formation.

The *stellate reticulum* comprises the cell mass between the internal and external enamel epithelia. The tissue comprises small stellate cells with long thin intercommunicating cytoplasmic processes, engulfed in a mucoid intercellular substance rich in sulphated mucopolysaccharides. The charged and non-charged polar functional groups attract and bind water, which accounts for the turgidity of this tissue.

During this cap stage of tooth development, the cells of the dental papilla become more densely condensed as a result of continued mitotic activity. In addition, the dental papilla becomes gradually surrounded by the enamel organ, due to continued proliferation at the cervical loop. During this phase, blood vessels and nerves begin to form in the dental papilla.

Bell stage

The bell stage reflects the continued proliferation of the enamel organ, primarily at the cervical loop. In addition, there is local differential proliferation of the primordial occlusal surface. As a result, the occlusal morphology of the future tooth is mapped out. At this stage, two cell types may be discerned in the internal enamel epithelium. The layer nearest the dental papilla comprises the ameloblastic cell layer. These elongated columnar cells have a basal nucleus, opposite to which are cytoplasmic elongations in the form of Tomes' processes. Between the ameloblastic cell layer and stellate reticulum, another epithelial cell layer develops, termed the stratum intermedium. Just prior to and during amelogenesis, these cells comprise numerous free ribosomes, a well-developed Golgi apparatus and a high concentration of dehydrogenase, alkaline phosphatase and ATPase activity. This indicates that the primary function of the stratum intermedium is protein synthesis and energy production. During enamel maturation, these cells may be seen to contain numerous autophagosomes which presumably function to rid the cells of unwanted intracellular components after the completion of amelogenesis.

Amelogenesis does not occur until there is an initial deposition of dentine, i.e. there is ectodermal/ectomesenchymal interaction during all phases of odontogenesis. The ameloblasts develop Tomes' processes at the time of initial amelogenesis. These processes are separated from the remainder of the cell by a terminal bar apparatus. Hydroxyapatite crystallites of enamel are formed in association with these processes. As amelogenesis progresses, the ameloblasts retreat from the advancing mineralization front.

Subsequent to the completion of enamel formation, the stellate reticulum and stratum intermedium become reduced, so the external enamel epithelium and ameloblastic cell layers become juxtaposed. These cell layers remain virtually intact, thereby preventing the newly formed enamel contacting the adjacent connective tissue: such contact leads to either enamel resorption or the superficial cementum formation over the enamel surface. These cell layers of the enamel organ are then termed the reduced enamel epithelium and fuse with the oral mucosa on tooth eruption into the oral cavity.

Enamel

Composition

The crowns of the teeth are invested by enamel, the hardest tissue of the body. Enamel is unlike other calcified tissues. It is of ectodermal origin, produced by ectodermal ameloblasts. Enamel comprises approximately 95% inorganic matter, 1% organic matter and 4% water by weight. The bulk of the inorganic phase comprises hydroxyapatite crystals which have a number of topically-incorporated ions on the superficial surface including fluoride, lead, iron and zinc.[2,3] Fluoride incorporation renders the superficial surface of enamel more resistant to dissolution, whereas increased carbonate ions lead to increased acid solubility. Most of the enamel water content is present as the water of hydration surrounding the hydroxyapatite crystallites, the remainder being associated with the organic matrix, thereby influencing enamel permeability.

The organic content of enamel varies with maturation. Proline and histidine decrease, whereas the relative proportions of glycine, serine, aspartic acid and hydroxyproline increase.[4] The acid mucopolysaccharides present in immature enamel are greatly diminished as enamel matures, whereas most of the hexoses and pentoses (galactose, glucose, fucose and xylose) are probably bound to protein. The citrate content of enamel may be important during mineralization in view of its capacity to chelate calcium ions.[5] Similarly, the lipid content decreases with enamel maturation and may have significance in calcification.

The physical properties of enamel are highly variable, reflecting marked variability of enamel thickness and composition in various regions of the tooth crown. Enamel is a hard substance (250–500 Knoop hardness number) with a high modulus of elasticity (much higher than that of dentine). When stressed, enamel tends to fracture, rather than deform elastically. By contrast, the underlying dentine tends to deform and rebound, thereby providing some shock absorption for the brittle enamel. Enamel is also selectively permeable, the pores probably comprising the interprismatic or sheath region, an area rich in organic matrix, lacking crystallites.

The outer surface of enamel is much less soluble than the bulk of enamel, probably reflecting the higher fluoride content and the absence of enamel rods characteristic of the bulk of the enamel. With the exception of the superficial enamel surface, enamel comprises a series of enamel rods (prisms) arranged in parallel. The keyhole appearance of these rods reflects the orientation of the component hexagonal apatite crystallites.[5] In the head region of the rods, the crystallites are orientated parallel to the long axis, whereas in the tail region, the crystallites deviate 65–70° and then fan out in the terminal portion. The discrete demarcation of adjacent enamel rods reflects the orientation of the component crystallites; there is a dramatic change in crystallite orientation between adjacent rods. By contrast, the interprismatic region (prism sheath) comprises mainly organic matrix, lacking crystallites. The component hydroxyapatite crystallites are larger than the crystals found in bone or dentine, but are highly variable. The enamel rods are orientated approximately perpendicular to the dentino-enamel junction and traverse the whole thickness of enamel in an oblique wavy fashion. As the incisal or cusp tip is approached, the rods assume a more vertical orientation, whereas near the cervical margin, they tend to be orientated apically.[6]

The brown striae of Retzius comprise incremental lines reflecting successive waves of enamel formation (ameloblast function). The quiescent periods of enamel formation result in striae formation and appear on histological sections as brown bands coursing obliquely in an occlusogingival direction. In both deciduous and first permanent molar teeth, one of these lines is more accentuated than the remainder, indicative of the physiological trauma resulting from birth (the neonatal line).

There are also a number of imperfections in the enamel.[7] Firstly, enamel lamellae comprise ribbon-like cracks within the enamel. They arise at the surface of the tooth and traverse to the dentino-enamel junction parallel to the long axis of the tooth. It is uncertain how these lamellae develop but they contain varied organic debris and may provide the line of least resistance for initial carious lesions.

Secondly, enamel tufts may be seen arising from the dentino-enamel junction and pass up to one-third the distance into the enamel substance. These enamel tufts comprise ribbon-like bands of hypocalcified enamel rods (prisms).

Thirdly, the dentino-enamel junction forming the interface between enamel and dentine presents as a scalloped border, with the convexities facing the dentine. Occasionally, odontoblastic processes traverse into the enamel, a feature denoted by terminal enlargements, termed enamel tufts.

Amelogenesis

As an example of mineralized matrix, enamel is unlike dentine, bone, cartilage or cementum. These latter mesenchymal tissues, in the mature state, comprise a substantial amount of collagenous protein which is impregnated by the mineral phase comprising a poorly crystalline calcium hydroxyapatite. The collagen makes its appearance at the earliest stages of tissue formation as the dominant organic component and is retained as such in the mature tissue. Alterations in matrix components do occur but the bulk of the initial collagen remains.

Enamel presents a very different picture in that the enamel matrix is almost lost from the tissue before final mineralization. This protein loss becomes apparent as the enamel reaches its full thickness and prior to enamel maturation. The tissue at this stage shows a great deal of porosity as the organic matrix is replaced by tissue fluid. The composition of the enamel matrix remains largely enigmatic. Although 80–90% comprise amelogenins unusually rich in proline, they do not contain hydroxyproline or collagen. Minor enamel proteins comprise enamelins which contain less proline glutamic acid and histidine but more acidic amino acids. The loss of matrix prior to enamel maturation is accompanied by a dramatic change in the amino acid composition, primarily indicative of selective loss of amelogenin, although there may also be some changes in the enamelin. The role of these complex enamel protein changes is largely speculative. Since the amelogenins occupy most of the tissue's volume, which is ultimately replaced by the mineral phase, they most effectively delineate space into which the hydroxyapatite crystals can grow. The enamelins, by contrast, occupy only a small volume of the tissue, and their more intimate association with the mineral phase suggests a nucleating function for the hydroxyapatite crystals. Dispersed in an orderly manner throughout the amelogenin matrix, they possibly serve to dictate the position and orientation of crystallites. Alternatively enamelins may impede crystal growth. Conceivably, controlled amelogenin removal provides a means for governing crystal growth so that the crystals grow simultaneously to a uniform size, rather than some growing at the expense of others. In addition, this could ensure that those crystals formed last, at the enamel surface, were also the last to grow, ensuring complete mineralization throughout the depth of the tissue.

Dentine

Composition

Dentine is a mineralized tissue of ectomesenchyme origin. Coronally, dentine is invested by enamel, whereas cervically and apically it is covered by cementum. The composition of dentine is similar to that of bone, with 70% by weight inorganic matter, 20% organic matter and 10% water. The inorganic component primarily comprises hydroxyapatite, with the inclusion of a number of trace elements. Proteins form the bulk of the organic components of dentine. The major protein is collagen, with minor amounts of phosphoproteins. The lipid component is more varied, comprising triglycerides; cholesterol esters; phosphatidylserine; phosphatidylinositol and phosphatidic acid. A number of hexoses, hexuronic acids and aminosugars are found in dentine as constituents of proteoglycans and glycoproteins, in addition to hyaluronic acid and chondroitin 6- and 4-sulphates.

Collagen is one of the principal components of the dentine matrix and appears first as large fibrils in the amorphous ground substance between the newly differentiated odontoblasts and the basement membrane supporting the internal enamel epithelium.

Procollagen molecules are first assembled at ribosomal sites on the rough endoplasmic reticulum of odontoblasts. They are then transported to the Golgi complex, glycosylated, and passed in the secretory vesicles to the cell surface. There, they are released as collagen molecules into the extracellular compartment. In the extracellular compartment, they aggregate together to form the characteristic collagen fibrils. The large diameter collagen fibrils first seen in dentinogenesis are aligned at right angles to the basement membrane supporting the internal enamel epithelium, where they intermingle with the aperiodic fibrils hanging from it.[8] These collagen fibrils and associated ground substances comprise the organic matrix of the first formed dentine. Subsequently, the odontoblasts continue to increase in size, gradually eliminating the intervening ground substance between them, i.e. they form a continuous cell layer at the periphery of the dental papilla.

Dentinogenesis

Mineralization of the organic matrix begins with the formation of small membrane-bound vesicles which are pinched off from the odontoblastic cell surface.[9,10] These vesicles are not only rich in calcium and phosphate ions but also alkaline phosphatase. They also contain hydroxyapatite crystals which subsequently burst through the vesicle walls to contact the extracellular collagen. The crystals are then aligned along these collagen fibrils, where they provide nucleation centres for the deposition of further crystallites. Thus, although odontoblasts are required for initial dentinal mineralization, further mineralization may proceed independently.

After the first layer of dentine has been produced, the collagen fibres of the organic matrix become smaller in diameter and arranged in a felt-like framework at right angles to the forming dentinal tubules. Mantle dentine is the term used for the first formed dentine, with the bulk of dentine being termed circumpulpal dentine. Mineralization of circumpulpal dentine occurs as a result of the spread of crystallite formation from the calcification foci in the mantle dentine. Matrix vesicles are not found in circumpulpal dentine.

Dentine formation in the tooth root occurs in a similar manner, except the initial large diameter collagen fibres are orientated parallel, rather than at right angles, to the basement membrane supporting the epithelial root sheath. The template for root dentine formation is provided by the epithelial root sheath of Hertwig, formed by fusion of the internal and external enamel epithelium at the level of the future cemento-enamel junction. Root dentine forms at a slower rate than that of the coronal region.

The bulk of dentine is occupied by dentinal tubules. Some odontoblastic processes of the odontoblasts traverse the length of these tubules, whereas others pass only a short distance in the tubules. Some of the dentinal tubules have numerous lateral branches, leading to the supposition that the odontoblastic processes provide a network throughout the circumpulpal dentine.

The dentine immediately surrounding the odontoblastic processes is more highly mineralized than the remainder of the dentine and is termed peritubular dentine. The dentinal tubules describe a sigmoid curve as they traverse from the pulp to the amelodentinal or cementodentinal junction. At the amelodentinal junction some of the odontoblastic processes pass into the enamel, resulting in enamel tuft formation. Sections of dentine demonstrate two forms of striations, one representing slight changes in dentinal tubule orientation (incremental lines of Owen) and the other, termed incremental lines of von Ebner, representing incremental lines of odontoblastic activity (similar to the brown striae of Retzius).

Microscopically, dentine is a heterogeneous tissue. The interface between inter- and peritubular dentine is well demarcated, owing to differences in mineralization. Fifty per cent of intertubular dentine is organic, mainly comprising collagen fibres. There are also zones of interglobular dentine which comprise regions of hypocalcification formed during the initial stages of dentinogenesis.

Odontoblasts

When dentine formation begins, the odontoblasts are tall columnar cells with abundant cytoplasm and well-developed cytoplasmic organelles. During dentine formation, the odontoblast migrates centrally. As this occurs, some of the odontoblastic short stubby processes in the region of the basement membrane become accentuated and persist as major cellular extensions. These are termed the odontoblastic processes. It is at the basal end of this process, where it joins the cell body, that many of the secretory products are released. With continued dentine deposition, this cell process becomes surrounded by dentine, thus forming the dentinal tubule. The S-shaped curvature of the dentinal tubules, seen in mature dentine, represents the fossilized course of the odontoblastic cell movement from the periphery to the tooth centre.[11]

Recent studies have shown that the odontoblast process may in fact pass only to a depth of 0.5–0.7 mm into dentine.[12,13] Around the process and beyond it, the tubules contain a serous-like fluid whose movement towards and away from the pulp may provide one of the mechanisms of dentine sensitivity.

The dentinal tubule is lined for much of its extent by peritubular dentine. This dentine is different from the adjacent intertubular dentine in that there are fewer collagen fibres and a significant (9%) greater degree of mineralization. Due to its different nature, peritubular dentine is more readily destroyed in the initial stages of caries. With increasing age, the dentinal tubules may become partly or completely obturated by continued growth of peritubular dentine. In particular, precipitation of mineral salts within the tubules is associated with persistent low-grade dentinal irritation, resulting in dentinal hypermineralization–sclerosis.[14]

Dentinal permeability

The major channels for solute diffusion across dentine are the dentinal tubules. Since dentine permeation is proportional to the product of tubule number and diameter, dentinal permeability increases rapidly as the pulp chamber is approached. The presence of a smear layer of cutting debris, on top of dentine cut during cavity preparation, decreases dentine permeability. Recent studies[15] have shown that dentine permeability is reduced within hours of cavity preparation and possibly reflects leakage of plasma proteins from the pulpal blood vessels. Possibly these plasma proteins subsequently permeate the dentinal tubules, where they are either adsorbed to the tubule walls or physically trapped in such a way as to reduce dentine permeability. In addition, dentine permeability may be reduced by mineral deposits, collagen fibrils, proteoglycans, bacteria, etc.

Cementum

Cementum is a specialized calcified connective tissue that covers the root surface. There have been few investigations into the physiology of cementum, possibly reflecting its close morphological and physical similarity to lamellar bone.[16,17] Cementum is, however, dissimilar to bone in a number of ways:

(1) It is avascular.
(2) It lacks nerve input.
(3) It does not usually undergo remodelling or resorption.
(4) Calcification does not usually involve extracellular mineralizing vesicles.

The component collagen fibres of the periodontal ligament are attached to the dentinal root surface by cementum. Cementum therefore functions as a component tooth supporting mechanism. Cemental apposition continues throughout the life of the tooth. In this way, the cementum provides a continuous site for periodontal ligament fibre attachment. This is an important function since the periodontal ligament collagen fibres undergo almost constant remodelling. In addition, such continuous cemental apposition compensates for the loss of substance due to occlusal tooth attrition. Ultimately, continued cemental apposition may lead to periapical foraminal obliteration.

The thin, highly calcified, cemental layer comprises two forms: acellular and cellular.

Acellular cementum

This comprises variable numbers of acellular layers separated by resting lines. It extends from the cemento-enamel junction, where it is thin, to the tooth apex, where it tends to increase in thickness. This tissue is produced at a very slow rate, so it is envisaged that the cementoblasts have time to migrate away before being actually incorporated into the matrix. This layer is also characterized by the incorporation of large numbers of Sharpey's fibres, derived from inclusion of the periodontal ligament fibres.

Cellular cementum

This is found towards the root apex, covering the acellular cementum and dentine. This relatively thick layer contains cementocytes in lacunae arranged in an analogous manner to osteocytes.[18] Cellular cementum is formed quite rapidly, resulting in the cementoblasts being incorporated into the matrix.

Since all cementum is avascular, nutrition from the periodontal ligament is derived by diffusion. As a consequence, some of the cementocytes in the deeper aspects of cementum may undergo necrosis. This does not appear to be functionally significant.

Cementogenesis occurs during root formation, i.e. during periodontal ligament formation. Cementoblasts are of ectomesenchymal origin (derived from the cells of the dental sac (follicle)). In structure and function, cementoblasts and osteoblasts are very similar. Soon after root dentinogenesis is initiated, the epithelial root sheath of Hertwig undergoes progressive degeneration until its continuity is destroyed, save for the remnants, termed epithelial rests of Malassez. At this time, root dentine is exposed for the first time to the cells of the dental follicle. Some of these cells abutting the dentine surface differentiate to cementoblasts, leading to the formation of precementum, and subsequently cementum, on the root surface. Just prior to epithelial root sheath fragmentation, an enameloid material is deposited on the dentine surface by the inner ectodermal cell layer of the epithelial root sheath. This very thin layer probably serves to anchor the cementum on to the dentine surface. (This enameloid layer is also known as intermediate or hyaline cementum.)

During the subsequent cementogenesis it is not unusual for some of the epithelial cells of Malassez to be incorporated into the cemental matrix. The process of cementogenesis is continuous, albeit with fluctuating phases of activity, i.e. cementum exhibits incremental lines.

In general, the inorganic content of cementum is similar to that of bone, with 50–60% by weight comprising hydroxyapatite crystals. The organic component mainly comprises Type I collagen (40–50%). This collagen may be derived from both fibroblasts and cementoblasts. Conceivably, the cementoblasts synthesize and secrete the intrinsic collagenous fibres, whereas the periodontal ligament fibroblasts produce the extrinsic cemental collagen fibres. The larger extrinsic fibres originate in the periodontal ligament and become incorporated into the cementum during cementogenesis. By contrast, the intrinsic fibres form the felt-like matrix of cementum.

Unlike bone, dentine or calcified cartilage, the initial calcification of cementum does not involve vesicle formation. In fact, the first cementum matrix is calcified by the spread of hydroxyapatite crystallites from the root dentine. Also, unlike bone, cementum rarely undergoes remodelling. Conceivably, this reflects the presence of an intrinsic osteoclastic inhibitor substance in the cemental matrix. Cementoclasts are rarely found adjacent to the cemental surface, although macrophages and osteoclastic cells have been reported, especially in the presence of excessive orthodontic forces.

Dental pulp

Composition

The pulp tissue is contained within the central space surrounded by the hard tissues of the tooth. The odontoblast normally lines the perimeter of this space. In the coronal aspect, the odontoblast is columnar in shape and there is marked crowding of the odontoblastic cell bodies. In fact, there are approximately 45 000 odontoblasts/mm^2 in the crown of a tooth, with their cell bodies aligned at slightly different levels. There are fewer odontoblasts in the root portion of the tooth so that the odontoblasts are consequently more regularly aligned and rather more flattened. The cell bodies of the odontoblasts appear to be joined by a series of complex junctions (gap junctions, zonulae occludens and zonulae adherens) that are prominent in the neck of the cell, just below the odontoblastic process.[19]

The odontoblastic process extends 0.5–0.75 mm into the dentine.[20] It differs from the cell body in that it is devoid of major organelles but contains numerous microfilaments and microtubules. The process's role in dentinogenesis is in the transport of the secretory vesicles and their release into the extracellular space. The collagen precursors are secreted by a merocrine-type activity, in which the vesicle membrane fuses with the plasma membrane of the process. Presumably the transport system also operates in reverse, to recycle membrane components and allow modification of the matrix during calcification. In fact, the odontoblast process probably plays a multiple role in the calcification of dentine:

1. Initiation of mineralization.
2. Transportation of calcium.
3. Modification of matrix composition and in changes that produce peritubular and secondary dentine.

Dentinal calcification is apparently not carried on within intracellular vesicles. A second pathway exists whereby calcium passes between odontoblasts and diffuses into the region of calcification through the extracellular fluid. Alternatively, the phospholipids may move within the plane of the odontoblastic membrane, carrying calcium with them.[21] The detailed mechanisms of dentinal calcification have, however, yet to be elucidated.[22]

The body of the pulp tissue comprises loose areolar connective tissue that supports the nerves and blood vessels. The fibroblast is the principal cell: it functions primarily to form or degrade collagen and ground substance, although it may transform to an odontoblast in emergency situations.[23] In young pulps the collagen is relatively sparse and appears mostly as single fibrils forming sheaths around the major nerve and vascular trunks. In addition, the pulp tissue contains undifferentiated mesenchymal cells. These are probably stem cells capable of differentiating to fibroblasts or odontoblasts depending upon the stimulation. These cells tend to occur mainly in the perivascular region and appear to be the first cells to undergo mitosis following pulpal stimulation.

Ground substance

The ground substance of the pulp comprises a number of substances including glycosaminoglycans, glycoproteins, glycolipids and water.

Proteoglycans

Proteoglycans are large macromolecules occurring primarily extracellularly in connective tissues. They comprise a central protein core to which side chains of glycosaminoglycan, and to a certain extent, oligosaccharide, are covalently linked. The high molecular weight and intense negative charge density are the primary determinants for the physiological properties of proteoglycans in a tissue.

The proteoglycans have an extended structure and occupy a large space in the tissue. The resilience of a connective tissue is therefore largely a function of its proteoglycans constituents, as is the diffusion and flow of molecules of different sizes. In a specific tissue, there may be several proteoglycan populations, each population being polydiverse with respect to protein core size and number of glycosaminoglycans side chains. This fact, coupled with the variability in degree of sulphation, causes both the size and charge of the molecules to vary, thus influencing their functional properties.[24]

At the onset of mineralization, there is considerable loss of glycosaminoglycans from the dental papilla ground substance adjacent to the odontoblasts. During active dentinogenesis, predentine matrix is deposited by the odontoblasts and, after a certain time lag, it is mineralized to dentine. The composition of predentine is partly altered metabolically, as well as by addition of protein constituents. These latter are added just in advance of the mineralization front.[25] Predentine matrix consists of collagen and proteoglycans and, during the time period before mineralization, extracellular collagen fibrillogenesis occurs. It is known the proteoglycans and glycosaminoglycans interact with collagen and can influence this fibrillogenesis, thereby to some extent controlling the organization of the tissue.

Fibronectin

Fibronectin is an extracellular glycoprotein found in connective tissues and basement membranes. It may act as a mediator to cell adhesion, both to other cells and to extracellular components. Fibronectin permeates the pulp as a felt network, especially adjacent to blood vessels. Fibronectin is, however, only present in the organic matrix from which mantle dentine forms.

Non-collagenous proteins

The non-collagenous proteins of dentine include phosphoproteins, γ-carboxyglutaminate-containing proteins, proteoglycans, acidic glycoproteins and plasma proteins. With the exception of proteoglycans and plasma proteins, these non-collagenous proteins are not present in predentine but are secreted by odontoblasts just in advance of the mineralization front. This implies that such proteins are essential components in the biochemical mechanisms behind mineral formation in dentine.

Collagen

Collagen, primarily Types I and III, is a major organic component in the dental pulp. By contrast, no Type III collagen is present in dentine. The general consensus holds that the collagen of pulp connective tissue is not a precursor to dentine collagen.

Reactive powers of the pulp

The dental pulp as a tissue remains metabolically active.[26,27] This is illustrated by the use of calcium hydroxide, which is a common component of medicaments used to cover the surface of recently cut dentine, particularly when a cavity is so deep that the underlying pulp tissue is exposed.[28] The initial effect of calcium hydroxide applied to exposed pulp is the development of a superficial three-layer necrosis. The beneficial effect of calcium hydroxide is regarded as the result of the chemical injury caused by the hydroxyl ions, limited by a zone of firm necrosis against the vital tissue and the toleration of calcium by the tissue. The firm necrosis causes slight irritation and stimulates the pulp to defence and repair. The sequence of tissue reactions include: vascular and inflammatory cell migration and proliferation to control and eliminate the irritating agent; repair, including migration and proliferation of mesenchymal and endothelial pulp cells and the formation of collagen. When the pulp tissue is protected from irritation, odontoblasts differentiate and the tissue formed assumes the appearance of dentine, i.e. the function of the pulp is normalized.

Mineralization of the collagen starts with dystrophic calcification of both the zone of firm necrosis and the degenerated cells in the adjacent tissue leading to mineral deposition on the newly formed collagen. The presence of calcium ions stimulates calcium carbonate precipitation in the wound area, thereby contributing to the initiation of mineralization. In a few instances, internal resorption of the inner dentinal wall of the pulp chamber may occur, sometime after the application of calcium hydroxide on exposed pulp tissue. This appears to occur only when the pulp tissue is previously inflamed or when there is a blood clot between the wound surface and the calcium hydroxide.

Review questions

1. Contrast the composition of enamel and dentine.
2. What are the components of the ground substance of dentine? Are they the same as those of the dental pulp?
3. Contrast the physiological properties of enamel and cementum.
4. Explain the changes that occur in the dental lamina resulting in tooth germ formation.

References

1. LE DOUARIN, N. (1980) Migration and differentiation of neural crest cells. *Curr. Top. Dev. Biol.*, **16**, 32–86
2. DRIESSENS, F.C. (1982) Mineral aspects of dentistry. *Monogr. Oral Sci.*, **10**, Basel: Karger
3. KLEBER, C.J. (1984) Aluminium and dental caries. *Clin. Prevent. Dent.*, **6**, 14–25
4. BURGESS, R.C. and MOLCLAREN, C. (1965) *Tooth Enamel, its Composition, Properties and Fundamental Structure*. Baltimore: Williams & Wilkins
5. MECKEL, A.H., GRIEBSTEIN, W.J. and NEAL, R.J. (1965) Structure of mature human dental enamel as observed by electron microscopy. *Arch. Oral Biol.*, **10**, 775–783
6. ROWE, W. and IRELAND, R.G. (1956) Enamel rod direction in the cervical third of primary teeth. *Proc. Am. Acad. Pedodont.*, **9**, 24–25
7. SHIELDS, E.D. (1983) A new classification of heritable human enamel defects and a discussion of dentin defects. *Birth Defects*, **19**, 107–127
8. PATTERSON, S.S. and MITCHELL, D.F. (1965) Calcific metamorphosis of the dental pulp. *Oral Surg.*, **20**, 94–101
9. ALMUDDARIS, M.F. and DOUGHERTY, W.J. (1979) The association of amorphous mineral deposits with the plasma membrane of pre- and young odontoblasts and matrix vesicles in rat incisor teeth. *Am. J. Anat.*, **155**, 223–224
10. APPLETON, J. and MORRIS, D.C. (1979) An ultrastructural investigation of the role of the odontoblast in matrix calcification using the potassium pyroantimonate osmium method for calcium localization. *Arch. Oral Biol.*, **24**, 467–475
11. OSBORN, J.W. (1967) A mechanistic view of dentinogenesis and its relation to the curvatures of the processes of the odontoblasts. *Arch. Oral Biol.*, **12**, 275–280
12. HOLLAND, G.R. (1976) The extent of the odontoblast process in the cat. *J. Anat.*, **121**, 133–149
13. GARBEROGLIO, R. and BRANNSTROM, M. (1976) Scanning electron microscopic investigation of human dentinal tubules. *Arch. Oral Biol.*, **21**, 355–362
14. MJOR, I.A. (1985) Dentin-predentin complex and its permeability: pathology and treatment overview. *J. Dent. Res.*, **64**, 621–627
15. PASHLEY, D.H. (1985) Dentin-predentin complex and its permeability: physiologic overview. *J. Dent. Res.*, **64**, 613–620
16. STAHL, S.S. (1985) Periodontal attachment in health and disease. *J. West Sec. Periodont.*, **33**, 147–157
17. VAN DE VELDEN, U. (1984) Effect of age on the periodontium. *J. Clin. Periodont.*, **11**, 281–294
18. LANGELAND, K. and LANGELAND, L.K. (1965) Pulp reactions to crown preparation, impression, temporary crown fixation and permanent cementation. *J. Prosthet. Dent.*, **15**, 129–143
19. GARANT, P.R. and SZABO, G. (1968) The fine structure of the mouse odontoblast. *Arch. Oral Biol.*, **13**, 857–876
20. BRANNSTROM, M. and GARBEROGLIO, R. (1967) The dentinal tubules and odontoblast processes. *Acta Odontol. Scand.*, **30**, 291–311
21. HOLLAND, G.R. (1985) The odontoblast process: form and function. *J. Dent. Res.*, **64**, 499–514
22. BAUME, L.J. (1980) The biology of pulp and dentine. *Monogr. Oral Sci.*, **8**, Basel: Karger
23. TORNECK, C.D. (1978) Intracellular destruction of collagen in the human dental pulp. *Arch. Oral Biol.*, **23**, 745–747
24. HEINEGARD, D. and PAULSSON, M. (1984) Structure and metabolism of proteoglycans. In *Extracellular Matrix Biochemistry*, edited by K.A. Piez and A.H. Reddi. New York: Elsevier
25. LINDHE, A. (1984) *Dentin and Dentinogenesis*, Vols. 1 & 2. Boca Raton, Fla: CRC Press
26. TROWBRIDGE, H.O. (1985) Intradental sensory units: physiological and clinical aspects. *J. Endod.*, **11**, 489–498
27. BERMAN, L.H. (1985) Dental sensation and hypersensitivity. *J. Periodont.*, **56**, 216–222
28. SCHRODER, U. (1985) Effects of calcium hydroxide-containing pulp-capping agents on pulp cell migration, proliferation and differentiation. *J. Dent. Res.*, **64**, 541–548

23

Hormones

Introduction

Hormones are secretory products of ductless (endocrine) glands released into the extracellular (interstitial) space, absorbed into the blood stream and transported by the circulatory system to target cells (organs). There, they interact with their target cells, via receptors, which comprise large protein molecules with specific binding sites. Hormones subserve four main functions:

(1) Under basal conditions, they play a critical role in homeostasis.
(2) They play a vital role in the body's stress response.
(3) They control growth.
(4) They are essential for reproduction.

There are three main groups of hormones, proteins (peptides), steroids and amino acids. With the exception of dopamine, the hypothalamic and pituitary hormones are proteins, along with those from the pancreas and gut. The gonads and adrenal glands are the main source of steroid hormones, whereas dopamine, noradrenaline, adrenaline and thyroid hormone are amino acids.

The biological processes leading to the formation of a hormone can be classified according to its chemical structure.

Protein and polypeptide hormones

In this process, the DNA acts as a template for the specific production of messenger, ribosomal and transfer RNA molecules. The DNA and RNA transcripts contain the genetic code which determines the amino acid hormonal sequence. After leaving the nucleus, the messenger RNA molecules migrate to the ribosomes on the rough endoplasmic reticulum, where translation occurs leading to protein synthesis. The transfer RNA molecules play a crucial role in transporting amino acids to the correct position on the messenger RNA template. Each transfer RNA has an amino acid attachment site and a template recognition site. Specific enzymes link particular amino acids to their own transfer RNA. The production of factors that hydrolyze the bond between the polypeptide and the transfer RNA halt the protein synthesis. The completed molecule is then transported to the Golgi apparatus to be packaged for eventual secretion by exocytosis.

Steroid hormones

Steroid hormones are synthesized by a specific series of enzyme-catalysed reactions, with cholesterol as a substrate. This is either synthesized *de novo* within the cell or taken up by the cell via specific low density lipoprotein receptors. Cholesterol is the precursor of the five main types of steroid hormone:

(1) Progestogens.
(2) Glucocorticoids.
(3) Mineralocorticoids.
(4) Androgens.
(5) Oesteogens.

The synthesis of steroid hormones is illustrated by ACTH. After the reaction of ACTH with a specific cell surface receptor, activation of adenylate cyclase leads to cyclic AMP production. This then activates a protein kinase cascade, resulting in increased cholesterol transport into the mitochondrion, where side-chain cleavage occurs leading to the formation of progenolone.

After hormonal release from the endocrine cells, they are transported to their site of action. If this is to adjacent cells, e.g. a paracrine effect, transport is usually effected by simple diffusion. When hormones are released into the blood, however, certain hormones have specific transport proteins.[1] Such hormones may circulate bound to these proteins, to prolong their life in the circulation, and then dissociate to produce the free, biologically active hormone. The hormone-binding complex also acts as a reservoir of stored hormone.

The mechanisms of hormone action can best be defined by classifying hormones into the following:

(1) *Water-soluble hormones:* the peptide hormones and the catecholamines. These hormones mainly rcact with specific receptors on the cell surface by a series of secondary messengers (*Table 23.1*). These are generated within a cell (e.g. cGMP), or enter its cytosol as a result of the original hormone/receptor interaction, and then mediate the cellular response (e.g. calcium ions).
(2) *Lipid-soluble hormones:* the steroids, thyroid hormone and 1,25-hydroxyvitamin D_3. After binding to cytoplasmic receptors, these hormones are translocated to the nucleus.[2] The receptors are activated when they are bound by the hormone (*see Table 23.1*). In the nucleus, they bind to the nuclear acceptors on DNA. This leads to specific messenger RNA synthesis and eventual ribosomal protein synthesis. (Thyroid hormones differ by not having specific cytoplasmic receptors.)

The endocrine system can be considered an effective process for small signal amplification. For example, neural input into the hypothalamus stimulates the release of small amounts of regulatory hormone into the pituitary portal system to reach the anterior pituitary cells. These then secrete larger amounts of a hormone to be released into the systemic circulation. The target gland then responds to the trophic hormone by producing even greater amounts of its secretory product. This cascade is, in turn, modulated by negative feedback control systems: the product of the pituitary can inhibit the release of the hypothalamic hormones (short loop feedback control) and the product of the target gland can control the secretion of the pituitary and hypothalamus (long-loop negative feedback control system).

Most hormonal systems respond rapidly to the initiating stimulus. A prerequisite for such a system is that the hormone, once it has had its effect, should be inactivated and excreted. Some hormones are excreted as both an inactive metabolite and as the active hormone (e.g. cortisol). Some hormones are activated by target tissues, which can also serve to inactivate them (e.g. testosterone). The liver is the major organ for hormonal inactivation, although some are metabolized by the kidney. After the initial metabolic transformations, hormones, e.g. steroids, are frequently made water-soluble by conjugation with glucuronide or sulphate, so they can be excreted in the bile or urine.

There are numerous types of hormone. In this chapter only those primarily of dental interest and importance are considered.

Table 23.1 Second messengers

Hormone	*Target organ*
Using cyclic AMP as second messenger:	
ACTH	Adrenal cortex
Luteinizing hormone	Ovary/testes
TSH	Thyroid
Parathyroid hormone	Bone
Calcitonin	Bone
Glucagon	Liver
Using calcium as second messenger:	
Angiotensin II	Adrenal cortex/smooth muscle
Adrenaline	Liver
Insulin	Muscle/fat
Hypothalamic releasing pituitary factors	

Thyroid gland

The functional unit of the thyroid gland is the follicle (acinus) surrounded by a rich capillary plexus. The follicular glandular epithelium varies with the degree of thyroid stimulating hormone (TSH) stimulation, whereas the follicular lumen is filled with a clear proteinaceous fluid called colloid. This is the major constituent of the thyroid mass. Microvilli extend into the colloid from the apical border: this is the iodination reaction site. The initial phase of thyroid hormone secretion (resorption of the colloid by endocytosis) also occurs at the apical border. The parafollicular (C) cells, which secrete calcitonin, do not border on the follicular lumen.

The thyroid cells perform parallel functions in the synthesis of thyroid hormone:[3,4]

(1) The synthesis of thyroglobulin substrate. This is a glycoprotein that serves as a matrix in which thyroid hormone is formed; it is also the storage form of thyroid hormone.
(2) The thyroid gland secretes two iodothyronine hormones derived from the amino acid tyrosine. The major secretory product is 3,5,3',5'-tetraiodothyronine (thyroxine; T_4) and 3,5,3'-tri-iodothyronine (T_3).

The extracellular binding proteins for thyroid hormone are in the plasma, while the storage form (thyroglobulin) is in the follicular lumen (colloid). Virtually all T_4 is bound to plasma proteins, with only 0.05% unbound (free). This portion of unbound thyroxine represents the biologically active hormone. Thyroxine is mainly associated with two of the three binding proteins: thyroxine-binding globulin binds 75% of the plasma T_4; thyroxine-binding pre-albumin binds 15–20% of the circulating T_4; 9% of the T_4 is bound to albumin.

Whereas 99.5% of tri-iodothyronine T_3 is bound to thyroxine-binding globulin, 0.5% is unbound. The lower affinity of T_3 for the plasma binding proteins, and so the higher concentration of unbound T_3, contribute to the greater biological activity of T_3.

Control of thyroid secretion[5]

Thyroid stimulating hormone stimulates the thyroid follicle to secrete thyroid hormone, most of which is bound to plasma protein carriers. Thus, thyroid stimulating hormone stimulates the synthesis of the iodothyronines. The circulating free T_3 and T_4 concentrations influence TSH release by exerting a negative feedback at the level of the anterior lobe of the pituitary, and probably the hypothalamus. Other regulators include oestrogens and somatostatin which enhance TSH secretion, whereas dopamine, bromocriptine and dihydroxyphenylethylamine (dopa) decrease the basal secretion of TSH. Thyroid function is also regulated by intrinsic control which maintains the concentration of thyroid hormone stores.

Any enlargement of the thyroid is called a goitre. The antithyroid substances that cause thyroid enlargement (termed goitrogens) include:

(1) Thionamides, which block the coupling of iodotyrosines.
(2) Iodide excess and deficiency.
(3) Perchlorate and thiocyanate, which block iodide trapping.

Goitrogens result in increased TSH synthesis, resulting in thyroid gland hypertrophy.

Metabolism of thyroid hormone[6–8]

T_4 is the iodothyronine found in highest concentration in the plasma and is the only one that arises solely from direct glandular secretion. Most of the T_3 present in plasma is derived from peripheral conversion of T_4 by monodeiodination, mainly in the liver and kidney. Thyroid hormone is metabolized by deiodination, deamination and by conjugation with glucuronic acid, with the conjugate then being secreted via the bile duct into the intestine. In normal individuals, T_4 and T_3 are excreted mainly in the faeces, with a small amount appearing in the urine.

Physiological effects of thyroid hormone

Thyroid hormone increases the basal metabolic rate of most cells in the body, except the gonads, brain, lymph nodes, thymus, lung, spleen, dermis and some of the accessory sex organs. An increase in basal metabolic rate is correlated with increased mitochondrial number and activity, in addition to increased sodium and potassium ion and ATPase activity. The increased basal metabolic rate accounts for the thyroid hormone thermogenic effect. Thyroid hormone is also essential for normal bone growth and maturation, in addition to neurological tissue maturation, especially the brain. Thyroid hormone is also necessary for lactation. Finally, thyroid hormone directly affects carbohydrate, lipid, protein and vitamin metabolism.

Carbohydrate metabolism

In physiological amounts, thyroid hormone potentiates the action of insulin and promotes glycogenesis and glucose utilization. In pharmacological amounts, thyroid hormone is a hyperglycaemic agent, in that it potentiates the adrenaline glycogenolytic effect, causing glycogen depletion. Thyroid hormone is also gluconeogenic in that it increases the availability of precursors (lactate and glycerol), whereas, in large doses, thyroid hormone promotes interstitial glucose absorption.

Protein metabolism

In physiological amounts, thyroid hormone has a potent protein anabolic effect, whereas it has a protein catabolic effect in large doses.

Fat metabolism

Thyroid hormone stimulates all aspects of lipid metabolism, although on a net basis, the lipolytic effect is greater than the lipogenic effect. There is an inverse relationship between thyroid hormone levels and plasma lipids in that elevated thyroid hormone levels are associated with decreases in blood triglycerides, phospholipids and cholesterol, whereas, at higher levels, there are increases in plasma free fatty acids and glycerol.

Vitamin metabolism

Thyroid hormone affects fat-soluble vitamins in that it is required for vitamin A synthesis from carotene and the conversion of vitamin A to retinene. As a result, the serum carotene is elevated and the skin becomes yellow in hypothyroid states.

Pathological effects of thyroid hormone[9–15]

Hypothyroidism

Inadequate thyroid hormone production (hypothyroidism) may reflect a variety of causes.

(1) Primary pathology:
  (a) developmental;
  (b) iodine deficiency;
  (c) irradition or thyroidectomy;
  (d) antithyroid drugs;
  (e) Hashimoto's thyroiditis;
  (f) idiopathic (cause unknown).
(2) Secondary pathology: hypopituitarism

Simple thyroid goitre is a condition occurring at any age where the diet is deficient in iodine. Provided the enlarged thyroid gland can produce sufficient thyroid hormone, no ill-effects occur, apart from the swelling in the midline of the neck which may compress the adjacent structures, e.g. the recurrent laryngeal nerve. Moreover, if sufficient iodine is administered to the patient, then the gland will regress.

Cretinism is the classic congenital maldevelopment condition of the thyroid. It is typified by delayed somatic, dental and mental development, dry skin and sparse hair, and a protuberant abdomen. The overall development of the skull is impaired, with relative overdevelopment of the maxilla compared with the mandible: this may reflect the lack of growth of the cranial base. There may also be retraction of the bridge of the nose with nasal flaring. The face may be very wide but fails to develop in a longitudinal direction. The tongue is enlarged and oedematous, often associated with protrusive malocclusion. The eruption rate of the teeth is delayed and the deciduous teeth are retained beyond the usual time of shedding. Enamel hypoplasia is an important sequel in this condition.

Juvenile hypothyroidism: the signs and symptoms of this condition depend on when thyroid function deteriorates. There is retardation of the eruption rates and shedding rates of the teeth, in addition to a slowing in the rates of skeletal and developmental maturation.

Adult hypothyroidism: impaired thyroid function results in the development of myxoedema. This is typified by physical and mental sluggishness, generalized oedema (especially of the facial region), bradycardia, constipation, slow speech, hoarse voice and an intolerance of cold.

Hyperthyroidism

Hyperthyroidism is associated with a variety of disorders, including Grave's disease, toxic adenoma and toxic nodular goitre. The manifestations of hyperthyroidism include:

(1) Diarrhoea and increased appetite, but associated with weight loss.
(2) Anxiety, irritability, hyperkinesia and tiredness.
(3) Fine intention tremor of the outstretched hands.
(4) Cardiac arrhythmias, or cardiac failure in severe cases.
(5) Exophthalmos and associated inflammation around the eyes.
(6) Increased heat intolerance, due to heat production and sweating.
(7) Generalized osteoporosis may occur and tends to be associated with increased alveolar bone resorption.

Endocrine pancreas

The endocrine pancreas consists of the islets of Langerhans, which comprise three cell types:

(1) α cells: comprise 25% of the islet cells and are the source of glucagon;
(2) β cells: comprise 60% of the islet cells and are associated with insulin synthesis;
(3) D cells: comprise 10% of the islet cells and are the source of somatostatin.

Unmyelinated postganglionic sympathetic and parasympathetic nerve fibres terminate close to the three cell types and modulate their secretions via neurotransmitters. The liberation of acetylcholine causes insulin release only when blood glucose levels are elevated: noradrenaline secretion, via α receptor activation, leads to the inhibition of insulin release. Despite the dual α- and β-adrenergic receptor system in the β cells, the α-adrenergic action of adrenaline predominates so that insulin secretion is inhibited. The release of insulin is mediated via β-adrenergic receptors. Acetylcholine also appears to inhibit somatostatin release, whereas noradrenaline stimulates somatostatin release.

The α, β and D cells are contiguous, one with another, forming a paracrine control system for the co-ordinated secretion of pancreatic polypeptides:

(1) Insulin inhibits α cell (glucagon) secretion, which increases peripheral glucose uptake and opposes glucagon-mediated glucose production.
(2) Glucagon stimulates β cell (insulin) secretion and D cell (somatostatin) secretion, which increases hepatic glucose production and opposes hepatic glucose storage.
(3) Somatostatin inhibits α cell (glucagon) and β cell (insulin) secretion, which produces hypoglycaemia and inhibition of glucose absorption.

The lowering of blood glucose levels (hypoglycaemia) by somatostatin in diabetic patients is probably due to both inhibition of glucagon secretion and to reduced intestinal glucose absorption. Other factors may also be involved, since hyper- and hypoglycaemia are of a varied aetiology (*Tables 23.2, 23.3*).

Table 23.2 Causes of hypercalcaemia

Occurrence	*Cause*
Common	Malignant states Primary hyperparathyroidism
Uncommon	Thyrotoxicosis Sarcoidosis Vitamin D poisoning
Rare	Acute renal failure Immobilization Addison's disease

Table 23.3 Classification of Hypoglycaemia

Inappropriate insulin secretion
- Insulin-secreting tumour
  - Benign
  - Malignant
- Islet hyperplasia
- Pluriglandular syndrome
- Neonatal hypoglycaemia
  - Infants of diabetic mothers
  - Erythroblastosis fetalis

Counter-regulatory hormonal insufficiency
- Pituitary
- Adrenocortical
- Thyroid
- In long-standing insulin-dependent diabetics

Hepatic disease
- Hepatocellular diseases
- Congestive cardiac failure
- Neoplasia
- Glycogen storage disease
- Defective gluconeogenesis
  - Alcohol-induced
  - Pyruvate carboxylase deficien

Reactive hypoglycaemia – induced by:
- Glucose, e.g. post-gastrectomy, peptic ulceration, early diabetes, idiopathic (unknown cause)
- Galactose, e.g. galactosaemia
- Fructose – hereditary fructose intolerance
- Leucine – leucine hypersensitivity

Miscellaneous
- Extra-pancreatic neoplasms
- Starvation
- Prolonged exercise
- End-stage renal disease
- Auto-immune insulin syndrome

Physiological effects of insulin[16–19] (*Table 23.4*)

Carbohydrate metabolism

Insulin acts on the liver to promote glucose uptake and inhibit glucose production and release. As the hepatocyte is permeable to glucose, glucose uptake in the liver is not rate-limiting. A control point in glucose metabolism occurs when metabolism is initiated by glucose phosphorylation to glucose 6-phosphate, which is catabolized by hexokinase and glucokinase. Hexokinase is saturated at normal plasma glucose concentrations and is not regulated by insulin. Glucokinase is only half saturated at blood glucose concentrations, however, so this enzyme is both insulin and glucose dependent. The phosphorylation of fructose 6-phosphate by phosphofructokinase is enhanced by insulin, with a decrease in phosphofructokinase activity favouring gluconeogenesis and glucose formation. Insulin diminishes hepatic glucose output by activating glycogen synthetase and by inhibiting gluconeogenesis. They key intermediary reaction in gluconeogenesis is between pyruvate and phosphoenolpyruvate, which requires the enzymes pyruvate carboxylase and phosphoenolpyruvate carboxykinase, the latter enzyme being inhibited in the presence of glucose and insulin.

An insulin-dependent diffusion mechanism for glucose occurs in both skeletal and cardiac muscle, and glucose transport across muscle cell membranes requires insulin. Insulin also activates glycogen synthetase and phosphofructokinase, which respectively cause glycogen synthesis and glucose utilization.

Table 23.4 Actions of insulin

Metabolism	*Anabolic effect (increase)*	*Catabolic effect (decrease)*
Carbohydrate	Glucose transport Glucose phosphorylation Glycogenesis Glycolysis Pentose phosphate shunt Pyruvate dehydrogenase activity	Gluconeogenesis Glycogenolysis
Lipid	Triglyceride synthesis Fatty acid synthesis Adipose tissue activity	Lipolysis Lipoprotein (liver) Lipase (muscle) Ketogenesis Fatty acid oxidation
Protein	Amino acid transport Protein synthesis	Protein degradation
Electrolytes	Cellular potassium uptake	

Insulin stimulates glucose transport and activates glycogen synthetase and phosphofructokinase activity.

Fat metabolism

When insulin and carbohydrate are available, the liver is quantitatively a more important site for fat synthesis than is adipose tissue. In the absence of insulin, the liver does not actively synthesize fatty acids but it is capable of esterifying fatty acids with glycerol, which is phosphorylated by glycerokinase. Also, in the absence of insulin, there is an increase in fat oxidation and ketone production. Insulin therefore has a potent antiketogenic effect. Insulin deficiency also decreases the formation of fatty acids in adipose tissue. The major effect of insulin-stimulated glucose uptake in fat cells is to provide α-glycerophosphate for esterification of free fatty acids. The lipolytic effect, in the absence of insulin, is due to an increase in the hormone-sensitive lipase, triglyceride lipase, whose activity is normally inhibited by insulin.

Protein metabolism

Insulin is an important protein anabolic hormone. In diabetic patients, the muscle uptake of amino acids is reduced and postprandial blood levels elevated. During severe insulin deficiency, hypoaminoacid-aemia is present. Insulin increases amino acid uptake into muscle and increases amino acid incorporation into protein. Insulin increases body protein stores by increasing tissue amino acid uptake and protein synthesis, and decreasing protein catabolism and amino acid oxidation.

Electrolyte metabolism

Insulin lowers serum potassium ion concentration due to stimulation of muscle and hepatic tissue potassium uptake. Insulin also has an antinatriuretic effect.

Pathological effects of insulin[20–24]

Hyposecretion of insulin (diabetes mellitus)

Diabetes mellitus is a complex disease which may reflect abnormal pancreatic or other organ malfunctions (*Table 23.5*). The manifestations of diabetes may reflect abnormal β cell secretory products, circulating insulin antagonists, or increased non-hormonal insulin antagonists (*Table 23.6*). The physiological basis of diabetes includes the following:

(1) Inhibition of hepatic gluconeogenesis, which decreases the hepatic requirement for amino acids.
(2) The protein anabolic effect of insulin reduces the output of amino acids from muscle, thereby decreasing the availability of glucogenic amino acids for gluconeogenesis.

Table 23.5 Classification of the various forms of diabetes mellitus

Primary
Type 1: insulin-dependent diabetes mellitus
Type 2: non-insulin-dependent diabetes mellitus
Secondary to other pathology
Pancreatic pathology, e.g. pancreatitis, cystic fibrosis
Excess endogenous hormonal insulin antagonists, e.g. growth hormone, glucocorticoids, catecholamines
Liver disease
Medication with corticosteroids, e.g. phenytoin, thiazide diuretics
Associated with genetic syndromes
Muscular dystrophies
Down's syndrome
Turner's syndrome
Klinefelter's syndrome

Table 23.6 Causes of insulin resistance

Abnormal β cell secretory products	
	Abnormal insulin molecule
	Incomplete proinsulin to insulin conversion
Circulating insulin antagonists	
	Insulin antibodies
	Antibodies to insulin receptor
	Increased anti-storage hormonal secretion, eg. GH, cortisol, glucagon, catecholamines
	Increased non-hormonal insulin antagonists, eg. ketone bodies

(3) Glucose uptake by muscle is stimulated, providing an energy source to spare fatty acids, the release of which is inhibited by the antilipolytic effect of insulin.
(4) Fat accumulation is enhanced by increased hepatic lipogenesis.
(5) The antilipolytic action of insulin at the level of the adipose cell reinforces the insulin-mediated inhibition of hepatic ketogenesis and gluconeogenesis by depriving the liver of precursor substrates for ketogenesis and an energy source (fatty acids) and cofactors (acetyl-CoA) necessary for gluconeogenesis.

Diabetes mellitus is a common condition that may occur at any age. In slowly developing diabetes there is progressive weakness, weight loss, increased thirst and the passage of large quantities of urine. The associated metabolic disturbances are linked with an increased prevalence for infections, especially periapical and periodontal infections.[25] The impaired tissue resistance is aggravated by the depression of ascorbic acid (vitamin C) metabolism and increased vitamin B requirements.

Table 23.7 Long-term diabetes complications

Microangiopathy	
	Increased basement membrane synthesis
	Protein glycosylation
Neuropathy	
	Protein glycosylation
	Decreased myo-inositol levels
	Increased sorbitol synthesis
Macroangiopathy	
	Hyperinsulinaemia
	Increased lipid levels/synthesis

In the poorly controlled diabetic patient there is progressive xerostomia, associated with a dry tongue and impaired mechanical salivary lavage. There is often inflammation of the oral mucosa (glossitis and mucositis) in addition to advanced periodontal disease, together with other more general complications[26] (*Table 23.7*).

Glucagon

The major site of action of glucagon is in the liver. It has a hyperglycaemic action, resulting primarily from stimulation of hepatic glycogenolysis. Glucagon is an important gluconeogenesis compound and the hyperglycaemic actions of adrenaline are amplified by its stimulation of glucagon secretion and its inhibition of insulin secretion. Glucagon is a lipolytic hormone which causes an elevation in fatty acid and glycerol plasma levels. Glucagon has a net proteolytic effect in the liver, together with many other functions (*Table 23.8*).

Table 23.8 Main actions of glucagon

Metabolism	*Effect*
Carbohydrate	Gluconeogenesis Glycogenolysis
Lipid	Ketogenesis Lipolysis (in absence of insulin)
Protein	Amino acid transport Ureagenesis

Parathyroid hormone, calcitonin and vitamin D[27–31]

Calcium ions are necessary for many physiological reactions, including:

(1) Activation of clotting enzymes in the plasma, as well as the enzymes involved in inflammation.
(2) Control of membrane excitation, with calcium ion influx occurring during the excitatory process of nerves and muscles.
(3) Stabilization of cell membranes and intercellular adhesion.
(4) Excitation–contraction coupling in muscular contraction, in addition to being essential in all excitation–secretion processes, e.g. hormonal release by endocrine cells.
(5) Formation of bones and teeth, in addition to milk production.

Calcium ions therefore function in most of the important physiological processes of the body, although there are problems when the level of plasma calcium is increased (hypercalcaemia) (*Table 23.9*).

Table 23.9 Symptoms of raised serum calcium

Tiredness	Nausea
Lethargy	Vomiting
Polyuria	Constipation
Nocturia	Mental confusion (coma when severe)
Thirst	Itching

More than 99% of the total body calcium is stored in the skeleton, with the skeleton also serving as a phosphorus storage depot (about 80% of the phosphorus is stored in the skeleton). Essentially, the total body calcium may be conceptualized as two major pools:

(1) Ninety-nine per cent of the total calcium consists of stable mature bone which is not available for rapid mobilization and not readily exchangeable.
(2) Less than 1% of the total calcium consists of labile bone which is readily exchangeable with the extracellular fluid and provides an immediate buffer to sudden changes in blood calcium ion concentrations.

The plasma concentration of total calcium is about 2.5 mmol/litre, comprising 45% ionized or free, 10% complexed with citrate ion, HCO_3^-, HPO_4^{2-}, and 45% bound to protein (mainly albumin). The sum of the ionized and complexed calcium comprises the diffusible fraction (55%) of calcium, whereas the protein-bound form constitutes the non-diffusible fraction (45%). Parathyroid hormone (parathormone), calcitonin and vitamin D regulate the serum-ionized calcium concentration.

Calcium ion regulation involves: three tissues – bone, intestine and kidney; three hormones – parathormone, calcitonin and activated vitamin D_3 (calciferol); and three cell types – osteoblasts, osteoclasts and osteocytes.

Parathormone is secreted by the parathyroid gland chief cells and is hypercalaemic in that it exerts its effects on the bone, intestine and kidney. When the plasma calcium ion concentration increases, parathormone secretion decreases, and vice versa.

Table 23.10 Causes of hypocalcaemia

Occurrence	*Cause*
Common	Renal failure Vitamin D deficiency states
Uncommon	Acute pancreatitis Hypomagnesaemia Hypoparathyroidism
Rare	Pseudohypoparathyroidism Aminoglycoside therapy

Table 23.11 Sites of malignant tumours associated with hypercalcaemia

Breast
Female genital tract
Larynx/pharynx
Lung
Renal tract

Parathormone mobilizes calcium and phosphate from the non-readily-exchangeable bone calcium ion pool, although other factors result in raised blood calcium levels (*Tables 23.10, 23.11*). Thus, by stimulating adenyl cyclase activity, parathormone enhances osteoclastic and osteocytic function, stimulates osteoclastic cell progenitors to form multinucleated osteoclastic cells and causes temporary suppression of osteoblastic cell activity.

Increased intestinal calcium absorption is mediated indirectly through increased 1,25-dihydroxyvitamin D_3 synthesis. Parathormone increases the calcium renal threshold by promoting the active reabsorption of calcium by the distal tubules. It inhibits phosphate reabsorption in the proximal tubules. Thus parathormone leads to hypercalcaemia and hypocalciuria, in addition to hypophosphataemia and hyperphosphaturia.

Calcitonin is secreted by the parafollicular cells (C cells) of the thyroid gland. It is the hypocalcaemic hormone of the body, exerting its effects on the bone, intestine and kidney. When the plasma calcium ion concentration increases, the secretion of calcitonin also increases, and vice versa.

The antihypercalcaemic effect of calcitonin is mainly due to direct inhibition of osteoclastic activity: an effect independent of the kidney, intestine and parathyroid gland activity. Calcitonin also inhibits intestinal calcium and phosphate absorption and promotes urinary phosphate, calcium, sodium and chloride ionic excretion.

Vitamin D_3 (calciferol) is the largest of the steroid hormones. Only the active metabolites (calcidiol 25-hydroxycholecalciferol, and calcitriol 1,25-dihydroxycholecalciferol) of this hormone exert biological activity, functioning in concert with parathormone on the bone, small intestine and kidney. Calciferol therefore acts synergistically with parathormone to cause bone dissolution through osteoclastic proliferation, i.e. increased osteoclastic activity by parathormone requires calciferol.

Calciferol is the principal factor in increased small intestinal calcium ion absorption and, to a lesser extent, increased phosphorus absorption. It also promotes distal renal tubular calcium ion reabsorption and proximal tubular HPO_4^{2-} reabsorption. Thus the renal effects of parathormone and calciferol are similar in that both promote calcium ion reabsorption but, whereas parathormone promotes phosphate diuresis, calciferol promotes phosphate reabsorption, with a phosphaturic effect at pharmacological levels.

Pathological changes

Hyperparathyroidism

Primary hyperparathyroidism is a disease where the parathyroid glands secrete excessive parathormone. It tends to be associated with radiological evidence of areas of poorly mineralized bone, with a giant cell tumour or cystic lesion in the jaws often being the first sign of this condition. Characteristically, the bones show evidence of osteoporosis with abortive attempts at bone repair and new bone formation, with the effects depending on the duration and intensity of the condition. In addition, there may be associated drifting and spacing of the teeth within the dental arch. As shown in *Table 23.12*, other factors may also be responsible for such changes.

Table 23.12 Causes of rickets/osteomalacia

Vitamin D deficiency:
Elderly
Asians
Liver disease
Gastrointestinal disease
Anticonvulsant therapy
Vitamin D-dependent rickets
Vitamin D-resistant rickets
Tumoral rickets
Hypophosphatasia

Hypoparathyroidism commonly occurs following surgical therapy to the thyroid gland. There may be aplasia or hypoplasia of the teeth, depending on the time of origin.

Adrenal medulla

The neuroectodermal chromaffin cells of the adrenal medulla are of neural crest origin. In effect, the adrenal medulla represents an enlarged and specialized sympathetic ganglion.[32,33] It is innervated by long sympathetic preganglionic cholinergic neurones that form synaptic connections with the chromaffin cells. Small chromaffin cell clumps may also occur along the aorta and the chain of sympathetic ganglia. Approximately 80% of the chromaffin granules synthesize adrenaline; the remaining 20% synthesize noradrenaline.

The adrenal medulla synthesizes and secretes biogenic amines. Acetyl choline, from the preganglionic nerve endings of the greater splanchic nerve synapsing at the chromaffin cells, provides the major physiological stimulus for catecholamine secretion (adrenaline and noradrenaline). Catecholamine secretion is also stimulated by angiotensin II, bradykinin and histamine.

The plasma half-life of adrenaline and noradrenaline is 1–3 min. The biological effects of these circulating catecholamines are terminated by the uptake from the circulation by sympathetic nerve endings, leading to non-enzymatic intraneuronal storage and mitochondrial monoamine oxidase inactivation. Catecholamines are also readily metabolized in the liver, kidney, gut and lung.

The effects of adrenomedullary and sympathetic nerve stimulation are generally similar. In some tissues, adrenaline and noradrenaline produce different effects, however, due to the existence of two types of receptors (*Table 23.13*):

(1) The α-adrenergic receptors are sensitive to adrenaline and noradrenaline, and are associated with the excitatory functions of the body, except for one inhibitory function, i.e. motility of the gut.
(2) The β-adrenergic receptors respond to adrenaline but are generally insensitive to noradrenaline. These receptors are associated with inhibitory functions, and one excitatory function, the myocardium.

Table 23.13 Effects of α- and β-adrenergic receptors

α-receptor stimulation (mediated via altered cellular calcium ion concentration)
Pupillary dilatation
Coronary artery constriction
Gut, kidney, muscle and skin arteriolar constriction
Venular constriction
Stomach, bowel, anal sphincter contraction
Ejaculation
Increased sweating
Increased thickness of salivary secretion
Decreased pancreatic function (exocrine and endocrine)
Alterness, fear, anxiety (CNS effects)
β-receptor stimulation (mediated via adenyl cyclase)
Increased cardiac output, via increased heart rate, increased heart contractility, decreased peripheral resistance
Coronary, skeletal muscle, renal, pulmonary arterial and arteriolar dilatation
Bronchial smooth muscle relaxation
Decreased motility of gut
Increased pancreatic endocrine and exocrine function
Increased glucogenolysis
Increased lipolysis with FFA release

Catecholamine hyposecretion produces little or no symptoms as catecholamine production from the sympathetic nerve endings appears to satisfy the normal biological requirements. Hypersecretion of catecholamines, usually due to chromaffin cell tumours, results in the following:

(1) Sustained or paroxysmal headaches.
(2) Sweating.
(3) Palpitations.
(4) Chest pain.
(5) Extreme anxiety with a sense of impending death.
(6) Skin pallor caused by vasoconstriction.
(7) Blurred vision.

Adrenal cortex[34–36]

The adrenal cortex is a mesodermal derivative and, therefore, as with all mesodermally derived endocrine glands, secretes steroid hormones. In the outer zona glomerulosa layer, aldosterone and corticosterone synthesis occurs, whereas in the two inner zona fasciculata and zona reticularis layers, cortisol and some DHEA are synthesized. The adrenal cortex therefore secretes the following:

(1) Two glucocorticoids – cortisol and corticosterone.
(2) One mineralocorticoid – aldosterone.
(3) Biosynthetic precursors of three end-products:
   (a) progesterone;
   (b) 11-deoxycorticosterone;
   (c) 11-deoxycortisol.
(4) Androgenic substances (DHEA and its sulphate ester).

The hypothalamus stimulates the anterior pituitary to secrete adrenocortical trophic hormone (ACTH) which stimulates adrenocortical hormonal secretion. Only cortisol has ACTH-suppressing activity, the negative feedback control operating at the level of the ventral diencephalon and pituitary gland. In addition, there are diurnal variations in ACTH secretion, leading to diurnal variations in plasma cortisol and 17-hydroxycorticosteroid excretion levels. The normal hypothalamic–hypophyseal–adrenocorticoid control system, however, can be overridden by stress, including:

Severe trauma	Infections
Pyrogens	Pain
Hypoglycaemia	Psychological stress
Acute anxiety	Cold exposure
Haemorrhage	Burns
Exercise	Histamine injection.

In such stressful conditions, ACTH secretion is stimulated despite the fact that systemic levels of cortisol are much higher than those required to inhibit ACTH secretion in unstressed conditions.[37]

Effects of glucocorticoids[38,39] *(Table 23.14)*

Of the naturally occurring steroids, only cortisol, cortisone, corticosterone and 11-dehydrocortisone have appreciable glucocorticoid activity. Full recovery from hypothalamic–hypophyseal–adrenocortical suppression may take up to a year following cessation of all steroid activity.

Anti-inflammatory effects

Glucocorticoids inhibit inflammatory and allergic reactions by:

(1) Stabilizing lysosomal membranes, thereby inhibiting proteolytic enzyme release.
(2) Decreasing capillary permeability, thereby inhibiting polymorphonuclear leucocyte, macrophage and lymphocyte emigration from vessel walls, in addition to inflammatory exudate.
(3) Reducing the number of circulating lymphocytes, monocytes, basophils and eosinophils, primarily through redistributing these cells from the vascular compartment into lymphoid tissues, e.g. spleen, lymph nodes and bone marrow. The reduction in the number of circulating basophils accounts for the reduction in allergic responses. Steroids also inhibit the ability of polymorphonuclear leucocytes to adhere to the vessel walls during inflammation.
(4) Causing involution of the lymph nodes, thymus and spleen, leading to decreased antibody production, thereby emphasizing the need for antibiotic coverage to prevent secondary infections.
(5) Causing an increase in total blood count, leading to polycythaemia (excessive numbers of circulating red blood corpuscles).

Renal effects

Glucocorticoids restore glomerular filtration rate and renal plasma flow to normal following adrenalectomy, in addition to facilitating free water and uric acid excretion.

Gastric effects

Cortisol increases gastric flow and gastric acid secretion but decreases gastric mucosal proliferation, thereby predisposing to peptic ulceration.

Psychoneural effects

Chronic high-dose glucocorticoids result in initial euphoria, followed by psychosis, paranoia and depression.

Table 23.14 Main glucocorticosteroid (glucocorticoid) actions

1. Maintain life
2. Carbohydrate metabolism: raise blood glucose through gluconeogenesis; stimulate glycogenolysis
3. Protein metabolism: increased breakdown/overall negative nitrogen balance
4. Suppression of inflammatory response
5. Increase in neutrophils
6. Decrease in eosinophils
7. Suppression of ACTH secretion
8. Required for excretion of water overload
9. Minor effects on sodium retention and potassium excretion

Vascular effect

In pharmacological doses, cortisol enhances the pressor effect of noradrenaline on vascular smooth muscle.

Antigrowth effects

Large doses of cortisol:

(1) Antagonize the effect of active vitamin D metabolites on the absorption of calcium from the gut.
(2) Inhibit fibroblastic proliferation.
(3) Cause collagenous degradation, thereby predisposing osteoporosis development and delayed wound healing.
(4) Cause long-term muscular weakness and atrophy.
(5) Suppress growth hormone secretion and inhibit somatic growth.

Metabolic effects

Cortisol is a carbohydrate-sparing hormone and therefore exerts an anti-insulin effect, leading to hyperglycaemia and insulin resistance. Glucocorticoids maintain blood glucose by promoting the conversion of amino acids to carbohydrates and the storage of carbohydrate as glycogen. Cortisol is hyperglycaemic mainly because of its gluconeogenic activity, which is related to its protein catabolic effect on extrahepatic tissues, especially muscle. The anti-insulin effect of cortisol results from blocking glucose transport in muscle and adipose tissue, i.e. adrenal diabetes. In addition glucocorticoids augment the activity of key gluconeogenic enzymes by the induction of hepatic enzyme synthesis. Cortisol also indirectly inhibits the activities of glycolytic enzymes, which accounts for its anti-insulin effects.

The most important gluconeogenic substrates are amino acids derived from proteolysis in skeletal muscle and extrahepatic tissues, including the protein matrix of bone. Glucocorticoids also inhibit the *de novo* synthesis of protein, termed the anti-anabolic effect. Glucocorticoids are also lipolytic hormones, reflecting in part the potentiation of the lipolytic effects of other hormones, including growth hormone, catecholamines, glucagon and thyroid hormone. Excessive amounts of cortisol lead to hyperlipaemia and hypercholesterolaemia.

Pathological changes[40,41]

Acute adrenal cortical insufficiency is relatively rare; it occurs in Waterhouse–Friderichsen syndrome. It occurs with bilateral adrenal haemorrhage following acute septicaemia. Chronic insufficiency of the adrenal cortex is termed Addison's disease and is associated with skin and oral mucosal bronzing, mucous membrane pigmentation, and general debility, including heart failure, vomiting, diarrhoea and severe anaemia.

Hyperfunction of the adrenal cortex in the child is termed adrenogenital syndrome and results from hyperplasia or tumours of the adrenal cortex. Depending on the age and sex of the affected patient, the clinical signs include pseudohermaphroditism, sexual precocity, and virilism in females and feminization in males. If the disease begins early, premature tooth eruption may occur.

Table 23.15 Common ectopic ACTH secretion sources

Lung
Oat-cell tumours of bronchus
Bronchial carcinoid tumours
Thymus/pancreas
Carcinoid tumours in foregut derivatives
Neuroectodermal origin tumours
Medullary carcinoma of thyroid
Phaeochromocytoma

Cushing's disease results from excess of adrenocorticoid hormone production, reflecting anomalous adrenal cortical or pituitary function. It is characterized by rapidly acquired adiposity of the upper portion of the body, including a buffalo hump at the back between the shoulders, facial 'mooning', a dusky plethoric appearance with purple striae formation, muscular weakness, vascular hypertension, glycosuria uncontrolled by insulin, and albuminuria. In children, there may be osteoporosis and premature arrest of epiphyseal growth, whereas, in the adult, there may be marked osteoporosis. It is important to remember that, in addition to the adrenal cortex, other tissues, especially malignant tumours, may also secrete excessive adrenal corticosteroid (*Table 23.15*).

Pituitary gland

The pituitary gland is anatomically close to the hypothalamus. The adenohypophysis is derived from the primitive gut by an upward extension of the stomodeum (Rathke's pouch) and is therefore of oral ectoderm origin. The neurohypophysis develops as a downward extension of the neural tube at the base of the hypothalamus and is of neuroectodermal origin.

Of the many different hormones produced by the anterior pituitary gland (*Table 23.16*), only growth hormone is considered, reflecting its primary importance to dentistry.

Table 23.16 Anterior pituitary hormones

Hormone	*Site/effects of action*	*Action*
GH	Liver	Somatomedin production
	Metabolic effects	Protein synthesis
		Anti-insulin effect
ACTH	Adrenal effects	Cortisol production
		Maintenance of adrenals
	Skin	Pigmentation
Prolactin	Breast	Lactation
TSH	Thyroid follicle	Thyroxine production
		Tri-iodothyronine production
LH	Ovarian follicle	Ovulation
		Corpus luteum
		Progesterone production
	Interstitial cells	Testosterone production
FSH	Ovarian follicle	Oestrogen production
	Seminiferous tubules	Spermatogenesis
LPH	?	?β-endorphin precursor

Growth hormone[42–46]

Growth hormone is synthesized by the acidophils of the anterior lobe of the pituitary, under the control of two hypothalamic hormones.

Somatotropin releasing factor is the putative releasing factor for growth hormone, which may be stimulated by:

(1) Adrenaline and noradrenaline.
(2) Insulin-induced hypoglycaemia.
(3) Increased plasma concentrations of amino acids.
(4) Decreased free fatty acid concentrations.
(5) Oestrogen.
(6) Exercise.
(7) Emotional stress.
(8) Stress due to fever, surgery, trauma, repeated venepucture.
(9) Fasting.

Growth hormone can limit its own secretion via a short-loop feedback mechanism that operates between the anterior lobe of the pituitary and median eminence. In addition, *somatostatin* inhibits the synthesis and release of growth hormone in addition to blocking the secretion of insulin, glucagon and gastrin, and inhibiting the intestinal adsorption of glucose. Cortisol not only leads to a reduction in growth hormone secretion, but also interferes with the metabolic actions of growth hormone. A decline in growth hormone secretion is observed in late pregnancy, and clinical diabetes is frequently associated with late pregnancy. The development of gestational diabetes is probably due to insulin antagonism caused by normal plasma concentrations of human placental lactogen.

Metabolic effects

The effects of growth hormone on skeletal growth are mediated by a family of polypeptides called somatomedins, which are synthesized in the liver as well as the kidney and muscle tissue. Growth hormone, through somatomedin, stimulates the proliferation of chondrocytes and osteoblasts. Growth hormone has predominantly anabolic effects on skeletal and cardiac muscle, where it stimulates the synthesis of protein, DNA and RNA, in addition to promoting amino acid transport. Growth hormone is also a diabetogenic hormone and, because of its anti-insulin effect, it tends to cause hyperglycaemia. Growth hormone also promotes urinary retention of calcium, phosphorus and sodium, and so has a role in mineral metabolism.

Growth retardation can occur when growth hormone levels are increased and the somatomedin levels are depressed, e.g. kwashiorkor. Both growth hormone and somatomedin levels are normal in the African pigmy but there is a decrease in the cellular receptors for growth hormone. Over-production of growth hormone during adolescence results in giantism, characterized by excessive long bone growth. Excessive growth hormone production during adulthood, after epiphyseal plate fusion, leads to acromegaly, characterized by:

(1) Mandibular prognathism.
(2) Paranasal sinus enlargement.
(3) Thickening and coarsening of the facial skin due to connective tissue proliferation and oedema.
(4) Renewed periosteal growth of the vertebrae and phalanges of the hands and feet.
(5) Soft tissue hypertrophy, leading to cardiomegaly, hepatomegaly, splenomegaly, renomegaly, etc.

By contrast, deficient growth hormone secretion in immature individuals leads to:

(1) Growth stunting (dwarfism).
(2) Sexual immaturity.

(3) Hypothyroidism.
(4) Adrenal insufficiency.

Such growth hormonal deficiency may reflect an isolated entity or a component of anterior pituitary deficiency.

Conclusions

Hormones affect virtually all the body tissues, including those of the craniofacial skeleton. Possibly the corticosteriods and the catecholamines are of greatest dental importance: corticosteroids, since these comprise a component of such a large number of drugs frequently prescribed for long periods of time, e.g. for rheumatoid arthritis; catecholamines, since all too high a proportion of our patients suffer from various anxiety neuroses when they sit in the dental chair.

In this chapter, the references have been very carefully selected from a vast literature: in fact, only review references have been included, since they provide a key to future reading on the various topics.

Review questions

1. Describe the relationship between hormonal and bone metabolism.
2. How does the administration of corticosteroids influence the general health of patients?
3. Why should a poorly controlled diabetic patient be of concern in dental treatment?
4. Why do hyperthyroid patients make poor dental patients?
5. Contrast the functions of adrenaline and noradrenaline.

References

1. GREEN, D.P. (1984) Are prehormones converted to hormones during secretion? *Med. Hypotheses*, **15**, 47–59
2. RINGOLD, G.M. (1985) Steroid hormone regulation of gene expression. *Ann. Rev. Pharmacol. Toxicol.*, **25**, 529–566
3. NUNEZ, J. (1982) Formation of thyroid hormones. *Vitam. Horm.*, **39**, 175–229
4. CODY, V. (1984) Thyroglobulin and thyroid hormone synthesis. *Endocrin. Rev.*, **10**, 73–88
5. VRIEND, J. (1983) Evidence for pineal gland modulation of the neuroendocrine–thyroid axis. *Neuroendocrinology*, **36**, 68–78
6. BIRO, J. (1983) Some theoretical questions of mechanisms of thyroid hormone action. *Med. Hypotheses*, **10**, 151–166
7. BAGCHI, N. (1982) Thyroid function in a diabetic population. *Spec. Top. Endocrinol. Metab.*, **3**, 45–55
8. HERZOG, V. (1984) Pathways of endocytosis in thyroid follicle cells. *Int. Rev. Cytol.*, **91**, 107–139
9. NUNEZ, J. (1984) Effects of thyroid hormones during brain differentiation. *Mol. Cell. Endocrinol.*, **37**, 125–132
10. KING, D.B. (1984) Thyroidal influence on body growth. *J. Exp. Zool.*, **232**, 453–460
11. LEVINE, S.N. (1983) Current concepts of thyroiditis. *Arch. Intern. Med.*, **143**, 1952–1956
12. FARRAR, W.B. (1983) Complications of thyroidectomy. *Surg. Clin. North Am.*, **63**, 1353–1361
13. DANFORTH, E. (1983) The role of thyroid hormones and insulin in the regulation of energy metabolism. *Am. J. Clin. Nutr.*, **38**, 1006–1017
14. CASTELLS, S. (1984) Thyroid function in juvenile diabetics. *Pediatr. Clin. North Am.*, **31**, 623–634
15. DE GROOT, L. (1983) Development of thyroid immunity. *Prog. Clin. Biol. Res.*, **116**, 1–22
16. WILSON, H.K. (1984) Understanding insulin: the old and the new. *Adv. Intern. Med.*, **29**, 357–384
17. MALAISE, W.J. (1983) Insulin release: the fuel concept. *Diabet. Metab.*, **9**, 313–320
18. HOWELL, S.L. (1984) The mechanism of insulin secretion. *Diabetologica*, **26**, 319–327
19. FAIN, J.N. (1984) Insulin secretion and action. *Metabolism*, **33**, 672–679
20. PRICE, M.J. (1984) Insulin and oral hypoglycemic agents. *Nurs. Clin. North Am.*, **18**, 687–706
21. ARKY, R.A. (1983) Prevention and therapy in diabetes mellitus. *Nutr. Rev.*, **41**, 165–173
22. KEREIAKES, D.J. (1984) The heart in diabetes. *West. J. Med.*, **140**, 583–593
23. LEBOVITZ, H.E. (1984) Etiology and pathogenesis of diabetes mellitus. *Pediatr. Clin. North Am.*, **31**, 521–530
24. GORELICK, F.S. (1983) Diabetes mellitus and the exocrine pancreas. *Yale J. Biol. Med.*, **56**, 271–275
25. MANOUCHEHR-POUR, M. (1983) Periodontal disease in juvenile and adult diabetic patients: a review of the literature. *J. Am. Dent. Assoc.*, **107**, 766–770
26. CZECH, M.P. (1984) New perspectives on the mechanism of insulin action. *Recent Prog. Horm. Res.*, **40**, 347–377
27. HABENER, J.F. (1984) Parathyroid hormone: biochemical aspects of biosynthesis, secretion, action and metabolism. *Physiol. Rev.*, **64**, 985–1053
28. GREENE, R.M. (1984) Role of cyclic AMP, prostaglandins and catecholamines during normal palate development. *Curr. Top. Dev. Biol.*, **19**, 65–79
29. BELL, N.H. (1985) Vitamin D-endocrine system. *J. Clin. Invest.*, **76**, 1-6
30. NORMAN, A.W. (1984) Hormonal actions of vitamin D. *Curr. Top. Cell Res.*, **24**, 35–49

31. MOORADIAN, A.D. (1984) Endocrine dysfunction in chronic renal failure. *Arch. Intern. Med.*, **144**, 351–352
32. UNGAR, A. (1983) Regulation of the adrenal medulla. *Physiol. Rev.*, **63**, 787–843
33. LIVETT, B.G. (1984) Adrenal medullary chromaffin cells *in vitro*. *Physiol. Rev.*, **64**, 1103–1161
34. BURCKHARDT, P. (1984) Corticosteroids and bone: a review. *Horm. Res.*, **20**, 59–64
35. RAMACHANDRAN, J. (1984) Corticotrophin receptors, cyclic AMP and steroidogenesis. *Endocrin. Res.*, **10**, 347–363
36. HORNSBY, P.J. (1984) Regulation of adrenocortical cell proliferation in culture. *Endocrin. Res.*, **10**, 259–281
37. BAHN, S.L. (1982) Glucocorticosteroids in dentistry. *J. Am. Dent. Assoc.*, **105**, 476–481
38. FISHER, A.A. (1983) Allergic reactions to topical corticosteroids or their vehicles. *Cutis*, **32**, 122, 129–132, 137
39. BAILIN, P.L. (1982) Cutaneous reactions to rheumatological drugs. *Clin. Rheum. Dis.*, **8**, 493–516
40. GUIN, J.D. (1984) Contact sensitivity to topical corticosteroids. *J. Am. Acad. Dermatol.*, **10**, 773–782
41. GABBLE, S.G. (1983) Drug therapy in autoimmune disease. *Clin. Obstet. Gynecol.*, **26**, 635–641
42. WASS, J.A. (1983) Growth hormone neuroregulation and the clinical relevance of somatostatin. *Clin. Endocrinol. Metab.*, **12**, 695–724
43. REICHLIN, S. (1983) Somatostatin. *N. Engl. J. Med.*, **309**, 1495–1501, 1556–1563
44. SCHUSDZIARRA, V. (1983) Somatostatin–physiological and pathophysiological aspects. *Scand. J. Gastroenterol. (Suppl.)*, **82**, 69–84
45. PALADIM, A.C. (1983) Molecular biology of growth hormone. *CRC Crit. Rev. Biochem.*, **15**, 25–56
46. SCANES, C.G. (1984) Growth hormone: its physiology and control. *J. Exp. Zool.*, **232**, 443–452

Index